NEUROMUSCULAR DISORDERS

Edited by **Ashraf Zaher**

Neuromuscular Disorders
Edited by Ashraf Zaher

Published by InTech
Janeza Trdine 9, 51000 Rijeka, Croatia

Publishing Process Manager Oliver Kurelic

Technical Editor Teodora Smiljanic

Cover Designer InTech Design Team

Additional hard copies can be obtained from orders@intechopen.com

Neuromuscular Disorders, Edited by Ashraf Zaher
p. cm.
ISBN 978-953-51-0696-8

For EU product safety concerns:
IN TECH d.o.o., Prolaz Marije Krucifikse Kozulić 3, 51000 Rijeka, Croatia,
info@intechopen.com or visit our website at intechopen.com.

Meet the editor

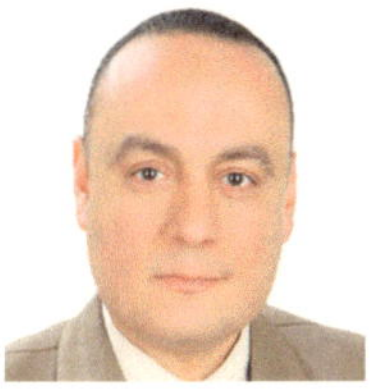

Dr Ashraf Zaher is an Associate Professor and Consultant of Neurology at Neurology department, school of Medicine, University of Mansoura, Egypt. He received his M.D, Ph.D. (2006), MSc (1999) and M.B.B.Ch (1993) from the School of Medicine, University of Mansoura, Egypt. His research interests include the EMG, NCV & Evoked Potentials "including Visual Evoked Potential, BAEP and P300", Neuromuscular Disorders, Cerebral Stroke and Epilepsy in which he had published many local and international researches. Professor Zaher has been teaching postgraduate and undergraduate Fifth year Medical Students "Both conventional and Manchester Program" and second year students at the Faculty of Nursing. He is also consulting in the Neurology field since 1999, and is a frequent contributor in many local and international conferences.

Contents

Preface XI

Chapter 1 **Integrins in the Development and Pathology of Skeletal Muscle 1**
Susan C. Brown, Ulrich Mueller and Francesco J. Conti

Chapter 2 **Facioscapulohumeral Muscular Dystrophy: From Clinical Data to Molecular Genetics and Return 21**
Monica Salani, Elisabetta Morini, Isabella Scionti and Rossella Tupler

Chapter 3 **AON-Mediated Exon Skipping for Duchenne Muscular Dystrophy 55**
Ingrid E. C. Verhaart and Annemieke Aartsma-Rus

Chapter 4 **Psychosocial Support Needs of Families of Boys with Duchenne Muscular Dystrophy 81**
Jean K. Mah and Doug Biggar

Chapter 5 **Comparison Between Courses of Home and Inpatients Mechanical Ventilation in Patients with Muscular Dystrophy in Japan 105**
Toshio Saito and Katsunori Tatara

Chapter 6 **Myopathy in Autoimmune Diseases – Primary Sjögren's Syndrome and Dermatomyositis 117**
Fumio Kaneko, Ari Togashi, Erika Nomura, Teiji Yamamoto and Hideo Sakuma

Chapter 7 **Dermatomyositis 129**
Fred van Gelderen

Chapter 8 **Interstitial Pneumonia in Dermatomyositis 143**
Tohru Takeuchi, Takuya Kotani and Shigeki Makino

Chapter 9 **IBMPFD and p97, the Structural and Molecular Basis for Functional Disruption 155**
Wai-Kwan Tang and Di Xia

Chapter 10 **Congenital Myasthenic Syndromes – Molecular Bases of Congenital Defects of Proteins at the Neuromuscular Junction 175**
Kinji Ohno, Mikako Ito and Andrew G. Engel

Chapter 11 **Motor Neuron Disease 201**
Hamdy N. El Tallawy

Chapter 12 **Spinal Muscular Atrophy 221**
Yasser Salem

Chapter 13 **Respiratory Muscle Aids in the Management of Neuromuscular Respiratory Impairment to Prevent Respiratory Failure and Need for Tracheostomy 235**
A. J. Hon and J. R. Bach

Chapter 14 **Neuromuscular Diseases in the Context of Psychology and Educational Science 253**
Andrea Pieter and Michael Fröhlich

Preface

Recent advances in the understanding of the genetics and basic mechanisms of neuromuscular diseases have been both rapid and spectacular. Furthermore, these advances have resulted in an expansion of the methods used for diagnosis—from routine clinical histologic and electrophysiologic tests to more specific techniques, such as biochemical and Western Blot analysis, and, most important, molecular genetic testing. These modern techniques have begun to replace more costly and painful procedures for some patients.

Although the goal of our specialty is to find cures or effective treatments for neuromuscular disorders, the management of symptoms to improve quality of life is still paramount. Ambulation and survival can be prolonged with well-planned rehabilitation programs, orthopaedic surgery, and proper early management of cardiac, respiratory, and gastrointestinal complications, particularly in patients with motor neuron diseases and muscular dystrophy. Prolonged survival has changed the care of these patients. For example, in the past patients with Duchenne muscular dystrophy generally died of respiratory failure before they developed symptomatic cardiac disease; now they are living longer and require aggressive treatment of their cardiac complications to further prolong their lives.

Many excellent textbooks and treatises dedicated to the understanding of the basic mechanisms of clinical and laboratory diagnoses of neuromuscular diseases also include discussions of treatment but this information is not comprehensive. In this text we aim to cover the current treatment and management of these subjects and to discuss promising experimental therapies.

The introductory chapter is a brief overview of the Integrins in the development and pathology of skeletal muscle—information that we hope will be helpful to young clinicians. The next several chapters discuss neuromuscular disorders and their general management, such as rehabilitation, orthopaedic surgery, and cardiac, gastrointestinal, and respiratory care. The balance of the chapters covers specific diseases as well as the basic mechanisms of these disorders.

The information in each chapter is intended to complement that in others, although occasionally there are minor repetitions. When possible, evidence-based treatment recommendations are given, particularly for the more common conditions, though we emphasize that the treatment of all patients should be individualized. For less common disorders, for which controlled trials have not yet been published, recommendations are based on published information and the authors' experience.

I am honored and grateful for the collaboration of an excellent group of renowned specialists. They have generously contributed their time and expertise to make what we hope is a textbook that is useful for all physicians who care for patients with neuromuscular disorders.

Ashraf Zaher, MD
Lecturer and Consultant of Neurology,
University of Mansoura, Mansoura,
Egypt

1

Integrins in the Development and Pathology of Skeletal Muscle

Susan C. Brown[1], Ulrich Mueller[2] and Francesco J. Conti[3,*]
[1]*Veterinary Basic Sciences, The Royal Veterinary College, London,*
[2]*Dorris Neuroscience Center and Department of Cell Biology,*
The Scripps Research Institute, CA,
[3]*Dubowitz Neuromuscular Centre, Institute of Child Health,*
University College London,
[1,3]*UK*
[2]*USA*

1. Introduction

1.1 Adhesion of muscle fibres to the extracellular matrix

Skeletal muscle is composed of many multinucleated myofibres each of which is surrounded by a connective tissue matrix that is essential for the function and the structural integrity of muscle. Apposed to each myofibre is a basement membrane, composed of a mixture of extracellular matrix (ECM) proteins, including collagen, fibronectin, glycoproteins (laminins, perlecan and nidogen) and proteoglycans. The proteins bind to multiple receptors expressed on the surface of muscle fibres: this is most notable at the level of the Z discs where an assembly of cytoskeletal proteins including dystrophin and integrins maintain continuity between the contractile apparatus, cytoskeleton and the ECM. This association of proteins is commonly referred to as the costamere, which is derived from the Latin word *costa,* meaning rib, because they encircle the whole muscle fibre and are arranged at regular intervals, thus conferring the appearance of a rib-like structure (Ervasti, 2003). Costameres are the means by which mechanical stress generated by contraction is diffused laterally across the myofibre. An additional structure where stress is transmitted to the ECM is the myotendinous junction (MTJ), where a connection to the tendon is made at the termini of muscle fibres (Tidball, 1991). This tight association between the muscle fibre and its surrounding matrix not only confers tensile strength to the entire muscle but also plays an important role in development, regeneration and synaptogenesis (Sanes, 2003). Indeed genetic defects in proteins that localise to the costameres and MTJs are a common cause of muscle disease, underscoring their importance in maintaining normal muscle function (Campbell and Stull, 2003).

The two main adhesion systems recognised in striated muscle are the dystrophin-associated protein complex (DPC) and the integrins. Each system is composed of transmembrane

---

* Corresponding Author

proteins that bind to the ECM, and of cytoplasmic proteins that connect to the cytoskeleton and transmit biochemical signals. The DPC is composed of several proteins, which include α- and β-dystroglycan that bind to laminin, dystrophin that connects to the cytoskeleton, and associated proteins such as sarcoglycans and neuronal nitric oxide synthase (nNOS). These proteins have the important function to confer mechanical integrity to the plasma membrane, which otherwise would break following muscle contraction. Indeed, this occurs in patients with mutations in DPC components, and present with several types of severe muscle disease, including Duchenne Muscular Dystrophy (DMD) and various forms of Limb Girdle Muscular Dystrophy (Bushby, 1999; Barresi and Campbell, 2006).

While integrins also establish a connection between the ECM and cytoskeletal and signalling proteins, the two complexes are biochemically distinct. As we will see below, integrins appear dispensable for the mechanical integrity of the sarcolemma, but have important functions during all stages of muscle development.

2. Integrins

Integrins are transmembrane receptors that connect via the extracellular domain to extracellular matrix (ECM) ligands such as collagen, laminin and fibronectin, and via the intracellular domain to the actin cytoskeleton and to a variety of signaling and adaptor proteins. Each integrin is a heterodimer composed of an α- and a β-subunit. In mammalian cells 18 α and 8 β subunits have been characterized, and are known to assemble to form 24 distinct integrin heterodimers, with the combination of α- and β- subunits determining ligand specificity. These play essential functions during development and in adult tissues. Accordingly, genetic ablation of individual subunits in mice leads to defects in tissues including brain, skin vasculature, lung, kidneys, inner ear, placenta, skeletal and cardiac muscle (Hynes, 2002).

The cytoplasmic domain of both the α- and β-integrin subunits is devoid of catalytic activity, but it binds to an array of proteins that mediate integrin effects on cell function. It is currently estimated that over 150 proteins are associated with integrin adhesion sites (Zaidel-Bar et al., 2007). Of these, we will discuss those that to date have been shown to be important in skeletal muscle. Some play structural roles, conferring mechanical integrity to myofibres by connecting integrins to the actin cytoskeleton, and others play signaling roles, by eliciting a biochemical response to mechanical stimuli caused by muscle contraction.

2.1 Developmental expression of integrins in skeletal muscle

Several integrins are expressed in myoblasts and muscle fibres, including αvβ3-integrin, α4-integrin (associated with β1 or β2), and β1-integrin with the α1, α2, α3, α5, α6, α7 or α9 subunits (Gullberg et al., 1998; Mayer, 2003; Thorsteinsdottir et al., 2011). Expression of these subunits is regulated, with regards both to the stage of muscle development and to the localization within muscle fibres (Thorsteinsdottir et al., 2011). Some integrin subunits (β1A, α4, α5, α6, α7b and αv) are detected in the somites and in myoblasts. During myotube formation, expression of most subunits is downregulated, and adult muscle fibres express the β1D subunit, paired with α7a, α7b, and α9. The subcellular distribution of these integrin subunits is also regulated: α7a is found at the MTJ, α7b at the sarcolemma, MTJ and neuromuscular junction (NMJ), α3- and αv-integrins are localized to the NMJ, and α9-integrin appears to be uniformly distributed along the sarcolemma (Wang et al., 1995; Martin et al., 1996). We will discuss here the functions identified for integrins in muscle, and refer the reader to recent reviews for details on the regulation of somitogenesis and NMJ formation by integrin-ECM interactions (Singhal and Martin, 2011; Thorsteinsdottir et al., 2011).

While the expression pattern of the different subunits is well characterized, the precise function of many remains to be addressed. Genetic ablation of integrins in mice has not always been informative in this regard. For instance, mice with an ablation of α1-, α9- and αv-integrins present no defects in skeletal muscle (Gardner et al., 1996; Bader et al., 1998; Huang et al., 2000). Mice with a genetic ablation of α3- and α6-integrins, die too early to study the long-term functions of integrins in skeletal muscle maintenance (Georges-Labouesse et al., 1996; Kreidberg et al., 1996). The distribution of laminin α5, which is the main ligand for α3-integrin, suggests a possible function in maturation of the muscle fibre and of the NMJ, since its initial expression throughout the basal lamina of developing myotubes becomes restricted to the NMJ in the first 3 weeks following birth (Nishimune et al., 2008). This is also consistent with α3-integrin expression being concentrated at the presynaptic NMJ (Martin et al., 1996).

Muscle defects have also been identified in mice with ablation of α5- and α7-integrins (Taverna et al., 1998; Mayer et al., 1997). α5-integrin is a receptor for fibronectin, and is expressed transiently during myotube differentiation. Ablation of α5-integrin in mice leads to early embryonic lethality with defects in mesoderm, vascular development and neural crest (Yang et al., 1993; Goh et al., 1997), but mice chimeric for this subunit survive postnatally and develop a form of muscular dystrophy (Taverna et al., 1998). No patients have been identified with mutations in α5-integrin possibly because, extrapolating from the data obtained in the mutant mouse models, null mutations are likely to be non viable. α7-integrin has been shown to play important functions in muscle in animal models and human patients, where mutations lead to a form of congenital muscular dystrophy (Mayer et al., 1997; Hayashi et al., 1998). Whilst it is possible that an in-depth analysis of the α-integrin subunit knockout mice would reveal muscle defects, for example in response to stressors such as exercise or mechanical damage, the apparent absence of a reported phenotype for some of these mice might be explained by redundancy. This possibility is supported by the generation of mice with a muscle specific ablation of the β1-subunit, which leads to the concomitant ablation of all αβ1-integrins (Schwander et al., 2003). These mice die shortly after birth, probably because of respiratory failure, with severe developmental defects in the muscle caused by impaired myoblast fusion and altered assembly of the sarcomere.

3. Integrins in skeletal muscle development

Fusion of myoblasts is essential for the formation of a syncytial myofibre, and it occurs in distinct steps: (i) migration of myoblasts to achieve cell proximity; (ii) contact between myoblasts and alignment of the plasma membranes; (iii) breakdown of the plasma membrane at the site of fusion, leading to the formation of fusion pores (iv) merging of the cytoplasmic contents (Chen et al., 2007). While the identity of the proteins leading to plasma membrane breakdown is unknown, studies in recent years have led to the identification of several components of the fusion machinery, most notably elucidating the importance of actin remodeling (Rochlin et al., 2010).

3.1 β1-integrin and talin

A direct involvement of integrins in the regulation of myoblast fusion in vertebrates has been obtained using genetically modified mice. Ablation of β1-integrin in developing muscle has revealed important functions in cell-cell fusion and assembly of the sarcomere (Schwander et al., 2003). β1-deficient mice died at birth, with histological analysis showing that many myoblasts failed to fuse. *In vitro* analysis showed that fusion defects could be rescued when wild-type and β1-deficient myoblasts were mixed, suggesting that heterophilic interactions of β1-integrin with an unidentified receptor may be important. Analysis of cultured myoblasts by electron microscopy showed that plasma membranes aligned properly, but fusion pores failed to open, indicating that integrins are not essential for the alignment of myoblasts, but affect a subsequent step in fusion. The analysis of mice lacking the integrin effectors talin 1 and talin 2 suggests that signaling to the cytoskeleton may be important in this respect.

Talin 1 and 2 are expressed by two distinct genes (*tln1* and *tln2*) and present a high degree of homology (74% identity in the amino acid sequence)(Senetar and McCann, 2005). They bind to cytoskeletal proteins such as actin and vinculin, and signaling effectors that include focal adhesion kinase (FAK) and PIPK1γ, which regulate the assembly of focal adhesions (Critchley, 2004). The two isoforms are essential to mediate β1-interin functions in myoblasts ablation of talin 1 and talin 2 in muscle (tln1/2-dKO) resulted in defects similar to those observed following ablation of β1-integrin: mice died shortly after birth, with abnormal development of the musculature, including defects in myoblast fusion, sarcomere assembly and in the clustering of α7-integrin, vinculin and integrin-linked kinase (ILK) at the MTJ (Conti et al., 2009). The tetraspanin CD9, which has been implicated in sperm-egg fusion (Kaji et al., 2000; Hemler, 2001), was mislocalised in β1-deficient muscle, but localized normally at the interface of tln1/2-dKO myoblasts, and integrin activation was also normal, suggesting that outside-in signaling mechanisms may be responsible for the fusion defects (Conti et al., 2009). In this respect, it is interesting to note that several of the proteins implicated in myoblast fusion are controlled by integrins, specifically, the Rho GTPases Rac1 and Cdc42, and associated proteins such as Dock180 (Laurin et al., 2008; Pajcini et al., 2008; Vasyutina et al., 2009). In mouse, vinculin, an actin- and talin-binding protein (see below) accumulates at the interface of fusing myoblasts, and genetic ablation of Rac and Cdc42 causes a reduction in this accumulation (Vasyutina et al., 2009). Furthermore, ablation of two other integrin effectors, FAK and filamin C, leads to compromised myoblast fusion (Dalkilic et al., 2006; Quach and Rando, 2006). These data are indicative of a possible involvement of integrins in regulating actin dynamics at the sites of fusion, although this still needs to be demonstrated directly.

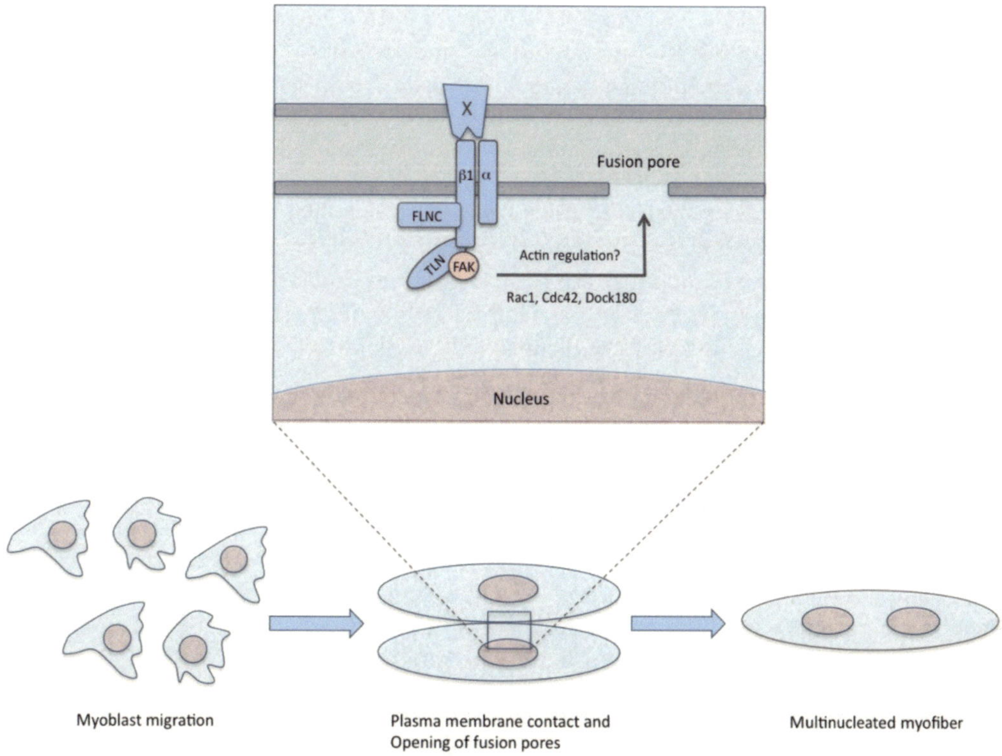

Fig. 1. **Integrins are essential for myoblast fusion.** Prior to fusion, migrating myoblasts elongate and make contact between their plasma membranes. Integrins localise at the cell interface, and are important for the formation of fusion pores, i.e. the breakdown of plasma membrane that precedes mixing of cytoplasmic content. In vitro experiments suggest that integrins interact heterophylically with an as yet unidentified counterreceptor (X in upper image). The mechanisms by which this occurs are unclear, but fusion defects are also observed following ablation of filamin C, talin 1 or talin 2, which are important actin regulators, suggesting that changes in cytoskeletal dynamics are important. Abbreviations: FLNC = filamin C; TLN = talin 1 or talin 2; FAK = focal adhesion kinase; α = as yet unidentified β1-integrin associated α-subunit. X = putative (unidentified) counter receptor for β1-integrin.

3.2 Filamin C

Filamins are actin binding proteins that cross-link actin filaments into orthogonal networks. They bind to over 30 proteins, including integrins and actin, through which they perform many functions, including modulation of cell adhesion to the ECM, cell migration, mechanical strengthening of the plasma membrane, and the activation of signaling networks. Mammalians express three filamin isoforms, termed filamin A, B and C. Filamins A and B are widely expressed, and play essential functions in the development of a variety of tissues. Expression of filamin C is mostly restricted to skeletal and cardiac muscle, where it localizes to the sarcolemma and to the Z-disk, and interacts with several proteins associated with muscular dystrophies, including calpain-3 and sarcoglycans (Zhou et al., 2010).

Downregulation of filamin C in C2C12 myoblasts via siRNA causes an impairment of cell-cell fusion, defective elongation of myotubes, and impaired gene expression during myoblast differentiation, including myogenin, caveolin 3 and α7-integrin (Dalkilic et al., 2006). An important function for filamin C in muscle differentiation was confirmed by analyzing mice in which its expression was genetically ablated. Filamin C-knockout mice died at birth likely because of respiratory failure, and presented with severe defects in myogenesis abnormal morphology of myofibres and a loss of muscle mass. While these defects partly overlap with those of β1-integrin and tln1/2-dKO mice, the phenotypes differ in that fusion and sarcomere defects are less pronounced, indicating that filamin C is not essential for β1-integrin function in muscle and that some of its effects are likely due to the interaction with other binding partners (Dalkilic et al., 2006).

Mutations in filamin C have been identified in patients with late-onset myopathies, characterized by progressive muscle weakness. Mutations in the C-terminal dimerization domain lead to myofibrillar myopathy, characterized by the accumulation of intracellular aggregates constituted of filamin C and various Z-disk associated proteins (Vorgerd et al., 2005; Lowe et al., 2007). The mutations are localized to the dimerization domain of filamin C, and cause the formation of a truncated protein that cannot form dimers, implying that dimerization is important for its function. Recently, mutations in filamin C have also been identified in patients with distal myopathies. These mutations are localized in the N-terminal actin-binding domain of filamin C, and induce increased actin binding. However, unlike the situation in patients where mutations are in the C-terminus, no protein aggregates accumulate in myofibres, suggesting that the pathological mechanisms differs from those observed in patients with mutations in the dimerization domain (Duff et al., 2011).

4. Structural connections of integrins to the cytoskeleton

Given the crucial functions played by integrins during skeletal muscle development, as determined by the studies in vitro and on animal models mentioned above, it is surprising that few defects in integrin function have been associated with muscle disease in patients. In fact, with the exception of α7-integrin and filamin C (Mayer et al., 1997), mutations in integrin effectors have been linked to defects in the heart but not in skeletal muscle. This is in contrast with the mutations in DPC, which have been identified as being the most common causes of muscular dystrophy (mutations the dystrophin gene alone affect approximately 1:3500 male births)(Goyenvalle et al., 2011). This could be due to mutations in integrins or integrin effectors being very rare, or to the pathology not being clearly identified, which would complicate the selection of patients for genetic screening. Although integrins and the DPC provide a similar link between laminin and the actin cytoskeleton, ablation of the two protein complexes leads to a different spectrum of muscle defects, and despite extensive analysis, the specific functions of each protein complex remain unclear.

4.1 α7β1-integrin

α7β1-integrin is a receptor for laminin in the basement membrane, localizes to costameres, NMJs and MTJs, and is the sole integrin known to be expressed in adult skeletal muscle (Bao et al., 1993; Martin et al., 1996). The intracellular domain of α7-integrin is spliced to produce two main isoforms, termed α7a and α7b. Their expression is tightly regulated during myoblast differentiation and muscle regeneration, and this regulation is conserved across mammals, suggesting that the specific roles played by these isoforms are important (Collo et al., 1993; Ziober et al., 1993; Cohn et al., 1999). The α7b isoform is expressed at higher levels in proliferating myoblasts and adult fibres, while the α7a isoform is expressed upon terminal differentiation. These α7-integrin splice variants bind with equal affinity to laminin, thus differences probably reside in binding to intracellular integrin effectors. It has been suggested that the splice variants may differ in the regulation of myoblast differentiation (Samson et al., 2007), as α7a interacts with Def-6, a guanine nucleotide exchange factor (GEF) for the Rho GTPase Rac-1 that has been implicated in the regulation of myoblast fusion. However, mice in which α7-integrin is ablated (α7-KO) are viable and present with normal muscle development, indicating that α7-integrin is not essential for myogenesis *in vivo* (Mayer et al., 1997). Instead, α7β1-integrin plays an important structural role in skeletal muscle by mediating a connection of actin to the sarcolemma at the MTJ. In α7-KO mice this connection fails, leaving a space filled with vesicular and amorphous material, and the mice developed a progressive myopathy, characterised by muscle weakness and a mild accumulation of centrally nucleated fibres (Mayer et al., 1997; Miosge et al., 1999). α7b-integrin has been shown have a protective effect against mechanical damage. Following exercise, expression of α7-integrin is upregulated in muscle, and exercise-induced damage is increased in α7-KO mice (Boppart et al., 2006). A protective function for α7-integrin is supported by studies in which the α7bX2 splice variant was overexpressed in mice. The transgenic mice showed a reduced activation of the MAPK pathway, associated with injury, and of AKT, mTOR and $p70^{s6k}$, associated with hypertrophy, and presented with reduced muscle damage in response to exercise (Boppart et al., 2008). It is interesting to note that α7β1-integrin is increased in the muscle of patients with DMD and of *mdx* mice (Hodges et al., 1997). Thus, upregulation of α7β1-integrin might be a natural mechanisms to increase the resistance of muscle to injury in the absence of dystrophin and indeed, enhanced α7-integrin expression alleviates muscular dystrophy in transgenic mice lacking dystrophin and utrophin (Burkin et al., 2001; Burkin et al., 2005).

Mutations in α7-integrin have been associated with muscle disease in humans: three Japanese patients were identified with a deficiency in α7-integrin, caused by deletion or frame-shift mutations in the *itga7* gene (Hayashi et al., 1998). Similar to the phenotype of α7-KO mice, the muscle in patients presented with no signs of necrosis and creatine kinase values that were only slightly elevated, indicating no major damage to the sarcolemma. However, the clinical phenotype was severe: patients presented with delayed motor milestones from early childhood, and in one case mental retardation. Follow up of one of the patients showed a severe progression of the disease, comparable to that of DMD, which led the patient to be wheelchair bound by the age of 12 (Nakashima et al., 2009). Thus, while the initial classification was that of a congenital myopathy, patients with a clinical presentation of congenital muscular dystrophy should also be considered for screening for integrin α7-deficiency. As no new patients have been diagnosed with a deficiency of α7-integrin since the initial identification, mutations appear to be rare.

4.2 Talin

Of the proteins that bind to the cytoplasmic domain of integrins, studies have revealed important functions for talin in mediating the connection to myofilaments at the MTJ. In

Drosophila, ablation of the talin gene (*mys*), induces detachment of actin filaments from the integrin cytoplasmic domain at muscle termini (Brown et al., 2002). Two talin isoforms are expressed in vertebrates, with talin 2 being most expressed in skeletal and cardiac muscle, while talin 1 is ubiquitous (Monkley et al., 2001). Muscle-specific ablation of talin 1 was achieved using conditional gene inactivation in muscle, as knockout of the talin 1 gene causes early embryonic lethality. In contrast, mice in which talin 2 was ablated were viable (Monkley et al., 2000; Conti et al., 2009). Both talin1-KO and talin2-KO mice presented with defects in skeletal muscle similar to those obtained following ablation of α7-integrin, consisting in structural failure at the MTJ, and a limited accumulation of centrally nucleated fibres, with no obvious damage to the sarcolemma. Consistent with the expression data, the phenotype was more severe in talin2-KO mice (Conti et al., 2008; Conti et al., 2009). Interestingly, adult muscle expresses a splice variant of integrin β1-integrin, termed β1D, which binds to F-actin with greater affinity than the ubiquitous β1A isoform (Belkin et al., 1997; van der Flier et al., 1997). The data suggest a model whereby a strong connection between the ECM and actin is established at the MTJ by complexes of α7β1D-integrin and talin 2, and, to a lesser extent, talin 1. In the absence of α7-integrin or of talin 2, stress induced by muscle contraction leads to mechanical failure at the MTJ.

4.3 Centrally nucleated fibres in myopathies

The reason for the accumulation of centrally nucleated fibres in muscles lacking integrins or talin is unclear. In muscular dystrophies, central nuclei are associated with regenerating fibres that are thought to form because the absence of DPC proteins causes fragility to the plasma membrane and necrosis of myofibres (Davies and Nowak, 2006). This does not occur when integrins are affected: patients with null mutations in the *itga7* gene have only mildly elevated plasma creatine kinase, and there is no evidence of damage to the sarcolemma in mice deficient in α7-integrin and talin 1 or 2 (Hayashi et al., 1998; Conti et al., 2008; Conti et al., 2009). Thus integrins appear dispensable for maintaining the structural integrity of the sarcolemma and other mechanisms must account for the presence of centrally nucleated fibres. One possibility is that cytoskeletal alterations might affect nuclear positioning. For example, internal nuclei were observed in mouse models lacking proteins that regulated actin organization and membrane trafficking, such as myotubularin 1, dynamin 2 and γ-actin, without evidence of damage to the sarcolemma (Buj-Bello et al., 2002; Bitoun et al., 2005; Sonnemann et al., 2006), but whether integrins regulate nuclear anchorage, it is at present unknown. Alternatively, integrins might be essential to provide survival signals to myofibres. In particular, signaling from FAK, which associates with talin, is important to suppress apoptosis in cultured cells (Lim et al., 2008). These signals might be perturbed in α7-KO and talin2-KO mice, leading to loss of myofibres and regeneration.

4.4 Vinculin

Vinculin is a ubiquitous component of focal adhesions that establishes a connection between integrins and an array of cytoskeletal proteins, including paxillin, talin, actin and the Arp2/3 complex, among others (Ziegler et al., 2006). In skeletal muscle, vinculin localizes to costameres, MTJ and NMJ (Bao et al., 1993), and in cardiac muscle, to costameres and intercalated disks (ICDs). Its expression levels are regulated by mechanical stress, and studies on cells in culture have revealed a function for vinculin in sensing mechanical stimuli and in reinforcing the connection of integrins to the actin cytoskeleton (Giannone et al., 2003; del Rio et al., 2009; Margadant et al., 2011). Cardiac myocyte-specific excision of the vinculin gene reveals an essential function for the structural integrity of the heart, where ICDs become disorganized and present with an altered distribution of the ICD proteins cadherins and connexin 43. Likely because of these defects, sudden death was found in about half of the transgenic mice, caused by ventricular tachycardia. The mice that survived developed dilated cardiomyopathy and died by 6 months of age (Zemljic-Harpf et al., 2007).

Mutations in the splice variant metavinculin, which includes an additional exon, have been identified in patients with dilated or hypertrophic cardiomyopathy, including deletions and missense mutations (Maeda et al., 1997; Olson et al., 2002; Vasile et al., 2006). A missense mutation in a vinculin-specific exon (L277M) was identified in a patient with hypertrophic cardiomyopathy, which led to a reduction in vinculin levels in ICDs (Vasile et al., 2006). Skeletal muscle problems were not reported for this patient, but the rarity of mutations in vinculin-specific exons, and the fact that the identified mutations are clustered in the metavinculin-specific exon, may be attributed to the fact that mutations in the ubiquitously expressed vinculin splice variant may lead to early lethality, as it occurs in mice (Xu et al., 1998).

5. Integrin signaling: Responses to mechanical stimuli

Integrins are important sensors of mechanical forces applied to cells (Geiger et al., 2009; Moore et al., 2010). For instance, the size of focal adhesions can be modulated by altering the stiffness of the ECM, actomyosin contractility, and by applying forces to specific integrin subunits (Giannone et al., 2003; Jiang et al., 2003; Moore et al., 2010). It is therefore significant that, in skeletal muscle, integrins are expressed specifically at costameres and MTJs, where mechanical stress generated by muscle contraction is transmitted through the plasma membrane to the ECM (Mayer, 2003). As we will see, integrins signaling is important for modultating hypertrophy in the heart in response to mechanical and soluble stimuli. Perhaps surprisingly, it is still unclear whether integrins are also important for regulating hypertrophy in skeletal muscle.

5.1 β1-integrin

No mutations in β1-integrin have been identified in patients, likely because compromised function would result in early lethality, as it occurs in the knockout mouse model (Fassler and Meyer, 1995; Schwander et al., 2003). However, mice with a heart-restricted ablation of β1-integrin present impaired contractility and develop ventricular fibrosis and cardiac hypertrophy in response to transverse aortic constriction (TAC, a procedure in which the lumen of the aorta is artificially restricted)(Shai et al., 2002). These data indicate that β1-integrins are essential for a normal response of cardiomyocytes to mechanical stress, and subsequent analysis identified several proteins associated with β1-integrin that mediate these effects.

5.2 Integrin-linked kinase (ILK)

ILK is closely associated to β1 and β3-integrins (Hannigan et al., 1996; Zervas et al., 2001; Wickstrom et al., 2010), and binds to several proteins that relay biochemical signals and regulate actin dynamics, including paxillin, α-and β-parvins and PKB. Ablation of ILK in invertebrates leads to detachment of myofibres at the MTJ, a phenotype similar to that obtained following ablation of talin (Zervas et al., 2001; Brown et al., 2002). Thus, in invertebrates, talin and ILK share a common function in the connection of actin to integrins at the MTJ. In vertebrates, however, MTJ defects following ablation of ILK differ from those observed in talin 1- or talin 2-KO mice. MTJ defects in ILK-deficient muscle consisted in discontinuities in the basal lamina and a detachment of actin filaments at the MTJ was not reported (Wang et al., 2008). ILK was important to stabilize MTJs in response to exercise, a process that might involve the relay of biochemical signals in association with the insulin growth factor receptor 1 (IGF-R1), which forms a complex with β1-integrins and plays a role during muscle repair (Musaro et al., 2001). IGF-R1 signaling was impaired in ILK-deficient muscle (Wang et al., 2008). Normally, in response to exercise, the insulin growth factor receptor 1R (IGF-1R) activates PKB/Akt, which in turn activates the kinase mTOR that is involved in the generation of new myofibrils. This activation was impaired in ILK-deficient muscle. Interestingly, β1-integrin was associated with IGF-R1, and this association increased in response to IGF-1. The data suggest a model whereby β1-integrin forms a complex with IGF-R1 that controls activation of ILK, the PKB/Akt and mTOR pathways to regulate skeletal muscle regeneration in response to exercise (Wang et al., 2008).

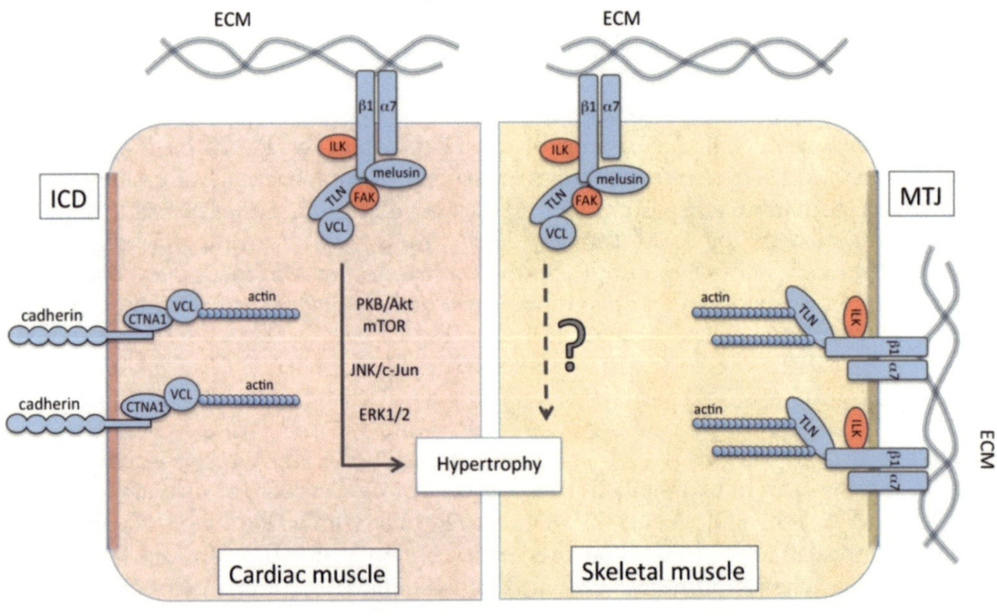

Fig. 2. **Integrin function in skeletal and cardiac muscle.** In skeletal muscle (right), integrins establish a connection between the ECM and actin filaments at the myotendinous junction (MTJ). In cardiac muscle (left), integrins activate hypetrophic signaling pathways, including PKB/AKT and mTOR, JNK/c-jun and ERK1/2, in response to mechanical and soluble stimuli. In addition, vinculin ablation leads to destabilization of intercalated disks (ICD). It is unclear at present whether integrins mediate hypertrophic responses in skeletal muscle. Abbreviations are: ECM = extracellular matrix; ILK = integrin-linked kinase; FAK = focal adhesion kinase; TLN = talin 1 or talin 2; VCL = vinculin; CTNA1 = α-catenin.

ILK is important for the sensing of mechanical stress in the heart. In the Zebrafish main squeeze (*msq*) mutant, isolated through a genetic screen, a missense mutation (L308P) was identified in the ILK gene (Bendig et al., 2006). Fish develop normally, but their hearts loose contractility, resulting in pericardial edema. The *msq* mutation disrupts the interaction with β-parvin, and morpholino-mediated knockdown of β-parvin phenocopies the ILK phenotype. These data suggests that the integrin-ILK-β-parvin complex is essential for transducing mechanical stimuli into signaling pathways important for cardiac contractility. In mice, conditional ablation of ILK in the heart causes dilated cardiomyopathy and sudden death in response to aortic pressure overload, with altered signaling from proteins involved in hypertrophy. A missense mutation in the ILK gene (A262V) has been identified in a patient affected by dilated cardiomyopathy (Knoll et al., 2007), and expression of ILK was elevated in patients affected by pathological cardiac hypertrophy, with a concomitant activation of signaling effectors associated with hypertrophic responses, including Rac, Cdc42, the ERK1/2 pathway and the kinase p70 S6 (Lu et al., 2006). It is at present unclear whether ILK plays any role in regulating hypertrophy in skeletal muscle.

5.3 Kindlin

Kindlin binds directly to β1-integrins and ILK. Three isoforms are expressed in vertebrates, named kindlin 1, 2 and 3. The main isoform expressed in skeletal and cardiac muscle is kindlin 2 (Ussar et al., 2006), which is localized at costameres and ICDs, again suggesting that it may play a structural role in areas of elevated mechanical stress (Dowling et al., 2008a). Mutations in kindlin 1 and 3 have been identified in patients affected by skin and immune disorders, respectively (Jobard et al., 2003; Siegel et al., 2003; Malinin et al., 2009; Svensson et al., 2009), but no mutations in kindlin 2 have been found in humans. *In vitro* studies have shown that kindlin 2 is important for differentiation of myoblasts (Dowling et al., 2008b), and knockdown of kindlin 2 in *Zebrafish* caused defective development of several organs, including skeletal and cardiac muscle, with disruption of ICDs and failure in the attachment of myofibrils to the membrane (Dowling et al., 2008a). Thus, kindlin 2 may be a good candidate gene for screening in patients affected by dilated cardiomyopathy or congenital myopathies.

5.4 FAK

Focal adhesion kinase (FAK) is closely associated with integrins, and following integrin engagement with ECM ligands, it becomes phosphorylated at tyrosine 397 (Y397). This creates a binding site for the SH2 domain of Src family kinases, and leads to the activation of several signaling effectors, including Rho and Rac, PI3K, Akt and the ERK1/2 signaling pathway (Franchini et al., 2009).

The tyrosine phosphorylation of FAK is rapidly increased following pressure overload in the rat heart (Franchini et al., 2000), and FAK activates hypertrophic signaling through PKB/AKT, the ERK1/2 and the JNK/c-JUN pathways. Additionally, FAK signaling regulates expression of the MEF2 transcription factors, which regulate the expression of several sarcomeric proteins (Nadruz et al., 2005). Insights on the function of FAK in striated muscle were obtained by generating mice with a conditional FAK ablation in cardiomyocytes. These mice developed defects that included thinner ventricular walls, ventricular septal defects and reduced cell numbers (DiMichele et al., 2006; Hakim et al.,

2007; Peng et al., 2008). However, the function of FAK in the postnatal heart is still unclear, as studies provide contrasting data on its function in cardiac hypertrophy, reporting either an increase in hypertrophy following mechanical or chemical stimuli (Peng et al., 2008), or an impaired hypertrophic response, with reduced expression of ANF and ERK1/2 (Hakim et al., 2007). The reason for the discrepancy is unclear, but it might be due to differences in the timing of FAK deletion, in the extent of aortic constriction, or in the genetic background of the mice.

The conditional inactivation of FAK in skeletal muscle has not been reported. In myoblasts, the application of mechanical forces to integrins results in FAK phosphorylation, and induction of hypertrophy in skeletal muscle leads to increased FAK expression and activation. Conversely, unloading of skeletal muscle leads to a sharp decrease in FAK activation (Fluck et al., 1999; Carson and Wei, 2000; Laser et al., 2000; Taylor et al., 2000; Gordon et al., 2001; Kovacic-Milivojevic et al., 2001). The inactivation of FAK in skeletal muscle would address its function and clarify whether its activity enhances or inhibits muscle hypertrophy.

5.5 Melusin

Melusin binds directly to β1-integrins and is expressed in skeletal and cardiac muscle, where it colocalises at costameres with integrins and vinculin (Brancaccio et al., 2003). Its domain structure includes in the N-terminus repeats of CHORD domain, which bind Zn2+, and in the C-terminus the integrin binding site and an acidic region resembling domains in calreticulin and calsequestrin that bind to calcium. In addition, while melusin is not endowed with catalytic activity, it includes binding sites for SH2- and SH3-domain proteins. The *itgb1 bp2* gene, encoding melusin, was inactivated in mice (Brancaccio et al., 2003). The mutant mice developed normally and were fertile. The basal structure and function of the heart were normal. However, when subjected to pressure overload via TAC, melusin-null mice presented with an impaired hypertrophic response, characterized by a reduction in myocyte cross-sectional area, ventricular wall thickness and induction of hypertrophic markers such as atrial neuretic factor and β-MHC. These changes led to an enlarged left ventricular chamber, a decrease in contractile function and eventually cardiac arrest, and may involve signaling through GSK3β and Akt, as phosphorylation in these proteins was reduced. Interestingly, unlike what is observed in FAK-deficient mice, infusion with angiotensin II or phenylephrine did not cause an aberrant hypertrophic response in melusin-null mice, indicating that melusin is required to specifically sense mechanical but not biohemical stimuli (Brancaccio et al., 2006; 2003). No overt defects in skeletal muscle were observed in melusing-knockout mice.

6. Conclusions and future perspectives

In recent years integrins have emerged as key players in skeletal muscle, both during development, where they are essential for somitogenesis, myoblast fusion and assembly of the sarcomere, and in the adult, where they play important structural roles, in particular in conferring mechanical integrity to the MTJ of skeletal muscle, and to ICDs in cardiac muscle in the heart. Key questions remain to be addressed. For instance, how do the functions of integrins differ from those of the DPC? While both protein complexes create a link between the ECM and the actin cytoskeleton, the assortment of proteins that are associated with each complex differs, and it is likely that specific signaling pathways elicit different biochemical responses. Studies in the heart indicate that integrins translate mechanical stimuli into hypertrophic responses. Are they important for regulating hypertrophy in skeletal muscle? It is also unclear how integrins regulate the process of myoblast fusion, for instance whether defects in the function of integrins lead to altered actin organization at sites of cell-cell fusion. Are signaling cascades activated by integrins important for the activation or recruitment of other effectors that mediate the breakdown of plasma membrane occurring during cell-cell fusion? Few patients affected by congenital myopathy have been identified with mutations in an integrin ($\alpha7$). It is unclear still how defects in integrin function lead to the observed muscle defects, as, unlike for the DPC, breakdown of the sarcolemma is not usually apparent. This may be elucidated with the identification of additional patients, and by an in-depth analysis of $\alpha7$-KO mice. Also, do mutations in other integrins or associated proteins underlie genetically undiagnosed cases of muscular dystrophy or congenital myopathy? Talin, kindlin and vinculin are good candidate genes, as genetic studies in animal models showed essential roles for these proteins in conferring structural integrity to skeletal or cardiac muscle.

7. Acknowledgements

We would like to thank Dr Yalda Jamshidi (St. George's University of London) and Dr Sarah Farmer (Institute of Child Health, UCL, London) for comments on the manuscript. This work was supported by funding from the Institute of Child Health and Great Ormond Street Hospitals Biomedical Research Centre (BRC 09DN09), Association Francaise contres les Myopathies (AFM 14572) (F.J.C.) and from the Muscular Dystrophy Association (S.C.B.).

8. References

Bader, B. L., Rayburn, H., Crowley, D. and Hynes, R. O. (1998) 'Extensive vasculogenesis, angiogenesis, and organogenesis precede lethality in mice lacking all alpha v integrins', *Cell* 95(4): 507-19.

Baker, L. P., Daggett, D. F. and Peng, H. B. (1994) 'Concentration of pp125 focal adhesion kinase (FAK) at the myotendinous junction', *Journal of cell science* 107 (Pt 6): 1485-97.

Bao, Z. Z., Lakonishok, M., Kaufman, S. and Horwitz, A. F. (1993) 'Alpha 7 beta 1 integrin is a component of the myotendinous junction on skeletal muscle', *Journal of cell science* 106 (Pt 2): 579-89.

Barresi, R. and Campbell, K. P. (2006) 'Dystroglycan: from biosynthesis to pathogenesis of human disease', *Journal of cell science* 119(Pt 2): 199-207.

Belkin, A. M., Retta, S. F., Pletjushkina, O. Y., Balzac, F., Silengo, L., Fassler, R., Koteliansky, V. E., Burridge, K. and Tarone, G. (1997) 'Muscle beta1D integrin reinforces the cytoskeleton-matrix link: modulation of integrin adhesive function by alternative splicing', *The Journal of cell biology* 139(6): 1583-95.

Bendig, G., Grimmler, M., Huttner, I. G., Wessels, G., Dahme, T., Just, S., Trano, N., Katus, H. A., Fishman, M. C. and Rottbauer, W. (2006) 'Integrin-linked kinase, a novel component of the cardiac mechanical stretch sensor, controls contractility in the zebrafish heart', *Genes & development* 20(17): 2361-72.

Bitoun, M., Maugenre, S., Jeannet, P. Y., Lacene, E., Ferrer, X., Laforet, P., Martin, J. J., Laporte, J., Lochmuller, H., Beggs, A. H. et al. (2005) 'Mutations in dynamin 2 cause dominant centronuclear myopathy', *Nature genetics* 37(11): 1207-9.

Boppart, M. D., Burkin, D. J. and Kaufman, S. J. (2006) 'Alpha7beta1-integrin regulates mechanotransduction and prevents skeletal muscle injury', *American journal of physiology. Cell physiology* 290(6): C1660-5.

Boppart, M. D., Volker, S. E., Alexander, N., Burkin, D. J. and Kaufman, S. J. (2008) 'Exercise promotes alpha7 integrin gene transcription and protection of skeletal muscle', *American journal of physiology. Regulatory, integrative and comparative physiology* 295(5): R1623-30.

Brancaccio, M., Fratta, L., Notte, A., Hirsch, E., Poulet, R., Guazzone, S., De Acetis, M., Vecchione, C., Marino, G., Altruda, F. et al. (2003) 'Melusin, a muscle-specific integrin beta1-interacting protein, is required to prevent cardiac failure in response to chronic pressure overload', *Nature medicine* 9(1): 68-75.

Brancaccio, M., Hirsch, E., Notte, A., Selvetella, G., Lembo, G. and Tarone, G. (2006) 'Integrin signalling: the tug-of-war in heart hypertrophy', *Cardiovascular research* 70(3): 422-33.

Brown, N. H., Gregory, S. L., Rickoll, W. L., Fessler, L. I., Prout, M., White, R. A. and Fristrom, J. W. (2002) 'Talin is essential for integrin function in Drosophila', *Developmental cell* 3(4): 569-79.

Buj-Bello, A., Laugel, V., Messaddeq, N., Zahreddine, H., Laporte, J., Pellissier, J. F. and Mandel, J. L. (2002) 'The lipid phosphatase myotubularin is essential for skeletal muscle maintenance but not for myogenesis in mice', *Proceedings of the National Academy of Sciences of the United States of America* 99(23): 15060-5.

Burkin, D. J., Wallace, G. Q., Milner, D. J., Chaney, E. J., Mulligan, J. A. and Kaufman, S. J. (2005) 'Transgenic expression of {alpha}7{beta}1 integrin maintains muscle integrity, increases regenerative capacity, promotes hypertrophy, and reduces cardiomyopathy in dystrophic mice', *The American journal of pathology* 166(1): 253-63.

Burkin, D. J., Wallace, G. Q., Nicol, K. J., Kaufman, D. J. and Kaufman, S. J. (2001) 'Enhanced expression of the alpha 7 beta 1 integrin reduces muscular dystrophy and restores viability in dystrophic mice', *The Journal of cell biology* 152(6): 1207-18.

Bushby, K. M. (1999) 'Making sense of the limb-girdle muscular dystrophies', *Brain : a journal of neurology* 122 (Pt 8): 1403-20.

Campbell, K. P. and Stull, J. T. (2003) 'Skeletal muscle basement membrane-sarcolemma-cytoskeleton interaction minireview series', *The Journal of biological chemistry* 278(15): 12599-600.

Carson, J. A. and Wei, L. (2000) 'Integrin signaling's potential for mediating gene expression in hypertrophying skeletal muscle', *Journal of applied physiology* 88(1): 337-43.

Chen, E. H., Grote, E., Mohler, W. and Vignery, A. (2007) 'Cell-cell fusion', *FEBS letters* 581(11): 2181-93.

Cohn, R. D., Mayer, U., Saher, G., Herrmann, R., van der Flier, A., Sonnenberg, A., Sorokin, L. and Voit, T. (1999) 'Secondary reduction of alpha7B integrin in laminin alpha2 deficient congenital muscular dystrophy supports an additional transmembrane link in skeletal muscle', *Journal of the neurological sciences* 163(2): 140-52.

Collo, G., Starr, L. and Quaranta, V. (1993) 'A new isoform of the laminin receptor integrin alpha 7 beta 1 is developmentally regulated in skeletal muscle', *The Journal of biological chemistry* 268(25): 19019-24.

Conti, F. J., Felder, A., Monkley, S., Schwander, M., Wood, M. R., Lieber, R., Critchley, D. and Muller, U. (2008) 'Progressive myopathy and defects in the maintenance of myotendinous junctions in mice that lack talin 1 in skeletal muscle', *Development* 135(11): 2043-53.

Conti, F. J., Monkley, S. J., Wood, M. R., Critchley, D. R. and Muller, U. (2009) 'Talin 1 and 2 are required for myoblast fusion, sarcomere assembly and the maintenance of myotendinous junctions', *Development* 136(21): 3597-606.

Critchley, D. R. (2004) 'Cytoskeletal proteins talin and vinculin in integrin-mediated adhesion', *Biochemical Society transactions* 32(Pt 5): 831-6.

Dalkilic, I., Schienda, J., Thompson, T. G. and Kunkel, L. M. (2006) 'Loss of Filamin C (FLNc) results in severe defects in myogenesis and myotube structure', *Molecular and cellular biology* 26(17): 6522-34.

Davies, K. E. and Nowak, K. J. (2006) 'Molecular mechanisms of muscular dystrophies: old and new players', *Nature reviews. Molecular cell biology* 7(10): 762-73.

del Rio, A., Perez-Jimenez, R., Liu, R., Roca-Cusachs, P., Fernandez, J. M. and Sheetz, M. P. (2009) 'Stretching single talin rod molecules activates vinculin binding', *Science* 323(5914): 638-41.

DiMichele, L. A., Doherty, J. T., Rojas, M., Beggs, H. E., Reichardt, L. F., Mack, C. P. and Taylor, J. M. (2006) 'Myocyte-restricted focal adhesion kinase deletion attenuates pressure overload-induced hypertrophy', *Circulation research* 99(6): 636-45.

Dowling, J. J., Gibbs, E., Russell, M., Goldman, D., Minarcik, J., Golden, J. A. and Feldman, E. L. (2008a) 'Kindlin-2 is an essential component of intercalated discs and is required for vertebrate cardiac structure and function', *Circulation research* 102(4): 423-31.

Dowling, J. J., Vreede, A. P., Kim, S., Golden, J. and Feldman, E. L. (2008b) 'Kindlin-2 is required for myocyte elongation and is essential for myogenesis', *BMC cell biology* 9: 36.

Duff, R. M., Tay, V., Hackman, P., Ravenscroft, G., McLean, C., Kennedy, P., Steinbach, A., Schoffler, W., van der Ven, P. F., Furst, D. O. et al. (2011) 'Mutations in the N-terminal actin-binding domain of filamin C cause a distal myopathy', *American journal of human genetics* 88(6): 729-40.

Ervasti, J. M. (2003) 'Costameres: the Achilles' heel of Herculean muscle', *The Journal of biological chemistry* 278(16): 13591-4.

Fassler, R. and Meyer, M. (1995) 'Consequences of lack of beta 1 integrin gene expression in mice', *Genes & development* 9(15): 1896-908.

Fluck, M., Carson, J. A., Gordon, S. E., Ziemiecki, A. and Booth, F. W. (1999) 'Focal adhesion proteins FAK and paxillin increase in hypertrophied skeletal muscle', *The American journal of physiology* 277(1 Pt 1): C152-62.

Franchini, K. G., Clemente, C. F. and Marin, T. M. (2009) 'Focal adhesion kinase signaling in cardiac hypertrophy and failure', *Brazilian journal of medical and biological research = Revista brasileira de pesquisas medicas e biologicas / Sociedade Brasileira de Biofisica ... [et al.]* 42(1): 44-52.

Franchini, K. G., Torsoni, A. S., Soares, P. H. and Saad, M. J. (2000) 'Early activation of the multicomponent signaling complex associated with focal adhesion kinase induced by pressure overload in the rat heart', *Circulation research* 87(7): 558-65.

Gardner, H., Kreidberg, J., Koteliansky, V. and Jaenisch, R. (1996) 'Deletion of integrin alpha 1 by homologous recombination permits normal murine development but gives rise to a specific deficit in cell adhesion', *Developmental biology* 175(2): 301-13.

Geiger, B., Spatz, J. P. and Bershadsky, A. D. (2009) 'Environmental sensing through focal adhesions', *Nature reviews. Molecular cell biology* 10(1): 21-33.

Georges-Labouesse, E., Messaddeq, N., Yehia, G., Cadalbert, L., Dierich, A. and Le Meur, M. (1996) 'Absence of integrin alpha 6 leads to epidermolysis bullosa and neonatal death in mice', *Nature genetics* 13(3): 370-3.

Giannone, G., Jiang, G., Sutton, D. H., Critchley, D. R. and Sheetz, M. P. (2003) 'Talin1 is critical for force-dependent reinforcement of initial integrin-cytoskeleton bonds but not tyrosine kinase activation', *The Journal of cell biology* 163(2): 409-19.

Gordon, S. E., Fluck, M. and Booth, F. W. (2001) 'Selected Contribution: Skeletal muscle focal adhesion kinase, paxillin, and serum response factor are loading dependent', *Journal of applied physiology* 90(3): 1174-83; discussion 1165.

Goyenvalle, A., Seto, J. T., Davies, K. E. and Chamberlain, J. (2011) 'Therapeutic approaches to muscular dystrophy', *Human molecular genetics* 20(R1): R69-78.

Gullberg, D., Velling, T., Lohikangas, L. and Tiger, C. F. (1998) 'Integrins during muscle development and in muscular dystrophies', *Frontiers in bioscience : a journal and virtual library* 3: D1039-50.

Hakim, Z. S., DiMichele, L. A., Doherty, J. T., Homeister, J. W., Beggs, H. E., Reichardt, L. F., Schwartz, R. J., Brackhan, J., Smithies, O., Mack, C. P. et al. (2007) 'Conditional deletion of focal adhesion kinase leads to defects in ventricular septation and outflow tract alignment', *Molecular and cellular biology* 27(15): 5352-64.

Hannigan, G. E., Leung-Hagesteijn, C., Fitz-Gibbon, L., Coppolino, M. G., Radeva, G., Filmus, J., Bell, J. C. and Dedhar, S. (1996) 'Regulation of cell adhesion and anchorage-dependent growth by a new beta 1-integrin-linked protein kinase', *Nature* 379(6560): 91-6.

Hayashi, Y. K., Chou, F. L., Engvall, E., Ogawa, M., Matsuda, C., Hirabayashi, S., Yokochi, K., Ziober, B. L., Kramer, R. H., Kaufman, S. J. et al. (1998) 'Mutations in the integrin alpha7 gene cause congenital myopathy', *Nature genetics* 19(1): 94-7.

Hemler, M. E. (2001) 'Specific tetraspanin functions', *The Journal of cell biology* 155(7): 1103-7.

Hodges, B. L., Hayashi, Y. K., Nonaka, I., Wang, W., Arahata, K. and Kaufman, S. J. (1997) 'Altered expression of the alpha7beta1 integrin in human and murine muscular dystrophies', *Journal of cell science* 110 (Pt 22): 2873-81.

Huang, X. Z., Wu, J. F., Ferrando, R., Lee, J. H., Wang, Y. L., Farese, R. V., Jr. and Sheppard, D. (2000) 'Fatal bilateral chylothorax in mice lacking the integrin alpha9beta1', *Molecular and cellular biology* 20(14): 5208-15.

Hynes, R. O. (2002) 'Integrins: bidirectional, allosteric signaling machines', *Cell* 110(6): 673-87.

Jiang, G., Giannone, G., Critchley, D. R., Fukumoto, E. and Sheetz, M. P. (2003) 'Two-piconewton slip bond between fibronectin and the cytoskeleton depends on talin', *Nature* 424(6946): 334-7.

Jobard, F., Bouadjar, B., Caux, F., Hadj-Rabia, S., Has, C., Matsuda, F., Weissenbach, J., Lathrop, M., Prud'homme, J. F. and Fischer, J. (2003) 'Identification of mutations in a new gene encoding a FERM family protein with a pleckstrin homology domain in Kindler syndrome', *Human molecular genetics* 12(8): 925-35.

Kaji, K., Oda, S., Shikano, T., Ohnuki, T., Uematsu, Y., Sakagami, J., Tada, N., Miyazaki, S. and Kudo, A. (2000) 'The gamete fusion process is defective in eggs of Cd9-deficient mice', *Nature genetics* 24(3): 279-82.

Knoll, R., Postel, R., Wang, J., Kratzner, R., Hennecke, G., Vacaru, A. M., Vakeel, P., Schubert, C., Murthy, K., Rana, B. K. et al. (2007) 'Laminin-alpha4 and integrin-linked kinase mutations cause human cardiomyopathy via simultaneous defects in cardiomyocytes and endothelial cells', *Circulation* 116(5): 515-25.

Kovacic-Milivojevic, B., Roediger, F., Almeida, E. A., Damsky, C. H., Gardner, D. G. and Ilic, D. (2001) 'Focal adhesion kinase and p130Cas mediate both sarcomeric organization and activation of genes associated with cardiac myocyte hypertrophy', *Molecular biology of the cell* 12(8): 2290-307.

Kreidberg, J. A., Donovan, M. J., Goldstein, S. L., Rennke, H., Shepherd, K., Jones, R. C. and Jaenisch, R. (1996) 'Alpha 3 beta 1 integrin has a crucial role in kidney and lung organogenesis', *Development* 122(11): 3537-47.

Laser, M., Willey, C. D., Jiang, W., Cooper, G. t., Menick, D. R., Zile, M. R. and Kuppuswamy, D. (2000) 'Integrin activation and focal complex formation in cardiac hypertrophy', *The Journal of biological chemistry* 275(45): 35624-30.

Laurin, M., Fradet, N., Blangy, A., Hall, A., Vuori, K. and Cote, J. F. (2008) 'The atypical Rac activator Dock180 (Dock1) regulates myoblast fusion in vivo', *Proceedings of the National Academy of Sciences of the United States of America* 105(40): 15446-51.

Lim, S. T., Mikolon, D., Stupack, D. G. and Schlaepfer, D. D. (2008) 'FERM control of FAK function: implications for cancer therapy', *Cell cycle* 7(15): 2306-14.

Lowe, T., Kley, R. A., van der Ven, P. F., Himmel, M., Huebner, A., Vorgerd, M. and Furst, D. O. (2007) 'The pathomechanism of filaminopathy: altered biochemical properties explain the cellular phenotype of a protein aggregation myopathy', *Human molecular genetics* 16(11): 1351-8.

Lu, H., Fedak, P. W., Dai, X., Du, C., Zhou, Y. Q., Henkelman, M., Mongroo, P. S., Lau, A., Yamabi, H., Hinek, A. et al. (2006) 'Integrin-linked kinase expression is elevated in human cardiac hypertrophy and induces hypertrophy in transgenic mice', *Circulation* 114(21): 2271-9.

Maeda, M., Holder, E., Lowes, B., Valent, S. and Bies, R. D. (1997) 'Dilated cardiomyopathy associated with deficiency of the cytoskeletal protein metavinculin', *Circulation* 95(1): 17-20.

Malinin, N. L., Zhang, L., Choi, J., Ciocea, A., Razorenova, O., Ma, Y. Q., Podrez, E. A., Tosi, M., Lennon, D. P., Caplan, A. I. et al. (2009) 'A point mutation in KINDLIN3 ablates activation of three integrin subfamilies in humans', *Nature medicine* 15(3): 313-8.

Margadant, F., Chew, L. L., Hu, X., Yu, H., Bate, N., Zhang, X. and Sheetz, M. (2011) 'Mechanotransduction in vivo by repeated talin stretch-relaxation events depends upon vinculin', *PLoS biology* 9(12): e1001223.

Martin, P. T., Kaufman, S. J., Kramer, R. H. and Sanes, J. R. (1996) 'Synaptic integrins in developing, adult, and mutant muscle: selective association of alpha1, alpha7A, and alpha7B integrins with the neuromuscular junction', *Developmental biology* 174(1): 125-39.

Mayer, U. (2003) 'Integrins: redundant or important players in skeletal muscle?', *The Journal of biological chemistry* 278(17): 14587-90.

Mayer, U., Saher, G., Fassler, R., Bornemann, A., Echtermeyer, F., von der Mark, H., Miosge, N., Poschl, E. and von der Mark, K. (1997) 'Absence of integrin alpha 7 causes a novel form of muscular dystrophy', *Nature genetics* 17(3): 318-23.

Miosge, N., Klenczar, C., Herken, R., Willem, M. and Mayer, U. (1999) 'Organization of the myotendinous junction is dependent on the presence of alpha7beta1 integrin', *Laboratory investigation; a journal of technical methods and pathology* 79(12): 1591-9.

Monkley, S. J., Pritchard, C. A. and Critchley, D. R. (2001) 'Analysis of the mammalian talin2 gene TLN2', *Biochemical and biophysical research communications* 286(5): 880-5.

Monkley, S. J., Zhou, X. H., Kinston, S. J., Giblett, S. M., Hemmings, L., Priddle, H., Brown, J. E., Pritchard, C. A., Critchley, D. R. and Fassler, R. (2000) 'Disruption of the talin gene arrests mouse development at the gastrulation stage', *Developmental dynamics : an official publication of the American Association of Anatomists* 219(4): 560-74.

Moore, S. W., Roca-Cusachs, P. and Sheetz, M. P. (2010) 'Stretchy proteins on stretchy substrates: the important elements of integrin-mediated rigidity sensing', *Developmental cell* 19(2): 194-206.

Musaro, A., McCullagh, K., Paul, A., Houghton, L., Dobrowolny, G., Molinaro, M., Barton, E. R., Sweeney, H. L. and Rosenthal, N. (2001) 'Localized Igf-1 transgene expression sustains hypertrophy and regeneration in senescent skeletal muscle', *Nature genetics* 27(2): 195-200.

Nadruz, W., Jr., Corat, M. A., Marin, T. M., Guimaraes Pereira, G. A. and Franchini, K. G. (2005) 'Focal adhesion kinase mediates MEF2 and c-Jun activation by stretch: role in the activation of the cardiac hypertrophic genetic program', *Cardiovascular research* 68(1): 87-97.

Nakashima, H., Kibe, T. and Yokochi, K. (2009) "Congenital muscular dystrophy caused by integrin alpha7 deficiency", *Developmental medicine and child neurology* 51(3): 245.

Nishimune, H., Valdez, G., Jarad, G., Moulson, C. L., Muller, U., Miner, J. H. and Sanes, J. R. (2008) 'Laminins promote postsynaptic maturation by an autocrine mechanism at the neuromuscular junction', *The Journal of cell biology* 182(6): 1201-15.

Olson, T. M., Illenberger, S., Kishimoto, N. Y., Huttelmaier, S., Keating, M. T. and Jockusch, B. M. (2002) 'Metavinculin mutations alter actin interaction in dilated cardiomyopathy', *Circulation* 105(4): 431-7.

Pajcini, K. V., Pomerantz, J. H., Alkan, O., Doyonnas, R. and Blau, H. M. (2008) 'Myoblasts and macrophages share molecular components that contribute to cell-cell fusion', *The Journal of cell biology* 180(5): 1005-19.

Peng, X., Wu, X., Druso, J. E., Wei, H., Park, A. Y., Kraus, M. S., Alcaraz, A., Chen, J., Chien, S., Cerione, R. A. et al. (2008) 'Cardiac developmental defects and eccentric right ventricular hypertrophy in cardiomyocyte focal adhesion kinase (FAK) conditional knockout mice', *Proceedings of the National Academy of Sciences of the United States of America* 105(18): 6638-43.

Quach, N. L. and Rando, T. A. (2006) 'Focal adhesion kinase is essential for costamerogenesis in cultured skeletal muscle cells', *Developmental biology* 293(1): 38-52.

Rochlin, K., Yu, S., Roy, S. and Baylies, M. K. (2010) 'Myoblast fusion: when it takes more to make one', *Developmental biology* 341(1): 66-83.

Samson, T., Will, C., Knoblauch, A., Sharek, L., von der Mark, K., Burridge, K. and Wixler, V. (2007) 'Def-6, a guanine nucleotide exchange factor for Rac1, interacts with the skeletal muscle integrin chain alpha7A and influences myoblast differentiation', *The Journal of biological chemistry* 282(21): 15730-42.

Sanes, J. R. (2003) 'The basement membrane/basal lamina of skeletal muscle', *The Journal of biological chemistry* 278(15): 12601-4.

Schwander, M., Leu, M., Stumm, M., Dorchies, O. M., Ruegg, U. T., Schittny, J. and Muller, U. (2003) 'Beta1 integrins regulate myoblast fusion and sarcomere assembly', *Developmental cell* 4(5): 673-85.

Senetar, M. A. and McCann, R. O. (2005) 'Gene duplication and functional divergence during evolution of the cytoskeletal linker protein talin', *Gene* 362: 141-52.

Shai, S. Y., Harpf, A. E., Babbitt, C. J., Jordan, M. C., Fishbein, M. C., Chen, J., Omura, M., Leil, T. A., Becker, K. D., Jiang, M. et al. (2002) 'Cardiac myocyte-specific excision of the beta1 integrin gene results in myocardial fibrosis and cardiac failure', *Circulation research* 90(4): 458-64.

Siegel, D. H., Ashton, G. H., Penagos, H. G., Lee, J. V., Feiler, H. S., Wilhelmsen, K. C., South, A. P., Smith, F. J., Prescott, A. R., Wessagowit, V. et al. (2003) 'Loss of kindlin-1, a human homolog of the Caenorhabditis elegans actin-extracellular-matrix linker protein UNC-112, causes Kindler syndrome', *American journal of human genetics* 73(1): 174-87.

Singhal, N. and Martin, P. T. (2011) 'Role of extracellular matrix proteins and their receptors in the development of the vertebrate neuromuscular junction', *Developmental neurobiology* 71(11): 982-1005.

Sonnemann, K. J., Fitzsimons, D. P., Patel, J. R., Liu, Y., Schneider, M. F., Moss, R. L. and Ervasti, J. M. (2006) 'Cytoplasmic gamma-actin is not required for skeletal muscle development but its absence leads to a progressive myopathy', *Developmental cell* 11(3): 387-97.

Svensson, L., Howarth, K., McDowall, A., Patzak, I., Evans, R., Ussar, S., Moser, M., Metin, A., Fried, M., Tomlinson, I. et al. (2009) 'Leukocyte adhesion deficiency-III is caused by mutations in KINDLIN3 affecting integrin activation', *Nature medicine* 15(3): 306-12.

Taverna, D., Disatnik, M. H., Rayburn, H., Bronson, R. T., Yang, J., Rando, T. A. and Hynes, R. O. (1998) 'Dystrophic muscle in mice chimeric for expression of alpha5 integrin', *The Journal of cell biology* 143(3): 849-59.

Taylor, J. M., Rovin, J. D. and Parsons, J. T. (2000) 'A role for focal adhesion kinase in phenylephrine-induced hypertrophy of rat ventricular cardiomyocytes', *The Journal of biological chemistry* 275(25): 19250-7.

Thorsteinsdottir, S., Deries, M., Cachaco, A. S. and Bajanca, F. (2011) 'The extracellular matrix dimension of skeletal muscle development', *Developmental biology* 354(2): 191-207.

Tidball, J. G. (1991) 'Force transmission across muscle cell membranes', *Journal of biomechanics* 24 Suppl 1: 43-52.

Ussar, S., Wang, H. V., Linder, S., Fassler, R. and Moser, M. (2006) 'The Kindlins: subcellular localization and expression during murine development', *Experimental cell research* 312(16): 3142-51.

van der Flier, A., Gaspar, A. C., Thorsteinsdottir, S., Baudoin, C., Groeneveld, E., Mummery, C. L. and Sonnenberg, A. (1997) 'Spatial and temporal expression of the beta1D integrin during mouse development', *Developmental dynamics : an official publication of the American Association of Anatomists* 210(4): 472-86.

Vasile, V. C., Will, M. L., Ommen, S. R., Edwards, W. D., Olson, T. M. and Ackerman, M. J. (2006) 'Identification of a metavinculin missense mutation, R975W, associated with both hypertrophic and dilated cardiomyopathy', *Molecular genetics and metabolism* 87(2): 169-74.

Vasyutina, E., Martarelli, B., Brakebusch, C., Wende, H. and Birchmeier, C. (2009) 'The small G-proteins Rac1 and Cdc42 are essential for myoblast fusion in the mouse', *Proceedings of the National Academy of Sciences of the United States of America* 106(22): 8935-40.

Vorgerd, M., van der Ven, P. F., Bruchertseifer, V., Lowe, T., Kley, R. A., Schroder, R., Lochmuller, H., Himmel, M., Koehler, K., Furst, D. O. et al. (2005) 'A mutation in the dimerization domain of filamin c causes a novel type of autosomal dominant myofibrillar myopathy', *American journal of human genetics* 77(2): 297-304.

Wang, A., Patrone, L., McDonald, J. A. and Sheppard, D. (1995) 'Expression of the integrin subunit alpha 9 in the murine embryo', *Developmental dynamics : an official publication of the American Association of Anatomists* 204(4): 421-31.

Wang, H. V., Chang, L. W., Brixius, K., Wickstrom, S. A., Montanez, E., Thievessen, I., Schwander, M., Muller, U., Bloch, W., Mayer, U. et al. (2008) 'Integrin-linked kinase stabilizes myotendinous junctions and protects muscle from stress-induced damage', *The Journal of cell biology* 180(5): 1037-49.

Wickstrom, S. A., Lange, A., Montanez, E. and Fassler, R. (2010) 'The ILK/PINCH/parvin complex: the kinase is dead, long live the pseudokinase!', *The EMBO journal* 29(2): 281-91.

Xu, W., Baribault, H. and Adamson, E. D. (1998) 'Vinculin knockout results in heart and brain defects during embryonic development', *Development* 125(2): 327-37.

Zaidel-Bar, R., Itzkovitz, S., Ma'ayan, A., Iyengar, R. and Geiger, B. (2007) 'Functional atlas of the integrin adhesome', *Nature cell biology* 9(8): 858-67.

Zemljic-Harpf, A. E., Miller, J. C., Henderson, S. A., Wright, A. T., Manso, A. M., Elsherif, L., Dalton, N. D., Thor, A. K., Perkins, G. A., McCulloch, A. D. et al. (2007) 'Cardiac-myocyte-specific excision of the vinculin gene disrupts cellular junctions, causing sudden death or dilated cardiomyopathy', *Molecular and cellular biology* 27(21): 7522-37.

Zervas, C. G., Gregory, S. L. and Brown, N. H. (2001) 'Drosophila integrin-linked kinase is required at sites of integrin adhesion to link the cytoskeleton to the plasma membrane', *The Journal of cell biology* 152(5): 1007-18.

Zhou, A. X., Hartwig, J. H. and Akyurek, L. M. (2010) 'Filamins in cell signaling, transcription and organ development', *Trends in cell biology* 20(2): 113-23.

Ziegler, W. H., Liddington, R. C. and Critchley, D. R. (2006) 'The structure and regulation of vinculin', *Trends in cell biology* 16(9): 453-60.

Ziober, B. L., Vu, M. P., Waleh, N., Crawford, J., Lin, C. S. and Kramer, R. H. (1993) 'Alternative extracellular and cytoplasmic domains of the integrin alpha 7 subunit are differentially expressed during development', *The Journal of biological chemistry* 268(35): 26773-83.

2

Facioscapulohumeral Muscular Dystrophy: From Clinical Data to Molecular Genetics and Return

Monica Salani[2], Elisabetta Morini[1], Isabella Scionti[1] and Rossella Tupler[1,2]
[1]*Universita' degli Studi di Modena e Reggio Emilia,*
[2]*University of Massachussets Medical School,*
[1]*Italy*
[2]*USA*

1. Introduction

Facioscapulohumeral muscular dystrophy (FSHD or Dejerine-Landouzy muscular dystrophy, OMIM #158900) is the third most common hereditary myopathy, with prevalence of 1 in 20,000 (Padberg, 1982; Mostacciuolo et al., 2009). This disease is characterized by the progressive wasting of a highly selective set of muscle groups (Padberg, 1982) and it has been traditionally classified as an autosomal dominant trait (Lunt, 1998; Padberg, 1992). FSHD genetic locus has been mapped on chromosome 4q35 by genetic linkage analysis (Wijmenga et al., 1990). Interestingly, this muscular dystrophy has not yet been related to a classical mutation within a protein-coding gene, but rather the disease has been associated with DNA rearrangements in a polymorphic genomic region consisting of an array of tandemly repeated 3.3 kb segments, named D4Z4 (Wijmenga et al., 1992b). D4Z4 contains an ORF encoding a putative homeobox protein called "DUX4." The existence of native transcripts of DUX4 from D4Z4 single repeats is still controversial (Gabriels et al., 1999; Hewitt et al., 1994; Lyle et al., 1995), although recent data show evidences of the presence of the DUX4 transcript from the last D4Z4 unit in FSHD myoblasts (Lemmers et al., 2010a). The number of D4Z4 repeats varies from 11 to 100 in the general population, whereas less than 11 repeats are usually present in sporadic and familial FSHD patients. A very low copy number of 4q35 D4Z4 repeats (1-3) often correlates with an earlier onset and more severe disease. However no FSHD-linked array has been found to have zero copies of the repeat unit (Tupler et al., 1996; van der Maarel et al., 2007) suggesting that the repeat itself plays a critical role in the disease. Alleles with 4-7 repeats are the most frequent in the FSHD population and are associated with the more common form of FSHD that usually presents in adulthood, whereas alleles with 8-10 repeats typically display milder disease phenotypes with reduced penetrance. Nearly identical and equally polymorphic D4Z4 sequences reside on the subtelomere of chromosome 10q (Bakker et al., 1995; Deidda et al., 1995). The proportion of individuals in the general population carrying 4q or 10q chromosome ends with repeat arrays entirely or partially transferred between both chromosomes, is considerable (van Deutekom et al., 1996b; Lemmers et al., 1998; van Overveld et al., 2000). Rearrangements between 4q and 10q subtelomeres occur in 20% of subjects and represent an additional complication to FSHD molecular diagnosis. However, only subjects with reduced number of D4Z4 repeats on chromosome 4, but not on chromosome 10, develop FSHD. Thus, molecular diagnosis of FSHD is, at this time, based on the analysis of the D4Z4 polymorphic alleles (Lunt, 1998; Tawil et al., 2010). Despite the identification of the genetic defect associated with FSHD, the pathologic effects of the reduction of D4Z4 elements remain largely unknown. The observation of the unique linkage of the disease with chromosome 4, led to the hypothesis that in *cis* DNA elements must be present on D4Z4 reduced alleles to explain disease onset. An element within D4Z4 has been shown to behave as a silencer that provides a binding site for a transcriptional repressing complex (Gabellini et al., 2002). These results suggest a model in which reduction of D4Z4 leads to the inappropriate transcriptional derepression of proximal chromosome 4-specific genes. Indeed, closely located genes such as FSHD Region Gene 2 (*FRG2*), FSHD Region Gene 1 (*FRG1*), and Adenine Nucleotide Translocator (*ANT1*), with high myopathic potential, were observed to be transcriptionally upregulated in FSHD muscle (Gabellini et al., 2002). However, studies testing this model obtained conflicting results with some showing support (Gabellini et al., 2002; Rijkers et al., 2004; Klooster et al., 2009; Bodega et al., 2009), and others not (Winokur et al., 2003b; Jang et al., 2003; Osborne et al., 2007; Masny et al., 2010). These discrepancies prevented a general consensus on the role of 4q35 genes upregulation in FSHD pathogenesis. Recently it has been proposed that FSHD arises from chromosomes bearing a short D4Z4 repeat array associated with a novel polyadenylation signal capable of stabilizing *DUX4* mRNA from the normally transcriptionally inactive DUX4 gene. However, there is reason to believe that this model does not account for all FSHD cases. For example, several studies described FSHD patients carrying full-length D4Z4 alleles that are clinically indistinguishable from FSHD subjects carrying D4Z4 reduced alleles. Conversely, there is a high percent of normal individuals, unrelated to any FSHD patients, with reduced D4Z4 alleles (Scionti et al., 2012b). Most importantly it has been recently showed that the polymorphism adding the polyadenylation signal to *DUX4* RNA, is common in the general population. Thus, just a portion of subjects carrying this molecular signature develops FSHD (Scionti et al., 2012b). Consequently, the number of D4Z4 repeats at 4q35 by itself or in association with a specific haplotype, does not to fully explain FSHD development. The non linear correlation between the number of D4Z4 elements and FSHD expression raises the question whether or when FSHD can be considered a simple autosomal dominant mendelian disorder, or if a more complex picture should be considered in clinical practice. Indeed, recent findings suggest that epigenetic modification at the disease locus, such as DNA methylation (de Greef et al., 2008), histone modifications (Zeng et al., 2009) or chromosomal architecture (Petrov et al., 2006) can be altered in FSHD patients, adding further levels of complexity. Undeniably, the incomplete knowledge of molecular mechanism(s) leading to FSHD onset has hampered the possibility of developing effective therapeutic strategies. This chapter aims to discuss the recent advances in our understanding of FSHD pathology viewed against its clinical heterogeneity, considering all the factors that can contribute to the complexity of this elusive disease.

2. FSHD Clinical features: Role of D4Z4 repeats reduction

2.1 Clinical features

Facioscapulohumeral muscular dystrophy is considered an autosomal dominant myopathy characterized by progressive atrophy and weakness of a highly selective set of muscle groups (Padberg, 1982). The onset of the disease is in the second/third decade of life and usually involves weakness of facial mimic muscles. The clinical presentation is characterized by an initially restricted distribution of weakness starting with asymptomatic facial weakness followed by scapular fixator, humeral, truncal, and lower extremity weakness. The onset of lower-extremity weakness is typically in the anterior leg compartment, presenting with footdrop. Extraocular and bulbar muscles are typically spared. Although facial weakness is perhaps the most recognizable aspect of FSHD, affected individuals from otherwise clinically typical families may have no or minimal facial weakness (Flanigan et al., 2004). Weak abdominal muscles result in a protuberant abdomen and contribute to the lumbar lordosis. Lower abdominal muscles are weaker than the upper abdominal muscles, causing a strikingly positive Beevor's sign, a physical finding fairly specific for FSHD. In advanced cases, hip girdle may be as affected or more than shoulder girdle muscles, making difficult the clinical distinction between FSHD and limb-girdle muscular dystrophy. A notable distinctive feature of FSHD is that muscle weakness displays an asymmetric distribution, which does not correlate with the handedness of the individual (Brouwer et al., 1992). The chronology of disease progression is unpredictable; for example, long periods of stability can be followed by sudden and dramatic worsening. In addition, there is a wide variability in the spectrum of disease among patients, ranging from subjects with very mild muscle weakness, who are almost unaware of being affected, to those who are wheelchair-dependent. This variability in disease penetrance was exemplified by a set of monozygotic male twins who carried the same genetic mutation but were affected by FSHD to a dramatically different extent (Tupler et al., 1998). Electromyography and histological analysis reveal non-specific myopathic changes associated, in some cases, with neurologic aspects. The creatine kinase (CK) level can be moderately increased or normal. Thus, diagnosis of FSHD is mainly based on the clinical phenotype in combination with a molecular test (Lunt et al 1995; Lunt, 1998). Ancillary features such as sensorineural deafness or retinal vasculopathy have been also reported in FSHD patients, but they are not to be considered decisive criteria for FSHD diagnosis (Fitzsimmons et al., 1987; Padberg et al., 1995; Trevisan et al., 2008).

2.2 Molecular diagnosis

The FSHD genetic defect does not reside in mutation of any protein-coding gene. Instead FSHD has been causally associated with reduction of the number of 3.3 kb DNA elements at the subtelomeric region of chromosome 4q. When digested with the restriction enzyme EcoRI the FSHD allele originates a fragment of 35 kb in size or shorter that can be detected by Southern analysis using the probe p13E-11 (Wijmenga et al., 1992b). The polymorphic genomic region, identified by probe p13E-11, consists of an array of tandem repeat 3.3-kb segments (hereafter referred to as D4Z4 repeats), such that the variation in the size of EcoRI fragments is due to variability in the number of D4Z4 repeats (van Deutekom et al., 1993) (Figure 1). Normal subjects carry p13E−11 EcoRI alleles longer than 50 kb (>10 D4Z4 units) originating from chromosome 4 whereas alleles of 35 kb or shorter (≤ 8 D4Z4 units) are present in the majority of either de novo or familial FSHD patients (Lunt, 1998). *De novo* reduced allele transmitted by an affected parent to the offspring co-segregate with the disorder (Griggs et al., 1993). New mutations account for a surprisingly high percentage of FSHD patients (10%−33%) (Padberg et al., 1995; Zatz et al., 1995). This high incidence can be partly explained by the presence of parental mosaicism for 4q short alleles that has been reported in 19% of *de novo* cases (Upadhyaya et al.; 1995, Köhler et al.; 1996, Lemmers et al.,

2004). The presence of somatic mosaicism for a rearrangement of D4Z4 was found in as much as 3% of the general population (van der Maarel et al., 2000), suggesting that the D4Z4 repeat is highly recombinogenic.

A complication of molecular testing by Southern analysis is represented by the presence of a polymorphic region recognized by probe p13E-11 at the subtelomeric region of chromosome 10q, which shares numerous homologies with the 4q subtelomere (Bakker et al., 1995; Deidda et al., 1996). The repeat element at 10q is 98% identical to D4Z4 at 4q, and the size of 10q EcoRI alleles varies between 11 and 300 kb (1-100 D4Z4 units). Moreover, 10% of these alleles are shorter than 35 kb (8 D4Z4 units) (Bakker et al., 1996; Bakker et al., 1995), overlapping the 4q alleles. Clearly these overlapping features can interfere with the molecular diagnosis of FSHD. Nevertheless the presence of a BlnI restriction site within the 3.3 kb element associated with chromosome 10q allows the discrimination between 4q and 10q alleles (Deidda et al., 1996). As a result, Southern blot hybridization of EcoRI and EcoRI/BlnI digested genomic DNA is used for the molecular diagnosis of FSHD (Lunt, 1998) (Figure 1).

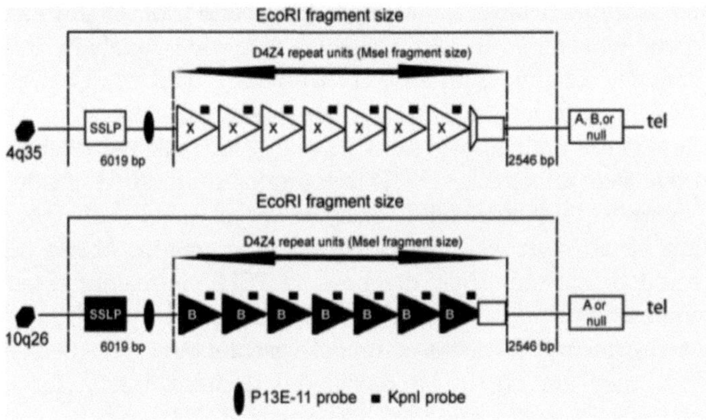

$$\frac{\text{[EcoRI fragment lenght - (6019 + 2546)]}}{\text{3.3 kb}} = \text{Number of D4Z4 repeats}$$

D4Z4 repeat units	EcoRI fragment approximate size
1U	12-13 kb
2U	14-16 kb
3U	17-20 kb
4U	21-23 kb
5U	24-26 kb
6U	27-30 kb
7U	31-33 kb
8U	34-36 kb
9U	37-39 kb
10U	40-43 kb

Fig. 1. **Schematic representation of Polymorphisms at the 4q and 10q subtelomeres.** Schematic representation of the method used to calculate D4Z4 repeat numbers from *Eco*RI-fragment sizes. Seven and eight D4Z4 repeats (31-36 kb *Eco*RI fragment size) were defined to be the upper diagnostic range for FSHD. D4Z4 repeat units on chromosomes 4 and 10 can be distinguished because all repeats on 10q contain *BlnI* restriction sites (**B**), while all D4Z4 repeats on 4q contain *XapI* restriction sites (**X**).

Through years, additional findings have emerged that need to be considered in the molecular diagnosis of FSHD. First, translocated 4-type repeats residing on chromosome 10q as well as translocated 10-type repeats residing on chromosome 4q are found in 10% of the population (van Deutekom et al., 1996b; van Overveld et al., 2000; Matsumura et al., 2002;). Therefore, FSHD-sized D4Z4 alleles may be attributed incorrectly to chromosome 10 and viceversa. Second, deletions at 4q encompassing the genomic sequence recognized by probe p13E-11 have been detected in FSHD cases. Thus D4Z4 short arrays might not be detected by using the standard diagnostic procedure. The frequency of such extended deletions has been estimated around 3% (Lemmers et al., 2003) and represents a possible caveat of FSHD molecular diagnosis. Third, 5-10% of subjects showing FSHD clinical features do not carry D4Z4 reduced alleles. Possible explanations for such anomalous cases include a different mechanism at 4q35, such as D4Z4 hypomethylation (De Greef et al, 2009) or the presence of other mutations not linked to the FSHD locus at 4q35. At present, no FSHD families linked to other chromosomal loci have been described. Figure 2 summarizes the diagnostic flow chart that should be used to study the 4q35 region in FSHD patients.

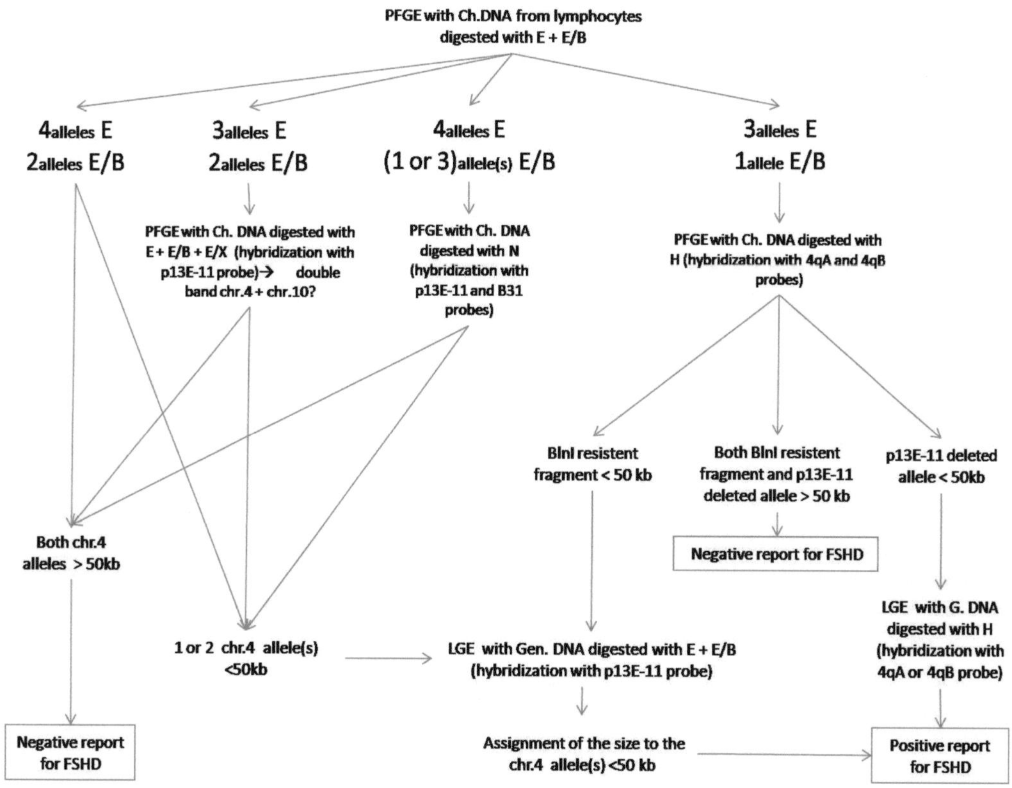

Fig. 2. **Schematic representation of FSHD diagnostic approach at 4q35 locus.**
Abbreviations: **Ch.DNA**: chromosomal DNA embedded in plugs; **Gen.DNA**: genomic DNA in solution; **PFGE**: Pulse Field Gel Electrophoresis; **LGE**: Linear Gel Electrophoresis; **E**: restriction enzyme EcoRI; **B**: restriction enzyme BlnI; **X**: restriction enzyme XapI; **N**: restriction enzyme NotI; **H**: restriction enzyme HindIII.

2.3 FSHD clinical ascertainment and molecular diagnosis: Necessity of standardized clinical examination

As said before, genomic studies conducted on groups of FSHD patients and families revealed the numerous difficulties that can be encountered in the molecular characterization of the 4q35 locus. Through years, the complexity of molecular diagnosis has been paralleled by the emerging complexity of FSHD clinical ascertainment. At present, criteria established in 1991, before the advent of molecular diagnosis (Padberg et al., 1991), and in 1998, following the ENMC workshop on FSHD (Lunt 1998), need probably to be reconsidered in light of the most recent observations.

2.3.1 Penetrance

Non-penetrance in FSHD was estimated to be less than 2% after the age of 50 years and more likely with allele sizes larger than 30 kb (Tawil et al., 1996). However, asymptomatic gene carriers seem to be more prominent in some families, and non-penetrance has even been found in carriers of 25 kb D4Z4 alleles (Ricci et al., 1999). In his work, Ricci et al. detected D4Z4 reduced alleles in several unaffected family members, named non-penetrant carriers, who are capable of transmitting the disease to their offspring. In addition reduced penetrance for D4Z4 reduced alleles was described in families in which patients heterozygous for FSHD alleles on both 4q chromosomes were present (Wohlgemuth et al., 2003; Tonini et al., 2004). Gender differences have been also described in FSHD, with males apparently more affected than females (Tonini et al., 2004). Nowadays correlation between penetrance of FSHD, length of the repeat array, age and sex is unsettled. Thus, the risk of developing the disease in correlation with D4Z4 allele sizes cannot be estimated and no prognostic tools are available. In addition several clinical reports describe patients displaying clinical and genetic features of FSHD associated with other documented muscle disorders including mitochondrial diseases (Chuenkongkaew et al., 2005; Filosto et al., 2008), glycogenosis (Nadaj-Pakleza et al., 2009), dystrophinopathies (Rudnik-Schoneborn et al., 2008). In all these cases the presence of the FSHD molecular defect seems to aggravate the clinical phenotype. Finally, phenotypic features of FSHD can be found in other myopathies (Oya et al., 2001; Saenz et al., 2005) as well as atypical phenotypes can be displayed by subjects carrying the FSHD molecular defect (Figueroa and Chapin, 2010; Tsuji et al., 2009; Zouvelou et al., 2009). All together these observations suggest that the variable penetrance observed in the FSHD population may be the result of the interaction of several factors. Indeed the presence of low-penetrant alleles suggests that susceptibility for FSHD is not only determined by the intrinsic properties of the diseased allele but also by additional factors that can be genetic, epigenetic and/or environmental factors. Identification of factors influencing FSHD clinical outcome remains one of the major challenges of FSHD research.

2.3.2 Severity of the disease and repeats number: Does a linear correlation exist?

An inverse relationship has been established between the D4Z4 repeat size and the severity and progression of the disease (Lunt et al., 1995; Ricci et al., 1999; Tawil et al., 1996; Zatz et al., 1998). In general, individuals with ≥11 repeats are healthy; in contrast, 1-3 D4Z4 repeats is associated with a severe form of disease that presents in childhood, 4-7 repeats with the most common form of FSHD, and 8-10 repeats with a milder disease and reduced penetrance. Nevertheless great variability of clinical expression has been described among FSHD patients even within the same family. Interestingly it has been suggested that patients harboring D4Z4 alleles of ≥35 kb (≥ 8 repeats) were less likely to present the classic FSHD phenotype as compared with patients with alleles of <35 kb (<8 repeats) (Felice and Whitaker, 2005). Several clinical reports described myopathic patients, carrying alleles of 38 kb (9 repeats) or larger, showing typical and atypical FSHD phenotypes (Vitelli et al., 1999; Felice et al., 2000; Felice and Moore, 2001; Butz et al., 2003; Krasnianski et al., 2003). However D4Z4 repeat arrays of size between 38-45 kb (9-11 repeats) were encountered in 3% of 200 control subjects in a Dutch study (van Overveld et al., 2000). These findings seems to indicate that in a substantial proportion of 38 to 45 kb-sized repeat arrays penetrance may be close to zero, but in some families 38−45 kb alleles are associated with myopathy (Butz et al., 2003). Remarkably D4Z4 repeat array of size between 21-34 kb (4-8 repeats) were found in 3% of 801 Italian and Brazilian samples of normal individuals unrelated to any FSHD patients, indicating that in this size-range, additional factors influence the disease expression (Scionti et al., 2012b). In conclusion the high variability in clinical expression makes difficult to establish a prognostic correlation between the number of the D4Z4 repeats and the severity of the disease. There is the necessity of clinical and molecular studies on large cohorts of FSHD patients and families to obtain significant information on FSHD development and generate useful prognostic information.

2.3.3 A standardized clinical evaluation tool: FSHD score

Based on the need of gaining statistically significant observations through large cohorts studies, a standardized clinical evaluation tool for patients with FSHD was created. The clinical protocol examines muscle groups specifically affected in FSHD. The test uses functional criteria, which allow expression of clinical severity in quantitative terms (Lamperti et al., 2010). The clinical examination results in an evaluation scale, which is divided into six independent sections that assess the strength and the functionality of (I) facial muscles (scored from 0 to 2); (II) scapular girdle muscles (scored from 0 to 3); (III) upper limb muscles (scored from 0 to 2); (IV) distal leg muscles (scored from 0 to 2); (V) pelvic girdle muscles (scored from 0 to 5); and (VI) abdominal muscles (scored from 0 to 1). The evaluation scale allows the functional quantification of muscle weakness in FSHD patients. This examination protocol, which is associated with a questionnaire that collects information on the clinical history of the subject, generates a disability score resulting from the sum of six independent scores of separately evaluated muscle regions, including the facial and abdominal muscles, which are specifically affected by FSHD. The total score can range from 0, when no signs of muscle weakness are present, to 15, when all muscle groups tested are severely impaired. The protocol represents a robust evaluation procedure for FSHD patients that can be performed easily in the medical office and is not influenced by the tester. The robustness of the clinical evaluation protocol provides a tool that can therefore be used by different neurologists in large cooperative clinical studies and allows translating what is called clinical impression of the progressive involvement of specific muscle groups into a number (Lamperti et al., 2010) (The FSHD clinical form and the FSHD evaluation scale form, as well as a visual guide to clinical assessment, are available online at www.fshd.it).

Use of the FSHD score can support studies for defining the natural history of the disease throughout time. Importantly, definition of the clinical involvement of specific muscle groups by a number permits identification and characterization of atypical cases and support the definition of clinical subcategories among FSHD patients.

By assessing the correlation between clinical severity, results of molecular analysis, and anamnestic records, the FSHD score can provide useful information for defining FSHD nosology.

3. Genomic characteristic of the 4q35 region: D4Z4 and role of specific polymorphisms

Since the discovery of the FSHD molecular defect (Wijmenga et al 1992b), many studies suggested the possibility that reduction of D4Z4 repeat units on chromosome 4 alone is not sufficient to FSHD development (Weiffenbach et al 1993; van Overveld et al., 2000; Lemmers et al., 2002, Lemmers et al., 2007). Thus, a detailed genomic characterization of the 4q35 region led to the identification of polymorphic regions flanking the D4Z4 repeat array which could contribute to FSHD onset.

3.1 Genetic variability and haplotypes

D4Z4 is part of a family of 3.3-kb repeats (D4Z4) are dispersed throughout the human genome and are generally found associated with regions of heterochromatin (Lyle et al.,1995). A homologue D4Z4 tandem array is present at the 10q telomere. This homology between the subtelomeric region of 10q and 4q is not confined to D4Z4 repeats but extends proximal 42 kb and distally to include the telomere (van Geel et al., 2002). However, despite the high level of sequence similarity (> 98% nucleotide identity) between the 10q and 4q subtelomeres, FSHD is associated only with the chromosome 4q (Bakker et al., 1995; Deidda et al., 1996). In the attempt of explaining the unique association between D4Z4 reduction of chromosome 4q and FSHD, a bi-allelic polymorphism was identified distal to the repeat array (van Geel et al., 2002). Two distinct polymorphic regions, named 4qA and 4qB, were observed at the distal end of chromosome 4q. Within 4qA there is a polymorphic 8-kb region of 68bp satellite DNA immediately distal to the D4Z4, and adjacent to this is a 1-kb divergent $(TTAGGG)_n$ array. None of these repeats is present within the 4qB sequence. In 4qB polymorphism, the last 3.3-kb repeat contains only the first 570 bp of a complete unit, whereas in 4qA the terminal repeat is a divergent 3.3-kb repeat named pLAM (van Deutekom et al., 1993). Sequence alignment and subsequent phylogenetic analysis of subtelomeric region of 10q showed a close relationship between 4qA sequences and 10q suggesting that the 4q subtelomere has been transferred onto chromosome 10q (van Geel et al., 2002). The distribution of these allelic variants is heterogeneous and depends on the studied population. Lemmers and colleagues (2004), analyzing 80 Dutch control individuals, have observed an almost equal frequencies of 4qA and 4qB alleles (42% and 58%, respectively), whereas in another study, conducted on 66 Italian control individuals, an overrepresentation of 4qA telomeres has been reported (68% for 4qA and 32% for 4qB) (Rossi et al., 2007). Proximal to the D4Z4 repeat array a simple sequence-length polymorphism (SSLP) has been described and those sequences are in a range between 157 bp and 180 bp (Figure 3).

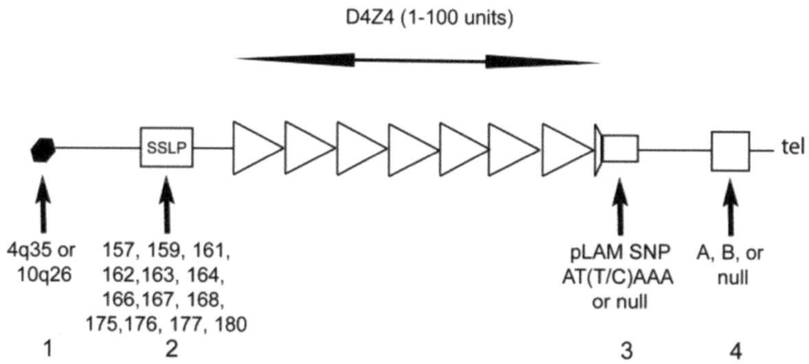

Fig. 3. The D4Z4 repeat array within the subtelomere of chromosomes 4q and 10q varies in size between 1 and 100 D4Z4 units (3.3-330 kb) and it is indicated with triangles. Elements that distinguish subjects include: 1. The chromosomal localization of the D4Z4 repeat, chromosome 4q35 or 10q26. 2. The Simple Sequence Length Polymorphism (SSLP). It is a combination of five Variable Number Tandem Repeats, an 8 bp insertion/deletion, and two SNPs localized 3.5 kb proximal to D4Z4 and vary in length between 157 and 182 bp. 3. Single nucleotide polymorphism AT(T/C)AAA (SNP) in the pLAM region. 4. A large sequence variation (termed 4qA or B) that is distal to D4Z4. In the 4qB variant the terminal 3.3-kb repeat contains only 570 bp of a complete repeat, whereas in the 4qA variant the terminal repeat is a divergent 3.3-kb repeat named pLAM. 4q chromosomes which do not hybridize to probes for A and B are termed "null" and their sequences vary from case to case.

A worldwide population (including African, European and Asian HAPMAP panels) analysis of 4q subtelomeric polymorphisms flanking the D4Z4 array revealed 17 distinct haplotypes on chromosome 4q (Lemmers et al., 2010b). On the basis of sequence similarities, all haplotypes were categorized in two groups: the major group 1 consists mainly of the haplotypes 4A159, 4A161 and 4B163, which are the most common in all three HAPMAP populations. The major group 2 contains other standard and nonstandard 4q haplotypes (4A166 and 4A168). Evolutionary studies showed that haplotypes 4A159 and 4A161 represent the oldest human D4Z4 haplotypes. Similarly, the 4A168 haplotype is most probably the oldest haplotype that belongs to major group 2. It has been hypothesized that all other haplotypes originate from only four discrete sequence-transfer events during human evolution (Lemmers et al., 2010b).

3.2 Permissive and non-permissive genetic background

Analysis of 4qter polymorphisms of 80 unrelated Dutch patients with FSHD revealed that D4Z4-reduced alleles are associated with the 4qA variant (Lemmers et al., 2002). Subsequently, by studying three families in which two D4Z4-reduced alleles segregate, it has been proposed that 4qB chromosomes carrying short D4Z4 repeats do not cause FSHD, since only subjects carrying D4Z4-reduced alleles associated with the 4qA polymorphism had FSHD (Lemmers et al., 2004). The almost exclusive association between FSHD disease-expression and the D4Z4-reduced allele of the 4qA type has been confirmed in a large cohort of 164 unrelated patients with FSHD from Turkey and the UK. Even though that study described FSHD patients lacking the 4qA/4qB end (Thomas et al., 2007). Subsequent studies led to the hypothesis that D4Z4 contraction on 4qA chromosome *per se* is not sufficient to cause disease. Analysis of SSLP proximal to the repeat array in 86 FSHD patients and 222 healthy controls revealed a unique association of FSHD with the 161 allele and the 4qA sequence. In particular the haplotype 4A166 associated with D4Z4-reduced alleles was detected in multiple unaffected relatives of two independent families and the 4B163 haplotype was associated with 17 FSHD-sized alleles carried in healthy subjects (Lemmers et al., 2007). On this basis it has been hypothesized that FSHD can develop only in a specific "permissive" chromosomal background represented by the haplotype 4A161. Following this hypothesis, proximal and distal sequences of 4A161 chromosome were compared to those of "non-permissive" ones, such as 4B163 and 10A166. This approach led to the identification of a single nucleotide polymorphism (SNP, AT(T/C)AAA) in the adjacent pLAM sequence, immediately distal to D4Z4 array. In particular 4A161 and two other uncommon permissive variants, 4A159 and 4A168 presented the ATTAAA variant, which has been interpreted as a polyadenylation signal able to stabilize the *DUX4* transcript (Figure 4a).

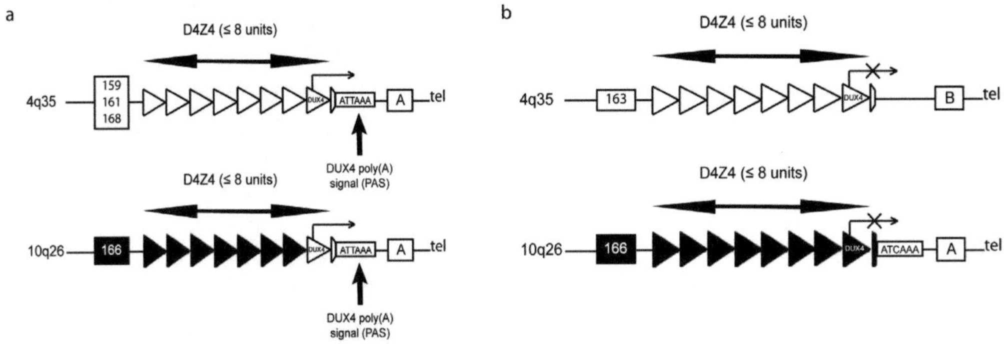

Fig. 4. **Schematic representation of the current view of permissive and not-permissive haplotype. a.** Permissive haplotypes **b.** Non-permissive haplotype. The ATTAAA variant creates a polyadenylation signal (PAS) that stabilizes the *DUX4* transcript and has been postulated to be the critical factor causing FSHD.

By contrast sequences associated with non-permissive chromosome 10A166 and 4B did not allow the expression of DUX4 (Lemmers et al., 2010a). Analysis of more than 300 unrelated FSHD patients and 5 families with one or more FSHD patients carrying D4Z4-reduced allele strongly supported the hypothesis that the last 4qA D4Z4 unit with the directly adjacent pLAM sequence including the ATTAAA is necessary to the FSHD development (Lemmers et al., 2010a). On this basis it has been proposed that FSHD arises through a toxic gain of function attributable to the stabilized distal *DUX4* transcript (Lemmers et al., 2010a) (Figure 4b). Despite the intriguing premise, the notion that FSHD is a fully-penetrant autosomal dominant disorder caused by the reduction of D4Z4 repeat number associated with 4A161PAS haplotype is challenged by recently published data. First a study conducted on 750 unrelated FSHD families from Italy revealed that the frequency of individuals carrying two D4Z4 reduced alleles (compound heterozygotes) is 2,7%, a frequency much higher than expected for a fully penetrant autosomal dominant disorder with prevalence of 1 in 20,000. Interestingly in these families with compound heterozygosity, 25% of relatives carrying D4Z4-reduced alleles and 4A161PAS are healthy (Scionti et al., 2012a). Second, characterization of 253 unrelated FSHD probands from the Italian National Registry for FSHD showed that only 127 of them (50.1%) carry D4Z4 alleles with 1-8 D4Z4 associated with 4A161PAS, whereas the remaining FSHD probands carry different haplotypes or alleles with greater number of D4Z4 repeats (Scionti et al., 2012b). Third, molecular analysis of 801 normal healthy subjects from Italy and Brazil showed that that 3% of individuals from the general population carry alleles with reduced number (4-8) of D4Z4 repeats on chromosome 4q and one third of these alleles occurs in combination with the 4A161PAS haplotype (Scionti et al., 2012b) All these findings challenge the hypothesis that 4APAS structure is necessary and sufficient for the development of FSHD. This discovery is not incompatible with evidence implicating DUX4 or other factors as important mediators of disease. Nonetheless, it does demonstrate that FSHD pathogenesis is more complex than currently thought.

4. One disease (too) many theories

After the genetic correlation between D4Z4 and FSHD the most difficult task has been to explain the role of D4Z4 in disease development. D4Z4 can directly cause FSHD through DUX4 expression; on the other end D4Z4 reduction might indirectly cause FSHD by exerting long distance effects. None of the proposed models entirely explain the mechanism leading to disease. In this regard the scientific community does not express undisputed consensus.

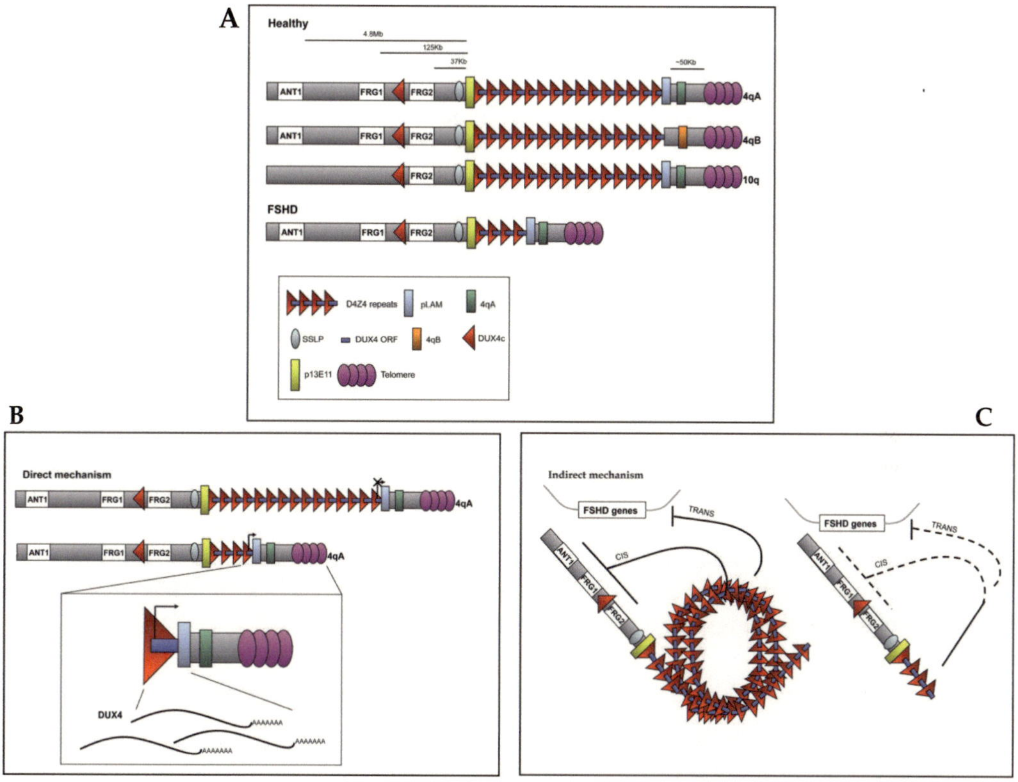

Fig. 5. **Models for the molecular basis of FSHD. A.** Healthy individuals carry 11-150 units of D4Z4, whereas FSHD patients have less than 11 repeats. **B. DIRECT MECHANISM**: reduction of D4Z4 repeat array leads to the synthesis of DUX4 transcript, which is normally not transcribed, through changes in D4Z4 heterochromatin and/or stabilization of DUX4 mRNA. **C. INDIRECT MECHANISM:** the reduction of D4Z4 repeats leads to modifications of the spatial and structural organization of chromatin generating changes of transcriptional control over the expression of candidate genes localized in *cis* or in *trans*.

In examining all the models that have been proposed it is important to remember essential points:

- 80-85% of FSHD patients carry a reduction in D4Z4 whereas loss of the whole array is not associated with FSHD;
- 15-20% of FSHD patients have a normal number of repeats;
- No specific 4q haplotype is associated with FSHD;
- 25% of relatives carrying D4Z4 alleles who are old than 56 years do not have FSHD;
- Healthy individuals bearing allele with reduced number of repeats (4-8 units) are present in 3% of the healthy population;
- Repeat reduction in the highly homologous D4Z4 copy on chromosome 10 is not associated with the FSHD;
- Penetrance of the FSHD is not complete and its severity does not clearly correlate with number of repeats;

Notably in all proposed models, epigenetic changes such as methylation or histone modifications are used as an additional level of complexity that might help interpreting the complex correlation between genotype and phenotype in FSHD. In this paragraph we will shortly describe the main mechanisms that have been proposed. In the following paragraphs all the factors that have been considered important for the disease onset will be explained in detail.

4.1 Direct mechanism: DUX4

The most recent model proposed to explain FSHD pathogenesis is based on the idea that the most distal copy of the *DUX4* gene, whose open reading frame is present in each D4Z4 repeat, is transcribed and the expression of this gene has a direct role in FSHD pathophysiology. At first it has been proposed that partial reduction of the D4Z4 repeat array results in destabilization of the D4Z4 heterochromatin and in the inappropriate upregulation of *DUX4* gene (Gabriels et al., 1999; Hewitt et al., 1994). However this hypothesis has never been proven. This model has been consequently modified introducing the concept of a "permissive" chromosomal background namely a single nucleotide polymorphism in the pLAM sequence that provides a polyadenylation signal (PAS) for the *DUX4* transcript. This should stabilize the *DUX4* transcript from the most distal D4Z4 unit on 4q chromosomes resulting in disease through a toxic gain-of-function mechanism (Lemmers et al., 2010b) (Figure 5A).

4.2 Indirect mechanism: Iindirect overexpression of candidate genes

All the other models proposed to explain the role of D4Z4-reduced alleles in FSHD pathogenesis, predict that D4Z4 reduction is able to generate a modification in the spatial and structural organization of chromatin at 4q35. As a consequence loss of transcriptional control over the expression of candidate genes, localized in *cis* or in *trans*, is generated (Figure 5B).

Cis-spreading model: 4q35 genes derepression

D4Z4 contains heterochromatic DNA elements. It was thus reasoned that D4Z4 and surrounding sequences would be strongly packed as heterochromatin. Based on this idea, it was hypothesized that loss of D4Z4 repeat would produce a local chromatin relaxation (i.e., loss of heterochromatinization) and, consequently, the transcriptional upregulation of genes nearby D4Z4, possibly in a distance-related manner (Hewitt et al., 1994; Winokur et al., 1994).

The identification of a repressor complex that binds to a specific 27 bp DNA element within D4Z4 (Gabellini et al., 2002) supports the *cis*-spreading model. Consistently, three 4qter genes (*FRG2, FRG1,* and *ANT1)* were found upregulated in muscle of FSHD patients (Gabellini et al., 2002).

Cis-looping model: 4q35 genes derepression

According to this model, D4Z4 is able to interact with target gene(s) by long-distance loops only when the D4Z4 contraction impairs the formation of normal D4Z4 intra-array loops. The hypothesis that normal-sized D4Z4 repeats form intra-array loops is supported by the size distribution of D4Z4 repeats which is multimodal, with equidistant peaks 65 kb apart (van Overveld et al., 2000).

Insulator model

D4Z4 is localized between the distal heterochromatic telomeric sequences and the euchromatic sequences more upstream. It has thus been proposed that it might act as an insulator (van Deutekom, 1996a). Reduction of the repeat arrays would impair the separation between domains, and, consequently, the spreading of heterochromatic would silence proximal genes in *cis*. This model is supported by the finding that D4Z4 itself acts as an insulator, which interferes with enhancer–promoter communication and protects from position effect (Ottaviani et al., 2009). Results obtained with different experimental approaches demonstrated that both, the transcriptional factor CTCF (CCCTC-Binding factor), and the A-type intermediate filament Lamins binding, are necessary for D4Z4 insulator function. In this model, FSHD contracted *D4Z4* array associates with CTCF and A-type Lamins at the nuclear periphery resulting in both *cis* and *trans* insulation of gene(s) physiologically interacting with the 4q35 terminal sequences (Ottaviani et al., 2010). This may lead to the miss regulation of these genes and to the FSHD phenotype.

Cis model: Nuclear localization

The FSHD genomic region at 4q35.2 is consistently and specifically localized at the nuclear envelope (Petrov et al., 2006; Ottaviani et al., 2009) in proliferating myoblasts, fibroblasts, lymphoblasts, and differentiated myotubes. Interestingly it is not the D4Z4 repeat itself that mediates interaction with the nuclear envelope but a chromosome 4 genomic regions just proximal to the D4Z4 repeat (D4S139) (Masny et al., 2004; Ottaviani et al., 2009). Since FSHD region is localized to the nuclear periphery, an alternative model for FSHD pathogenesis has been proposed. In this model improper interaction with transcription factors or chromatin modifiers at the nuclear envelope could induce aberrant expression of genes localized in *cis* or in *trans*. However a differential localization of normal or FSHD alleles to the nuclear periphery has not been observed (Masny et al., 2004).

Trans-effect model: Genome wide effect

It has been also postulated that reduction of D4Z4 might have a more genome-wide effects, affecting other pathways, such the slow-to-fast fiber differentiation pathway (Celegato et al., 2006) and the response to oxidative stress and myogenic differentiation pathway (Winokur et al., 2003b). Because D4Z4 can be regarded as a docking platform for protein factors, loss of repeats may generate a local imbalance in the availability of D4Z4 proteins in the cell, and/or lead to new interaction with different proteins at the disease allele.

5. Direct role of D4Z4: The double homeobox gene 4 (DUX4)

The D4Z4 unit has been completely sequenced (Hewitt et al., 1994; Winokur et al., 1994 Lee et al., 1995). Each D4Z4 repeat unit contains an ORF with a double homeobox putatively encoding the DUX4 protein. *DUX4* belongs to a family of highly homologous genes scattered throughout the genome. One almost identical copy, named *DUX4c*, is located 42 kb proximal to the repeat array. Based on the presence of the molecular signature 4A-PAS, which should allow the stabilization of the mRNA from the distal copy of the *DUX4* gene; it has been proposed that FSHD arises through a toxic gain-of-function mechanism attributable to the pathological expression of *DUX4* mRNA (Lemmers et al., 2010a). More detailed analysis of *DUX4* expression shows that the *DUX4* pre-mRNA can be alternatively spliced and apparently, the FSHD muscle expresses a different splice form of *DUX4* mRNA compared to control muscle (Snider et al., 2010). It is important to note that *DUX4* is a rare transcript and the amount of *DUX4* has been estimated in one copy per cell. To explain how such low expression level of *DUX4* can cause FSHD, it has been proposed that in FSHD muscle the DUX4 protein may exert its toxic effect in a small subset of nuclei, which express a relatively abundant amount of *DUX4* transcript. The possible toxic effect of DUX4 has been inferred on the basis of in vitro and in vivo studies (Kowaljow et al., 2007; Bosnakovski et al., 2008; Wallace et al., 2011) in which *DUX4* was expressed at very high levels. Thus in order to explain FSHD pathogenesis, it is difficult to reconcile those experimental observations with the very limited amount of *DUX4* detected in human muscle cells.

6. 4q35 genes in FSHD phatogenesis: Role of genes overexpression

Although the exact molecular mechanism responsible for FSHD is unknown, it is a common agreement that reduction of D4Z4 elements might cause up-regulation of gene(s) in *cis*. A few genes have been considered as good candidates for FSHD based on their localization and/or function.

This section will critically discuss function and potential role of 4q35 candidate genes in FSHD development.

6.1 FSHD region gene 2 (FRG2)

FSHD Region Gene 2 (*FRG2*) was originally identified by *in silico* gene prediction (Van Geel et al., 1999) as a region of 3 kb 37 kb proximal to the D4Z4 repeat array. Predicted exons are preceded by a putative muscle specific promoter. *FRG2* gene is composed of four exons and encodes an mRNA of 2084 bp with two alternative polyadenylation sites. The *FRG2* ORF encodes a putative protein of 278 amino acids. The FRG2 protein does not show significant homology to known proteins (Rijkers et al., 2004). Alternative splicing creates an additional alanine codon (Rijkers et al., 2004). Even though *FRG2* has been shown to be nuclear, (Rijkers et al., 2004) its sequence contains not only two potential nuclear localization signals (NLS) but also a peroxisomal targeting signal (PTS1) at the carboxyterminal end of the protein (Swinkels et al., 1992). Copies of *FRG2* are dispersed throughout the genome, prevalently located in subtelomeric or pericentromeric regions (Winokur et al., 1994; van Geel et al., 1999; van Geel et al., 2002). However, only the *FRG2* copies on chromosomes 4 and 10 show a 98% identity, differing for just five nucleotide mismatches in the ORF (Rijkers et al., 2004). Experiments demonstrated that the *FRG2* promoter is sensitive to the presence of D4Z4 repeat units making *FRG2* an interesting candidate gene for FSHD pathophysiology (Rijkers et al., 2004). Indeed it has been shown that overexpression of *FRG2* is obtained by suppressing the activity of the D4Z4 recognition complex (DRC) (Gabellini et al., 2002). Moreover data suggests that in muscle biopsies from FSHD patients, *FRG2* overexpression inversely correlates with D4Z4 repeat number (Gabellini et al., 2002). However the overexpression of *FRG2* in FSHD is still controversial. If there is a general agreement that mRNA is virtually absent in most of human tissue, there is no consensus regarding the expression of *FRG2* in FSHD patients' samples. *FRG2* overexpression was reported in differentiating, but not proliferating myoblasts of FSHD patients (Rijkers et al., 2004). The overexpression of *FRG2* in FSHD myotubes has not been fully confirmed in other works (Arashiro et al., 2009; Cheli et al., 2011; Masny et al., 2010; Osborne et al., 2007). The different outcomes of expression studies may be explained by the intrinsic difficulties in detecting *FRG2* mRNA due to its low expression level and by the presence in the genome of multiple copies of *FRG2*. Moreover *FRG2* is not represented in the gene arrays currently used for RNA expression studies. Whether *FRG2* is involved in FSHD pathogenesis still remains in discussion. Indeed muscle-specific overexpression of *FRG2* in mice does not result in an aberrant phenotype (Figure 6A) (Gabellini et al., 2006), and FSHD patient with proximal deletion encompassing FRG2 have been found (Lemmers et al., 2003). Nevertheless it is worth mentioning that *FRG2* appears late in the evolution together with D4Z4 repeats and it is not present in the mice genome making the mice model for *FRG2* overexpression not conclusive. The function of this protein is still unknown.

6.2 FSHD region gene 1 (*FRG1*)

In the human genome *FRG1* gene is located 125 kb centromeric to D4Z4 array on chromosome 4. As for many other genes from the 4q subtelomeric region, several copies of FRG1 are present in the human genome (van Deutekom et al., 1996c). The *FRG1* copy on chromosome 4 encodes a 258-amino acid protein. Although the FRG1 protein does not share significant overall homology to any known protein, it contains two nuclear localization signals in the N-terminal region (NLSs, aa 22-25 and 29-32), a bipartite NLS in the C-terminal region (aa 253-261) and a single fascin-like domain (aa 58-176), indicative of an actin-binding protein (Figure 6B), one potential RNA-binding domain (22-35 aa) homologous to several RNA-binding proteins (RBPs). FRG1 protein is highly conserved among invertebrates and vertebrates: human FRG1 shares 42% identity with *C. elegans*, 81% identity with *Xenopus* and 97% identity with mouse protein (Figure 6B). The high level of conservation throughout species suggests that FRG1 might have a very important function that is preserved during the evolution.

Since its discovery, FSHD Region Gene 1 (*FRG1*) has been considered a candidate gene for FSHD (Van Deutekom et al., 1996c). Analysis of its expression level in muscle tissues obtained from FSHD patients and healthy subjects showed that *FRG1* was abnormally up-regulated in FSHD affected muscles. Significantly, in lymphocytes from FSHD patients, its expression was equivalent to that observed in normal tissue, indicating that this over-expression in FSHD is muscle-specific (Gabellini et al., 2002). Consistent with this evidence,

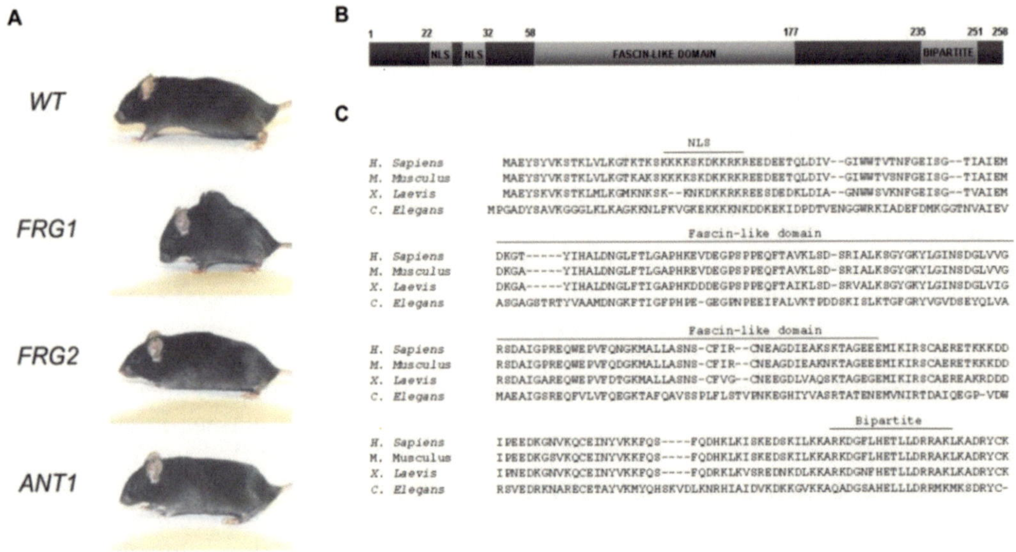

Fig. 6. **FSHD Region Gene 1 (FRG1). A.** WT and FRG1, FRG2 and ANT1 transgenic mice. Only FRG1 transgenic mice develop a muscular dystrophy with features of the human disease. **B**. FRG1 protein domains **C.** Alignament of FRG1 homologs: human FRG1 shares 42% identity with *C. elegans*, 81% identity with *Xenopus* and 97% identity with mouse.

transgenic mice over-expressing *FRG1* develop a muscular dystrophy with features of the human disease (Figure 6A). Importantly the myopathic features of these mice are corrected by the use of RNA interference to target and reduce FRG1 level in the affected muscles. Interestingly, the same result was obtained by two groups using two different experimental approaches (Wallace et al., 2011; Bortolanza et al., 2011). Furthermore, in muscles of *FRG1* transgenic mice and FSHD patients, specific pre-mRNAs undergo aberrant alternative splicing. Collectively, these results suggest that FSHD might results from inappropriate over-expression of *FRG1* in skeletal muscle, which leads to abnormal alternative splicing of specific pre-mRNAs (Gabellini et al., 2006).

Recent studies show the crucial role of FRG1 in maintaining proper muscle structure and function (Hanel et al., 2011; Hanel et al., 2009; Liu et al., 2010). In *C. elegans*, frg1 protein localized both in nuclei and in the dense bodies that are homologous to vertebrate Z-disk. Interestingly *frg1* overexpression in this invertebrate model disrupts the body-wall musculature and the muscular organization (Liu et al., 2010). In *Xenopus* both knock down and overexpression of *frg1* resulted in defective growth and morphogenesis of the myotome indicating that precise levels of *frg1* must be maintained for normal muscle morphology (Hanel et al., 2009). Together these results strongly suggest an evolutionary conserved function of *FRG1* in muscular development. Additional evidences support the role of *FRG1* in muscle cell biology. *FRG1* expression increases during myogenic differentiation. Its activation is paralleled by chromatin remodeling at the *FRG1* promoter with loss of the polycomb repressor complex and replacement of the H3K27 trimethylation (H3K27me3) repression marker with the H3K4 trimethylation (H3K4me3) activation marker (Bodega et al., 2009). Interestingly the physical interaction between *FRG1* promoter and D4Z4 array has been shown (Petrov et al., 2008). In this context replacement of H3K27me3 by H3K4me3 during myoblasts differentiation might indicate that chromatin structure undergoes dynamic changes during myogenic differentiation that lead to the loosening of the FRG1/4q-D4Z4 array loop in myotubes. Consistently, *FRG1* over-expression was detected in the early stages of differentiation in FSHD myoblasts in comparison with control myoblasts (Bodega et al., 2009).

FRG1 molecular function has not been elucidated yet. Several observations suggest that it could be involved in RNA processing. FRG1 is a nuclear protein that localizes in Cajal bodies, in nucleoli and in nuclear speckles, sites where RNA processing takes place (van Koningsbruggen et al., 2004). Its interaction with RNA has been demonstrated *in vitro* and *in vivo* (Sun et al., 2011). Proteomic studies found FRG1 as a component of purified spliceosomes (Rappsilber et al., 2002; Bessonov et al., 2010). Moreover in muscle of *FRG1* over-expressing transgenic mice, specific pre-mRNAs undergo aberrant alternative splicing (Gabellini et al., 2006). Studies showed that FRG1 has nuclear and cytoplasmic localizations. Interestingly in human muscle sections, FRG1 localizes with Z-disc (Hanel et al., 2011) an element of muscle sarcomere. In a muscle cells ribosomes are available at sarcomere for local synthesis of contractile proteins providing a mechanism to quickly respond to changes in the extra-cellular environment. It would be interesting to test wheter FRG1 is involved in Z line targeting and/or translation of specific m-RNAs. Despite the interest in FRG1 as candidate for FSHD pathogenesis has diminished because expression studies failed to detect *FRG1* consistently overexpressed in FSHD biopsies (Gabellini et al., 2002; Jiang et al., 2003; Winokur et al., 2003b; Dixit et al., 2007; Osborne et al., 2007; Arashiro et al., 2009), experimental evidences point at the critical role of *FRG1* in muscle development and indicate the presence of negative regulatory mechanisms on its expression, which is released in a myogenic-specific manner. On this basis *FRG1* remains a very suitable candidate gene for FSHD pathophysiology.

6.3 Adenine Nucleotide Translocator (ANT1)

The Adenine Nucleotide Translocator gene (*ANT1*) is located approximately 4 Mb centromeric to the tandem array and encodes a 298-amino acid protein. This protein is a member of integral membrane transport molecules family that are among the most abundant constituents of the inner mitochondria membrane (IMM), responsible for the transport of adenine nucleotides across the inner mitochondrial membrane, importing ADP for oxidative phosphorylation and exporting ATP to the cytosol (Klingenberg and Aquila, 1982). There are three different ANT genes in humans, *ANT1*, *ANT2*, and *ANT3*. These genes share 88% amino acid sequence identity and are characterized by a distinct tissue specific expression patterns (Levy et al., 2000; Stepien et al., 1992). *ANT1* is the predominant isoform expressed in the mitochondria of heart and skeletal muscle tissue. In addition to regulating adenine nucleotide pools, ANT1 functions as a component of the mitochondrial permeability transition pore (PTP), which is essential for the release of pro-apoptotic proteins during the activation of the intrinsic-apoptosis pathway (Bauer et al., 1999; Sharer et al., 2002). *ANT1* overexpression seems critical in inducing programmed cell death in different eukaryotic cell lines (Bauer et al., 1999). Although mice overexpressing *ANT1* do not show evident dystrophic phenotype (Figure 6A) (Gabellini et al., 2006), an increased amount of ANT1 protein was detected in both unaffected and affected FSHD muscles in comparison to healthy controls (Laoudj-Chenivesse et al., 2005). Even though both increase of oxidative stress and *ANT1* overexpression are proposed to be early events in the development of FSHD, it remains unclear if these are sequential or parallel processes (Winokur et al., 2003a).

7. Epigenetic and FSHD: Role of methylation and chromatine structure

Several clinical features, such as penetrance variability, gender bias in severity, asymmetric muscle wasting, and discordance in monozygotic twins, suggest that FSHD development involves epigenetic factors that can influence gene expression through local modification of chromatin structure.

7.1 DNA methylation

C5 methylation of cytosine, the most common epigenetic modification of mammalian DNA is known to be involved in development, X-chromosome inactivation, imprinting, and gene silencing (Robertson and Wolffe, 2000). CpG methylation can affect occupancy of specific genomic regions since several transcription factors and chromatin-binding proteins, such as CTCF and Yin Yang 1 (YY1), are sensitive to it (Hark et al., 2000; Kim et al., 2003). Each D4Z4 repeat unit harbors two classes of GC-rich sequences, namely the low copy-repeats hhspm3 and LSau. This type of repetitive DNA is predominantly found in heterochromatic regions of the genome (Hewitt et al., 1994). On this basis, it has been hypothesized that D4Z4 repeat reduction might induce changes in chromatin conformation leading to inappropriate expression of 4q35 genes. The first study of DNA methylation at the D4Z4 repeat array did not show a change in this epigenetic marker in FSHD tissues. D4Z4 was found highly methylated in both normal and FSHD lymphoblasts, as well as in somatic tissues, including skeletal muscle. Nevertheless the study did not discriminate between the methylation status of the repeat array at chromosome 4 or chromosome 10 (Tsien et al., 2001). A subsequent study, revealed a significant hypomethylation of three different CpG dinucleotides of the D4Z4-reduced allele in lymphoblasts and muscle biopsies from FSHD patients (van Overveld et al., 2003). Importantly, low methylation levels at D4Z4 were observed at both chromosome 4 and 10 in the so-called phenotypic FSHD patients. These patients are clinically indistinguishable from 4q-linked FSHD patients but do not carry any D4Z4-reduced (de Greef et al, 2009). However, methylation levels can vary substantially between individuals. Generally, patients with residual repeat sizes between 10 and 19 kb (1-3 D4Z4 units) are severely affected and show very low DNA methylation levels, whereas FSHD patients with repeat sizes between 20 and 31 kb (4-6 D4Z4 units) show inter-individual variation in both clinical severity and D4Z4 hypomethylation (van Overveld et al., 2005). In addition, non-penetrant carriers show the same D4Z4 hypomethylation as their affected relatives and strong D4Z4 hypomethylation is also reported in patients with immunodeficiency, centromeric instability and facial anomalies syndrome (ICF) without any myopatic symptoms (Xu et al., 1999; Kondo et al., 2000; van Overveld et al., 2003). Currently, the role of D4Z4 hypomethylation in FSHD pathogenesis remains elusive.

7.2 Histone modification

Chromatin conformation results from the interaction between DNA and histone proteins and the involvement of other chromosomal proteins. The basic structural unit of chromatin is the nucleosome that consists of 146 bp of DNA wrapped around a protein octamer of core histone proteins (Kornberg et al., 1974; Finch et al., 1977). Histone proteins may be posttranslational modified, by acetylation, methylation, phosphorylation, ubiquitination, SUMOylation and ADP-ribosylation (Bernstein et al., 2007). Modified histones are likely to control the structure and/or function of the chromatin fiber, with different modifications yielding distinct functional consequences. Furthermore, recruitment of chromatin-associating proteins may depend upon the recognition of a specific histone modification pattern (Strahl and Allis, 2000; Peterson and Laniel, 2004). Extracellular and intracellular stimuli may change these patterns of modification, making the chromatin itself an integrator of various signaling pathways, ultimately affecting basic cellular processes such as transcription or replication (Cheung et al., 2000; Nightingale et al., 2006). *In vivo*, chromatin exists as fibers with differing degrees of compaction. The morphologically distinct classes of chromatin within the nucleus of higher eukaryotes are heterochromatin, which is more compacted and generally transcriptionally inactive, and euchromatin, wich is less compacted and generally transcriptionally active (Frenster et al., 1963). Although D4Z4 unit harbors two classes of repetitive DNA, hhspm3 and LSau, both of which are found predominantly in heterochromatic domains of the genome, FSHD locus at 4qter does not share some of the common properties of heterochromatin. For instance it does not co-localize with DAPI-intense loci or it does not replicate in late S-phase. A recent study on D4Z4 histone modification seems to indicate that the repeat array may be organized in distinct domains, some characterized by transcriptionally repressive heterochromatin and others by transcriptionally permissive euchromatin (Zeng et al., 2009). These results indicate that the D4Z4 locus might display a chromatin structure more similar to euchromatin and favor the hypothesis that this region might be more dynamic than expected. Interestingly loss of marks of unexpressed heterochromatin such as histone H3K9me3 was observed in both FSHD with or without D4Z4 contraction. This phenomenon seems to be strictly associated with FSHD phenotype; in fact it was not found in ICF syndrome, despite its apparent similarity to FSHD with regard to D4Z4 DNA hypomethylation, or in other types of muscular dystrophies tested (Zeng et al., 2009). H3K9 methylation at D4Z4 is specifically mediated by the histone methyltransferase SUV39H1 (Zeng et al., 2009), which interacts with MyoD to suppress MyoD-dependent muscle gene expression (Mal, 2006). Interestingly, the heterochromatin binding protein HP1, which mediates transcriptional silencing (Bannister et al., 2001; Bernard et al., 2001), and the sister chromatid cohesion complex, cohesin, bind to D4Z4 in an H3K9me3-dependent manner and their recruitment is seriously compromised in FSHD (Zeng et al., 2009). These data support the indirect mechanism (Figure 5 C) where loss of repeats generates structural and functional modification, possibly through epigenetic changes in the histone pattern, which in turn might have an effect on transcriptional regulation in *cis* and/or in *trans*. It is reasonable to anticipate that future studies on the possible chromatin organization involving D4Z4 and its changes in FSHD may provide critical insight into the mechanism of FSHD pathogenesis.

7.3 Long distance effect: A repressor complex binding D4Z4

The alteration of 4q35 gene expression observed in FSHD affected muscle (Gabellini et al., 2002) raised the question whether D4Z4 was directly involved in transcriptional control of 4q35 genes. The analysis of the interaction between D4Z4 and nuclear proteins revealed the presence of a 27 bp binding site (DBE, D4Z4 Binding Element) able to recruit a multi-protein complex in vitro and in vivo comprising of YY1, HMGB2 and nucleolin, termed D4Z4 Recognition Complex (DRC) (Gabellini et al., 2002). The ubiquitous transcription factor Yin Yang 1 (YY1) is a recruiter of polycomb group proteins (PcG), which are responsible for chromatin remodelling and epigenetic silencing in many fundamental biological processes. YY1, exerts its effects on genes involved in normal biologic processes such as embryogenesis, differentiation, replication, and cellular proliferation. Its ability to initiate, activate, or repress transcription depends upon context (Gordon et al., 2006). Furthermore, the activity of YY1 is modulated by histone deacetylases and histone acetyltransferases (Yao et al., 2001). HMGB2 is a member of one of the three families of high mobility group (HMG) proteins (Bustin, 1999; Bianchi and Beltrame, 2000;Agresti and Bianchi, 2003). It has been proposed that HMGB2 might be involved in the organization and/or maintenance of heterochromatic regions through the SP100-mediated interaction with HP1 (Lehming et al., 1998). The third component of the DRC, nucleolin, is an abundant nucleolar protein, which has been implicated in chromatin structure, ribosomal RNA (rRNA) transcription, rRNA maturation, ribosome assembly and nucleo-cytoplasmic transport. To address whether the level of the DRC components influenced transcription of 4q35 genes, antisense experiments to decrease intracellular levels of DRC components were performed. These experiments showed that depletion of YY1, HMGB2 or nucleolin results in overexpression of the 4q35 gene *FRG2*, which is silent in normal cells and tissues (Gabellini et al., 2002). Accumulating evidences indicate that gene regulation can be affected by physical interaction between two distant chromosomal regions in *cis* and in *trans* in mammalian cells (Tolhuis et al., 2002; Horike et al., 2005; Spilianakis et al., 2005; Lomvardas et al., 2006). Thus the DRC might exerts is inhibitory activity either modifying the chromatin structure or acting directly on 4q35 genes promoters through a physical interaction mediated by the formation of a cromatin loop (Gabellini et al., 2002; Pirozhkova et al., 2008). The physical interaction between D4Z4 and FRG1 has been demonstrated (Pirozhkova et al., 2008; Bodega et al., 2009) in normal myoblast by Chromosome conformation capture (3C), which is a technique that identifies long distance intra- and inter-chromosomal interactions (Dekker et al., 2002). Interestingly chromatin seems to undergo remodeling during myogenic differentiation. It has been shown that in normal myoblasts, the *FRG1* gene is repressed and its promoter physically interacts with the D4Z4 array; upon differentiation, *FRG1* gene is expressed and the chromatin loop between FRG1 promoter and D4Z4 is relaxed (Bodega et al.2009). Consistent with the observed mis-regulation of FRG1, a small reduction in the D4Z4–FRG1 promoter interaction was observed in FSHD myoblasts compared with controls (Bodega et al., 2009). Different findings obtained with 3C analysis described the formation of loops between other elements in the FSHD locus (DUX4c and the 4qA/B marker) and the FRG1 promoter (Pirozhkova et al., 2008). These data indicate that the tridimensional structure of the FSHD locus is complex and composite, probably more than one sequence elements (for example, D4Z4, DUX4c,4qA/B) or more than one chromatin modification factor might be required to obtain a fine regulation of *FRG1* gene expression during muscle differentiation (Petrov et al., 2006; Pirozhkova et al., 2008).

7.4 Subnuclear localization of 4q35

The nucleoplasm is a high defined and structured compartment and chromosomes occupy specific and distinct territories. These chromosome territories are related to gene density, transcriptional activity, replication timing, and chromosome size (Sun HB et al., 2000; Tanabe et al., 2002). The nucleoplasm is separated from the cytoplasm by the nuclear envelope (NE), consisting of an inner (INM) and outer nuclear membrane (ONM), (Gerace et al., 1988). Chromosome 4qter is preferentially localized in the outer nuclear periphery (Masny et al., 2004; Tam et al., 2004) although mammalian telomeres, including 10qter, are usually dispersed in the inner part of the nucleus (Ludérus et al., 1996; Nagele et al., 2001; Amrichová et al., 2003; Weierich et al., 2003). Sequences proximal to D4Z4, and not the repeat array itself, seem to be required to localize the 4q telomere at the periphery (Masny et al., 2004). These sequences are not found at 10qter and this may explain the different nuclear localization of 10qter. Recently, Ottaviani et al. (2009) identified an 80-bp sequence inside the D4Z4 unit that can trigger perinuclear positioning of artificial telomeres in a CTCF- and lamin A-dependent manner. Furthermore in cells lacking the *lamin A* gene, chromosome 4 telomeres are dispersed (Masny et al., 2004). In addition, lamin A is shown to be associated with D4Z4 in vivo by chromatin immunoprecipitation and the perinuclear localization of 4qter is largely lost in fibroblasts lacking lamin A/C (Ottaviani et al., 2009). Although Fluoresece In Situ Hybridization (FISH) analyses showed no change in the chromosome 4 localization, between FSHD and healthy subjects, the peripheral environment of the FSHD 4q35 allele may be altered because of modification in chromatin structure at D4Z4. This nuclear lamina alteration might produce a change in the binding of specific proteins, thereby contribute to the aberrant 4q35 gene expression reported in FSHD (Masny et al., 2004; Tam et al., 2004; Ottaviani et al., 2009).

8. Conclusions

D4Z4 repeat contraction in patients with FSHD was discovered almost 20 years ago, nevertheless the exact molecular mechanism causing the FSHD phenotype has still not been elucidated and the search for a unifying model that can explain all the clinical features that have been observed in time has been frustrated. No histological or biochemical markers are available to independently confirm a specific FSHD diagnosis that remains mainly clinical. The molecular test primarily used for FSHD diagnosis was based on the initial observation that 95% of FSHD patients carry a reduction of integral numbers of D4Z4 repeats at 4q35 with full penetrance (Van Deutekom et al., 2003). However the wide use of this test revealed several exceptions to the original assumption. Through the years the threshold size of D4Z4 alleles has been increased from the original 28 kb (6 D4Z4 repeats) (Wimenga et al., 1999b) to 35 kb (8 D4Z4 repeats) (Van Deutekom et al., 2003), with FSHD cases carrying D4Z4 alleles of 38-41 kb (9-11 D4Z4 repeats) considered borderline alleles (Butz et al., 2003; Vitelli et al., 1999). A further analysis of genotype-phenotype correlation led in time to the identification of subjects carrying D4Z4 reduced alleles with no sign of muscle weakness in FSHD families (Ricci et al., 1999; Tonini et al., 2004) as well as in normal controls (Van Overveld et al., 2000; Weiffenbach et al., 1992). The genotype-phenotype correlation conducted more recently on a large scale using a standardized method of evaluation allowed to estimate that 1) 20% of FSHD patients carry full-length D4Z4 alleles, 2) over 25% of relatives carrying D4Z4 reduced alleles do not have FSHD, 3) 3% of healthy subjects from the general population carry D4Z4 reduced alleles 4) no specific 4q haplotype is uniquely associated with FSHD. Remarkably, these studies established as a general rule rather than an exception that detection of a D4Z4 reduced allele is not sufficient to predict FSHD (Scionti et al., 2012a; Scionti et al., 2012b). Over the years, the molecular etiology of FSHD has remained enigmatic, and the literature is filled with claims of causes that fail to be confirmed by other groups. Indeed, this might be expected if the clinical manifestation of FSHD symptoms is not only dependent on the structure/haplotype of D4Z4 contractions. This does not exclude an important pathogenic role for DUX4 or other candidate factors, but do establish a complex mechanism beyond current understanding indicating that a profound re-thinking of the genetic disease mechanism and modes of inheritance of FSHD is required.

In-depth examination of disease points to a more complex genetic etiology in which D4Z4 reduction might play a significant role only in association with other determinants, including genetic, epigenetic and environmental factors. Indeed, it is possible that in the heterozygous state a D4Z4 reduction might produce a predisposing condition that requires other epigenetic mechanisms or mutations in additional genes, both in *cis* and in *trans,* to cause overt myopathy. Finally it is also plausible that drugs or toxic agents might contribute to the disease onset and clinical variability. It is likely that, all mechanisms described above may contribute to the diverse phenotypic expression observed in carrier of D4Z4 reduced alleles. One of the major challenges for clinicians and researchers involved in FSHD studies will be to establish the weight that each single factor has in FSHD development. Particular attention should be paid to the relevance of epigenetics in the pathogenesis of FSHD. At the 4q subtelomere chromatin is normally tightly packed, probably as facultative heterochromatin. However this region can be highly dynamic as demonstrated by the fact that in patients with FSHD, this chromatin structure becomes more open. As a consequence, regulation of candidate genes can be influenced by proteins that may bind to or be released from D4Z4. One of the major goals for future FSHD research will be to integrate these disease mechanisms into a single model that can be used to explain the clinical data and to improve the molecular diagnosis; both steps are essential to develop effective therapeutic strategies.

9. References

Agresti A. & Bianchi M. E. (2003) HMGB proteins and gene expression. *Curr. Opin. Genet. Dev.* 13: 170–178

Amrichova, J., Lukasova, E., Kozubek, S., & Kozubek, M. (2003). Nuclear and territorial topography of chromosome telomeres in human lymphocytes. *Exp Cell Res 289,* 11-26.

Arashiro, P., Eisenberg, I., Kho, A.T., Cerqueira, A.M., Canovas, M., Silva, H.C., Pavanello, R.C., Verjovski-Almeida, S., Kunkel, L.M., & Zatz, M. (2009). Transcriptional regulation differs in affected facioscapulohumeral muscular dystrophy patients compared to asymptomatic related carriers. *Proc Natl Acad Sci U S A* 106, 6220-6225.

Bakker, E., Van der Wielen, M.J., Voorhoeve, E., Ippel, P.F., Padberg, G.W., Frants, R.R., & Wijmenga, C. (1996). Diagnostic, predictive, and prenatal testing for facioscapulohumeral muscular dystrophy: diagnostic approach for sporadic and familial cases. *J Med Genet* 33, 29-35.

Bakker, E., Wijmenga, C., Vossen, R.H., Padberg, G.W., Hewitt, J., van der Wielen, M., Rasmussen, K., & Frants, R.R. (1995). The FSHD-linked locus D4F104S1 (p13E-11) on 4q35 has a homologue on 10qter. *Muscle Nerve* 2, S39-44.

Bannister, A.J., Zegerman, P., Partridge, J.F., Miska, E.A., Thomas, J.O., Allshire, R.C., & Kouzarides, T. (2001). Selective recognition of methylated lysine 9 on histone H3 by the HP1 chromo domain. *Nature* 410, 120-124.

Bauer, M.K., Schubert, A., Rocks, O., & Grimm, S. (1999). Adenine nucleotide translocase-1, a component of the permeability transition pore, can dominantly induce apoptosis. *J Cell Biol 147*, 1493-1502.

Bernard, P., Maure, J.F., Partridge, J.F., Genier, S., Javerzat, J.P., & Allshire, R.C. (2001). Requirement of heterochromatin for cohesion at centromeres. *Science* 294, 2539-2542.

Bernstein, B.E., Meissner, A., & Lander, E.S. (2007). The mammalian epigenome. *Cell* 128, 669-681.

Bessonov, S., Anokhina, M., Krasauskas, A., Golas, M.M., Sander, B., Will, C.L., Urlaub, H., Stark, H., & Luhrmann, R. (2010). Characterization of purified human Bact spliceosomal complexes reveals compositional and morphological changes during spliceosome activation and first step catalysis. *RNA* 16, 2384-2403.

Bianchi M. E. & Beltrame M. (2000) Upwardly mobile proteins. Workshop: the role of HMG proteins in chromatin structure,gene expression and neoplasia. *EMBO Rep.* 1: 109–114

Bodega, B., Ramirez, G.D., Grasser, F., Cheli, S., Brunelli, S., Mora, M., Meneveri, R., Marozzi, A., Mueller, S., Battaglioli, E., *et al.* (2009). Remodeling of the chromatin structure of the facioscapulohumeral muscular dystrophy (FSHD) locus and upregulation of FSHD-related gene 1 (FRG1) expression during human myogenic differentiation. *BMC Biol* 7, 41.

Bortolanza, S., Nonis, A., Sanvito, F., Maciotta S., Sitia, G., Wei, J., Torrente, Y., Di Serio, C., Chamberlain, J.R. & Gabellini D. (2011). AAV6-mediated systemic shRNA delivery reverses disease in a mouse model of facioscapulohumeral muscular dystrophy. *Mol Ther.* 11:2055-64

Bosnakovski, D., Xu, Z., Gang, E.J., Galindo, C.L., Liu, M., Simsek, T., Garner, H.R., Agha-Mohammadi, S., Tassin, A., Coppee, F., *et al.* (2008). An isogenetic myoblast expression screen identifies DUX4-mediated FSHD-associated molecular pathologies. *EMBO J. 27*, 2766-2779.

Brouwer, O.F., Padberg, G.W., van der Ploeg, R.J., Ruys, C.J., & Brand, R. (1992). The influence of handedness on the distribution of muscular weakness of the arm in facioscapulohumeral muscular dystrophy. *Brain* 115 (Pt 5), 1587-1598.

Bustin M. (1999) Regulation of DNA-dependent activities by the functional motifs of the High-Mobility-Group chromosomal proteins. *Mol. Cell. Biol.* 19: 5237–5246

Butz, M., Koch, M.C., Muller-Felber, W., Lemmers, R.J., van der Maarel, S.M., & Schreiber, H. (2003). Facioscapulohumeral muscular dystrophy. Phenotype-genotype correlation in patients with borderline D4Z4 repeat numbers. *J Neurol* 250, 932-937.

Celegato, B., Capitanio, D., Pescatori, M., Romualdi, C., Pacchioni, B., Cagnin, S., Vigano, A., Colantoni, L., Begum, S., Ricci, E., *et al.* (2006). Parallel protein and transcript profiles of FSHD patient muscles correlate to the D4Z4 arrangement and reveal a common impairment of slow to fast fibre differentiation and a general deregulation of MyoD-dependent genes. *Proteomics* 6, 5303-5321.

Cheli, S., Francois, S., Bodega, B., Ferrari, F., Tenedini, E., Roncaglia, E., Ferrari, S., Ginelli, E., & Meneveri, R. (2011). Expression Profiling of FSHD-1 and FSHD-2 Cells during

Myogenic Differentiation Evidences Common & Distinctive Gene Dysregulation Patterns. *PLoS One* 6, e20966.

Cheung, P., Allis, C.D., & Sassone-Corsi, P. (2000). Signaling to chromatin through histone modifications. *Cell* 103, 263-271.

Chuenkongkaew, W.L., Lertrit, P., Limwongse, C., Nilanont, Y., Boonyapisit, K., Sangruchi, T., Chirapapaisan, N., & Suphavilai, R. (2005). An unusual family with Leber's hereditary optic neuropathy and facioscapulohumeral muscular dystrophy. *Eur J Neurol* 12, 388-391.

de Greef, J.C., Frants, R.R., & van der Maarel, S.M. (2008). Epigenetic mechanisms of facioscapulohumeral muscular dystrophy. Mutat Res 647, 94-102.

de Greef, J.C., Lemmers, R.J., van Engelen, B.G., Sacconi, S., Venance, S.L., Frants, R.R., Tawil, R., & van der Maarel, S.M. (2009). Common epigenetic changes of D4Z4 in contraction-dependent and contraction-independent FSHD. *Hum Mutat* 30, 1449-1459.

Deidda, G., Cacurri, S., Grisanti, P., Vigneti, E., Piazzo, N., & Felicetti, L. (1995). Physical mapping evidence for a duplicated region on chromosome 10qter showing high homology with the facioscapulohumeral muscular dystrophy locus on chromosome 4qter. *Eur J Hum Genet* 3, 155-167.

Deidda, G., Cacurri, S., Piazzo, N., & Felicetti, L. (1996). Direct detection of 4q35 rearrangements implicated in facioscapulohumeral muscular dystrophy (FSHD). *J Med Genet* 33, 361-365.

Dekker, J., Rippe, K., Dekker, M., & Kleckner, N. (2002). Capturing chromosome conformation. *Science* 295, 1306-1311.

Dixit, M., Ansseau, E., Tassin, A., Winokur, S., Shi, R., Qian, H., Sauvage, S., Matteotti, C., van Acker, A.M., Leo, O., *et al.* (2007). DUX4, a candidate gene of facioscapulohumeral muscular dystrophy, encodes a transcriptional activator of PITX1. *Proc Natl Acad Sci U S A 104,* 18157-18162.

Felice, K.J., & Moore, S.A. (2001). Unusual clinical presentations in patients harboring the facioscapulohumeral dystrophy 4q35 deletion. *Muscle Nerve* 24, 352-356.

Felice, K.J., & Whitaker, C.H. (2005). The Clinical Features of Facioscapulohumeral Muscular Dystrophy Associated With Borderline (>/=35 kb) 4q35 EcoRI Fragments. *J Clin Neuromuscul Dis* 6, 119-126.

Felice, K.J., North, W.A., Moore, S.A., & Mathews, K.D. (2000). FSH dystrophy 4q35 deletion in patients presenting with facial-sparing scapular myopathy. *Neurology* 54, 1927-1931.

Figueroa, J.J., & Chapin, J.E. (2010). Isolated facial diplegia and very late-onset myopathy in two siblings: atypical presentations of facioscapulohumeral dystrophy. *J Neurol* 257, 444-446.

Filosto, M., Tonin, P., Scarpelli, M., Savio, C., Greco, F., Mancuso, M., Vattemi, G., Govoni, V., Rizzuto, N., Tupler, R., *et al.* (2008). Novel mitochondrial tRNA Leu(CUN) transition and D4Z4 partial deletion in a patient with a facioscapulohumeral phenotype. *Neuromuscul Disord* 18, 204-209.

Finch, J.T., Lutter, L.C., Rhodes, D., Brown, R.S., Rushton, B., Levitt, M. & Klug, A. (1977) Structure of nucleosome core particle of chromatin. *Nature* 269: 29-36

Fitzsimons, R.B., Gurwin, E.B., & Bird, A.C. (1987). Retinal vascular abnormalities in facioscapulohumeral muscular dystrophy. A general association with genetic and therapeutic implications. *Brain* 110 (Pt 3), 631-648.

Flanigan, K. M. in *Myology* (eds Engel, A. & Franzini-Armstrong, C.) 1123–1133 (McGraw Hill Professional, New York, 2004)

Frenster, J.H., Allfrey, V.G., & Mirsky, A.E. (1963). Repressed and Active Chromatin Isolated from Interphase Lymphocytes. *Proc Natl Acad Sci U S A* 50, 1026-1032.

Gabellini, D., D'Antona, G., Moggio, M., Prelle, A., Zecca, C., Adami, R., Angeletti, B., Ciscato, P., Pellegrino, M.A., Bottinelli, R., *et al.* (2006). Facioscapulohumeral muscular dystrophy in mice overexpressing FRG1. *Nature* 439, 973-977.

Gabellini, D., Green, M.R., & Tupler, R. (2002). Inappropriate gene activation in FSHD: a repressor complex binds a chromosomal repeat deleted in dystrophic muscle. *Cell* 110, 339-348.

Gabriels, J., Beckers, M.C., Ding, H., De Vriese, A., Plaisance, S., van der Maarel, S.M., Padberg, G.W., Frants, R.R., Hewitt, J.E., Collen, D., *et al.* (1999). Nucleotide sequence of the partially deleted D4Z4 locus in a patient with FSHD identifies a putative gene within each 3.3 kb element. *Gene* 236, 25-32.

Gerace, L., & Burke, B. (1988). Functional organization of the nuclear envelope. *Annu Rev Cell Biol* 4, 335-374.

Gordon, S., Akopyan, G., Garban, H., & Bonavida, B. (2006). Transcription factor YY1: structure, function, and therapeutic implications in cancer biology. *Oncogene* 25, 1125-1142.

Griggs, R.C., Tawil, R., Storvick, D., Mendell, J.R., & Altherr, M.R. (1993). Genetics of facioscapulohumeral muscular dystrophy: new mutations in sporadic cases. *Neurology* 43, 2369-2372.

Hanel, M.L., Sun, C.Y., Jones, T.I., Long, S.W., Zanotti, S., Milner, D., & Jones, P.L. (2011). Facioscapulohumeral muscular dystrophy (FSHD) region gene 1 (FRG1) is a dynamic nuclear and sarcomeric protein. *Differentiation* 81, 107-118.

Hanel, M.L., Wuebbles, R.D., & Jones, P.L. (2009). Muscular dystrophy candidate gene FRG1 is critical for muscle development. *Dev Dyn* 238, 1502-1512.

Hark, A.T., Schoenherr, C.J., Katz, D.J., Ingram, R.S., Levorse, J.M., & Tilghman, S.M. (2000). CTCF mediates methylation-sensitive enhancer-blocking activity at the H19/Igf2 locus. *Nature* 405, 486-489.

Hewitt, J.E., Lyle, R., Clark, L.N., Valleley, E.M., Wright, T.J., Wijmenga, C., van Deutekom, J.C., Francis, F., Sharpe, P.T., Hofker, M., *et al.* (1994). Analysis of the tandem repeat locus D4Z4 associated with facioscapulohumeral muscular dystrophy. *Hum Mol Genet* 3, 1287-1295.

Horike, S., Cai, S., Miyano, M., Cheng, J.F., & Kohwi-Shigematsu, T. (2005). Loss of silent-chromatin looping and impaired imprinting of DLX5 in Rett syndrome. *Nat Genet* 37, 31-40.

Jiang, G., Yang, F., van Overveld, P.G., Vedanarayanan, V., van der Maarel, S., & Ehrlich, M. (2003). Testing the position-effect variegation hypothesis for facioscapulohumeral muscular dystrophy by analysis of histone modification and gene expression in subtelomeric 4q. *Hum Mol Genet* 12, 2909-2921.

Kohler, J., Rupilius, B., Otto, M., Bathke, K., & Koch, M.C. (1996). Germline mosaicism in 4q35 facioscapulohumeral muscular dystrophy (FSHD1A) occurring predominantly in oogenesis. *Hum Genet* 98, 485-490.

Kornberg, R.D. (1974) Chromatin structure: a repeating unit of histones and DNA. *Science* 184, 868-871.

Kowaljow, V., Marcowycz, A., Ansseau, E., Conde, C.B., Sauvage, S., Matteotti, C., Arias, C., Corona, E.D., Nunez, N.G., Leo, O., *et al.* (2007). The DUX4 gene at the FSHD1A locus encodes a pro-apoptotic protein. *Neuromuscul Disord* 17, 611-623.

Kim, J., Kollhoff, A., Bergmann, A., & Stubbs, L. (2003). Methylation-sensitive binding of transcription factor YY1 to an insulator sequence within the paternally expressed imprinted gene, Peg3. *Hum Mol Genet* 12, 233-245.

Klooster, R., Straasheijm, K., Shah, B., Sowden, J., Frants, R., Thornton, C., Tawil, R., & van der Maarel, S. (2009). Comprehensive expression analysis of FSHD candidate genes at the mRNA and protein level. *Eur J Hum Genet 17*, 1615-1624.

Klingenberg, M., & Aquila, H. (1982). Some characteristics of the isolated ADP/ATP carrier. Tokai J Exp Clin Med *7 Suppl*, 43-49.

Kondo, T., Bobek, M.P., Kuick, R., Lamb, B., Zhu, X., Narayan, A., Bourc'his, D., Viegas-Pequignot, E., Ehrlich, M., & Hanash, S.M. (2000). Whole-genome methylation scan in ICF syndrome: hypomethylation of non-satellite DNA repeats D4Z4 and NBL2. *Hum Mol Genet* 9, 597-604.

Krasnianski, M., Eger, K., Neudecker, S., Jakubiczka, S., & Zierz, S. (2003). Atypical phenotypes in patients with facioscapulohumeral muscular dystrophy 4q35 deletion. *Arch Neurol* 60, 1421-1425.

Lamperti, C., Fabbri, G., Vercelli, L., D'Amico, R., Frusciante, R., Bonifazi, E., Fiorillo, C., Borsato, C., Cao, M., Servida, M., *et al.* (2010). A standardized clinical evaluation of patients affected by facioscapulohumeral muscular dystrophy: The FSHD clinical score. *Muscle Nerve* 42, 213-217.

Laoudj-Chenivesse, D., Carnac, G., Bisbal, C., Hugon, G., Bouillot, S., Desnuelle, C., Vassetzky, Y., & Fernandez, A. (2005). Increased levels of adenine nucleotide translocator 1 protein and response to oxidative stress are early events in facioscapulohumeral muscular dystrophy muscle. *J Mol Med* (Berl) 83, 216-224.

Lee, J.H., Goto, K., Matsuda, C., & Arahata, K. (1995). Characterization of a tandemly repeated 3.3-kb KpnI unit in the facioscapulohumeral muscular dystrophy (FSHD) gene region on chromosome 4q35. *Muscle Nerve* 2, S6-13.

Lehming, N., Le Saux, A., Schuller, J., & Ptashne, M. (1998). Chromatin components as part of a putative transcriptional repressing complex. *Proc Natl Acad Sci U S A* 95, 7322-7326.

Lemmers, R.J., de Kievit, P., Sandkuijl, L., Padberg, G.W., van Ommen, G.J., Frants, R.R., & van der Maarel, S.M. (2002). Facioscapulohumeral muscular dystrophy is uniquely associated with one of the two variants of the 4q subtelomere. Nat Genet *32*, 235-236.

Lemmers, R.J., Osborn, M., Haaf, T., Rogers, M., Frants, R.R., Padberg, G.W., Cooper, D.N., van der Maarel, S.M., & Upadhyaya, M. (2003). D4F104S1 deletion in facioscapulohumeral muscular dystrophy: phenotype, size, and detection. *Neurology* 61, 178-183.

Lemmers, R.J., van der Maarel, S.M., van Deutekom, J.C., van der Wielen, M.J., Deidda, G., Dauwerse, H.G., Hewitt, J., Hofker, M., Bakker, E., Padberg, G.W., *et al.* (1998). Inter- and intrachromosomal sub-telomeric rearrangements on 4q35: implications for facioscapulohumeral muscular dystrophy (FSHD) aetiology and diagnosis. *Hum Mol Genet* 7, 1207-1214.

Lemmers, R.J.L., de Kievit, P., van Geel, M., van der Wielen, M.J., Bakker, E., Padberg, G.W., Frants, R.R., & van der Maarel, S.M. (2001). Complete allele information in the diagnosis of facioscapulohumeral muscular dystrophy by triple DNA analysis. *Ann Neurol* 50, 816-819.

Lemmers, R.J., van der Wielen, M.J., Bakker, E., Padberg, G.W., Frants, R.R., & van der Maarel, S.M. (2004). Somatic mosaicism in FSHD often goes undetected. Ann Neurol *55*, 845-850.

Lemmers, R.J., Wohlgemuth, M., van der Gaag, K.J., van der Vliet, P.J., van Teijlingen, C.M., de Knijff, P., Padberg, G.W., Frants, R.R., & van der Maarel, S.M. (2007). Specific sequence variations within the 4q35 region are associated with facioscapulohumeral muscular dystrophy. *Am J Hum Genet 81*, 884-894.

Lemmers, R.J., van der Vliet, P.J., Klooster, R., Sacconi, S., Camano, P., Dauwerse, J.G., Snider, L., Straasheijm, K.R., van Ommen, G.J., Padberg, G.W., *et al.* (2010a). A unifying genetic model for facioscapulohumeral muscular dystrophy. *Science 329*, 1650-1653.

Lemmers, R.J., van der Vliet, P.J., van der Gaag, K.J., Zuniga, S., Frants, R.R., de Knijff, P., & van der Maarel, S.M. (2010b). Worldwide population analysis of the 4q and 10q subtelomeres identifies only four discrete interchromosomal sequence transfers in human evolution. Am J Hum Genet *86*, 364-377.

Levy, S.E., Chen, Y.S., Graham, B.H., & Wallace, D.C. (2000). Expression and sequence analysis of the mouse adenine nucleotide translocase 1 and 2 genes. *Gene 254*, 57-66.

Liu, Q., Jones, T.I., Tang, V.W., Brieher, W.M., & Jones, P.L. (2010). Facioscapulohumeral muscular dystrophy region gene-1 (FRG-1) is an actin-bundling protein associated with muscle-attachment sites. *J Cell Sci 123*, 1116-1123.

Lomvardas, S., Barnea, G., Pisapia, D.J., Mendelsohn, M., Kirkland, J., & Axel, R. (2006). Interchromosomal interactions and olfactory receptor choice. *Cell* 126, 403-413.

Luderus, M.E., van Steensel, B., Chong, L., Sibon, O.C., Cremers, F.F., & de Lange, T. (1996). Structure, subnuclear distribution, and nuclear matrix association of the mammalian telomeric complex. *J Cell Biol 135*, 867-881.

Lunt, P.W., Jardine, P.E., Koch, M.C., Maynard, J., Osborn, M., Williams, M., Harper, P.S., & Upadhyaya, M. (1995). Correlation between fragment size at D4F104S1 and age at onset or at wheelchair use, with a possible generational effect, accounts for much phenotypic variation in 4q35-facioscapulohumeral muscular dystrophy (FSHD). *Hum Mol Genet* 4, 951-958.

Lunt, P.W. (1998). 44th ENMC International Workshop: Facioscapulohumeral Muscular Dystrophy: Molecular Studies 19-21 July 1996, Naarden, The Netherlands. *Neuromuscul Disord* 8, 126-130.

Lyle, R., Wright, T.J., Clark, L.N., & Hewitt, J.E. (1995). The FSHD-associated repeat, D4Z4, is a member of a dispersed family of homeobox-containing repeats, subsets of which are clustered on the short arms of the acrocentric chromosomes. *Genomics* 28, 389-397.

Mal, A.K. (2006). Histone methyltransferase Suv39h1 represses MyoD-stimulated myogenic differentiation. *EMBO J* 25, 3323-3334.

Masny, P.S., Bengtsson, U., Chung, S.A., Martin, J.H., van Engelen, B., van der Maarel, S.M., & Winokur, S.T. (2004). Localization of 4q35.2 to the nuclear periphery: is FSHD a nuclear envelope disease? *Hum Mol Genet* 13, 1857-1871.

Masny, P.S., Chan, O.Y., de Greef, J.C., Bengtsson, U., Ehrlich, M., Tawil, R., Lock, L.F., Hewitt, J.E., Stocksdale, J., Martin, J.H., *et al.* (2010). Analysis of allele-specific RNA transcription in FSHD by RNA-DNA FISH in single myonuclei. *Eur J Hum Genet* 18, 448-456.

Matsumura, T., Goto, K., Yamanaka, G., Lee, J.H., Zhang, C., Hayashi, Y.K., & Arahata, K. (2002). Chromosome 4q;10q translocations; comparison with different ethnic populations and FSHD patients. *BMC Neurol* 2, 7.

Mostacciuolo, M.L., Pastorello, E., Vazza, G., Miorin, M., Angelini, C., Tomelleri, G., Galluzzi, G. & Trevisan, C.P. (2009). Facioscapulohumeral muscular dystrophy: epidemiological and molecular study in a north-east Italian population sample. *Clin Genet.* 2009 Jun;75(6):550-5

Nadaj-Pakleza, A.A., Vincitorio, C.M., Laforet, P., Eymard, B., Dion, E., Teijeira, S., Vietez, I., Jeanpierre, M., Navarro, C., & Stojkovic, T. (2009). Permanent muscle weakness in McArdle disease. *Muscle Nerve* 40, 350-357.

Nagele, R.G., Velasco, A.Q., Anderson, W.J., McMahon, D.J., Thomson, Z., Fazekas, J., Wind, K., & Lee, H. (2001). Telomere associations in interphase nuclei: possible role in maintenance of interphase chromosome topology. *J Cell Sci 114*, 377-388.

Nightingale, K.P., O'Neill, L.P., & Turner, B.M. (2006). Histone modifications: signalling receptors and potential elements of a heritable epigenetic code. *Curr Opin Genet Dev* 16, 125-136.

Osborne, R.J., Welle, S., Venance, S.L., Thornton, C.A., & Tawil, R. (2007). Expression profile of FSHD supports a link between retinal vasculopathy and muscular dystrophy. *Neurology* 68, 569-577.

Ottaviani, A., Schluth-Bolard, C., Gilson, E., & Magdinier, F. (2010). D4Z4 as a prototype of CTCF and lamins-dependent insulator in human cells. *Nucleus* 1, 30-36.

Ottaviani, A., Schluth-Bolard, C., Rival-Gervier, S., Boussouar, A., Rondier, D., Foerster, A.M., Morere, J., Bauwens, S., Gazzo, S., Callet-Bauchu, E., *et al.* (2009). Identification of a perinuclear positioning element in human subtelomeres that requires A-type lamins and CTCF. *EMBO J* 28, 2428-2436.

Oya, Y., Morita, H., Ogawa, M., Nonaka, I., Tsujino, S., & Kawai, M. (2001). [Adult form of acid maltase deficiency presenting with pattern of muscle weakness resembling facioscapulohumeral dystrophy]. *Rinsho Shinkeigaku* 41, 390-396.

Padberg, G. (1982). Facioscapulohumeral disease. Leiden University The Netherlands.

Padberg, G.W. (1992). Why cells die in facioscapulohumeral muscular dystrophy. Clin Neurol Neurosurg 94 Suppl, S21-24.

Padberg, G.W., Frants, R.R., Brouwer, O.F., Wijmenga, C., Bakker, E., & Sandkuijl, L.A. (1995). Facioscapulohumeral muscular dystrophy in the Dutch population. *Muscle Nerve* 2, S81-84.

Padberg, G.W., Lunt, P.W., Koch, M., & Fardeau, M. (1991). Diagnostic criteria for facioscapulohumeral muscular dystrophy. *Neuromuscul Disord* 1, 231-234.

Peterson, C.L., & Laniel, M.A. (2004). Histones and histone modifications. *Curr Biol* 14, R546-551.

Petrov, A., Allinne, J., Pirozhkova, I., Laoudj, D., Lipinski, M., & Vassetzky, Y.S. (2008). A nuclear matrix attachment site in the 4q35 locus has an enhancer-blocking activity in vivo: implications for the facio-scapulo-humeral dystrophy. *Genome Res 18*, 39-45.

Petrov, A., Pirozhkova, I., Carnac, G., Laoudj, D., Lipinski, M., & Vassetzky, Y.S. (2006). Chromatin loop domain organization within the 4q35 locus in facioscapulohumeral dystrophy patients versus normal human myoblasts. *Proc Natl Acad Sci U S A* 103, 6982-6987.

Pirozhkova, I., Petrov, A., Dmitriev, P., Laoudj, D., Lipinski, M., & Vassetzky, Y. (2008). A functional role for 4qA/B in the structural rearrangement of the 4q35 region and in the regulation of FRG1 and ANT1 in facioscapulohumeral dystrophy. *PLoS One* 3, e3389.

Rappsilber, J., Ryder, U., Lamond, A.I., & Mann, M. (2002). Large-scale proteomic analysis of the human spliceosome. *Genome Res* 12, 1231-1245.

Ricci, E., Galluzzi, G., Deidda, G., Cacurri, S., Colantoni, L., Merico, B., Piazzo, N., Servidei, S., Vigneti, E., Pasceri, V., *et al.* (1999). Progress in the molecular diagnosis of facioscapulohumeral muscular dystrophy and correlation between the number of KpnI repeats at the 4q35 locus and clinical phenotype. *Ann Neurol* 45, 751-757.

Rijkers, T., Deidda, G., van Koningsbruggen, S., van Geel, M., Lemmers, R.J., van Deutekom, J.C., Figlewicz, D., Hewitt, J.E., Padberg, G.W., Frants, R.R., *et al.* (2004). FRG2, an FSHD candidate gene, is transcriptionally upregulated in differentiating primary myoblast cultures of FSHD patients. *J Med Genet* 41, 826-836.

Robertson, K.D., & Wolffe, A.P. (2000). DNA methylation in health and disease. *Nat Rev Genet 1,* 11-19.Rudnik-Schoneborn, S., Weis, J., Kress, W., Hausler, M., and Zerres, K. (2008). Becker's muscular dystrophy aggravating facioscapulohumeral muscular dystrophy--double trouble as an explanation for an atypical phenotype. *Neuromuscul Disord* 18, 881-885.

Rossi, M., Ricci, E., Colantoni, L., Galluzzi, G., Frusciante, R., Tonali, P.A., & Felicetti, L. (2007). The Facioscapulohumeral muscular dystrophy region on 4qter and the homologous locus on 10qter evolved independently under different evolutionary pressure. BMC Med Genet *8*, 8.

Rudnik-Schoneborn, S., Weis, J., Kress, W., Hausler, M., & Zerres, K. (2008). Becker's muscular dystrophy aggravating facioscapulohumeral muscular dystrophy--double trouble as an explanation for an atypical phenotype. *Neuromuscul Disord* 18, 881-885.

Saenz, A., Leturcq, F., Cobo, A.M., Poza, J.J., Ferrer, X., Otaegui, D., Camano, P., Urtasun, M., Vilchez, J., Gutierrez-Rivas, E., *et al.* (2005). LGMD2A: genotype-phenotype correlations based on a large mutational survey on the calpain 3 gene. *Brain* 128, 732-742.

Scionti, I., Fabbri, G., Fiorillo, C., Ricci, G., Greco, F., D'Amico, R., Tremanini, A., Vercelli, L., Tomelleri, G., Cao, M., Santoro, L., Percesepe, A., & Tupler, R. (2012a). Facioscapulohumeral muscular dystrophy: new insights from compound heterozygotes and implication for prenatal genetic counselling.*JMG* january 2012

Scionti, I., Greco, F., Ricci, G., Govi, M., Arashiro, P., Vercelli, L., Berardinelli, A., Angelini, C., Antonini, G., Cao, M., Di Muzio, A., Moggio, M., Morandi, L., Ricci, E., Rodolico, C., Ruggero, L., Santoro, L., Siciliano, G., Tomelleri, G., Trevisan, CP., Galluzzi, G., Wright, W., Zatz, M., & Tupler, R. (2012b). Large scale population analysis challenges
the current criteria for the molecular diagnosis of fascioscapulohumeral muscular dystrophy (FSHD). *AJHG* Paper accepted.

Sharer, J.D., Shern, J.F., Van Valkenburgh, H., Wallace, D.C., & Kahn, R.A. (2002). ARL2 and BART enter mitochondria and bind the adenine nucleotide transporter. *Mol Biol Cell 13*, 71-83.

Snider, L., Geng, L.N., Lemmers, R.J., Kyba, M., Ware, C.B., Nelson, A.M., Tawil, R., Filippova, G.N., van der Maarel, S.M., Tapscott, S.J., *et al.* (2010). Facioscapulohumeral dystrophy: incomplete suppression of a retrotransposed gene. PLoS Genet *6*, e1001181.

Spilianakis, C.G., Lalioti, M.D., Town, T., Lee, G.R., & Flavell, R.A. (2005). Interchromosomal associations between alternatively expressed loci. *Nature* 435, 637-645.

Stepien, G., Torroni, A., Chung, A.B., Hodge, J.A., & Wallace, D.C. (1992). Differential expression of adenine nucleotide translocator isoforms in mammalian tissues and during muscle cell differentiation. *J Biol Chem 267*, 14592-14597.

Strahl, B.D., & Allis, C.D. (2000). The language of covalent histone modifications. *Nature* 403, 41-45.

Sun, C.Y., van Koningsbruggen, S., Long, S.W., Straasheijm, K., Klooster, R., Jones, T.I., Bellini, M., Levesque, L., Brieher, W.M., van der Maarel, S.M., *et al.* (2011). Facioscapulohumeral Muscular Dystrophy Region Gene 1 Is a Dynamic RNA-Associated and Actin-Bundling Protein. *J Mol Biol.*

Sun, H.B., Shen, J., & Yokota, H. (2000). Size-dependent positioning of human chromosomes in interphase nuclei. *Biophys J 79*, 184-190.

Swinkels, B.W., Gould, S.J., & Subramani, S. (1992). Targeting efficiencies of various permutations of the consensus C-terminal tripeptide peroxisomal targeting signal. *FEBS* Lett 305, 133-136.

Tam, R., Smith, K.P., & Lawrence, J.B. (2004). The 4q subtelomere harboring the FSHD locus is specifically anchored with peripheral heterochromatin unlike most human telomeres. *J Cell Biol 167*, 269-279.

Tanabe, H., Habermann, F.A., Solovei, I., Cremer, M., & Cremer, T. (2002). Non-random radial arrangements of interphase chromosome territories: evolutionary considerations and functional implications. *Mutat Res 504*, 37-45.

Tawil, R., Forrester, J., Griggs, R.C., Mendell, J., Kissel, J., McDermott, M., King, W., Weiffenbach, B., & Figlewicz, D. (1996). Evidence for anticipation and association of deletion size with severity in facioscapulohumeral muscular dystrophy. The FSH-DY Group. *Ann Neurol* 39, 744-748.

Tawil, R., van der Maarel, S., Padberg, G.W., & van Engelen, B.G. (2010). 171st ENMC international workshop: Standards of care and management of facioscapulohumeral muscular dystrophy. *Neuromuscul Disord* 20, 471-475.

Thomas, N.S., Wiseman, K., Spurlock, G., MacDonald, M., Ustek, D., & Upadhyaya, M. (2007). A large patient study confirming that facioscapulohumeral muscular dystrophy (FSHD) disease expression is almost exclusively associated with an FSHD locus located on a 4qA-defined 4qter subtelomere. J Med Genet *44*, 215-218.

Tolhuis, B., Palstra, R.J., Splinter, E., Grosveld, F., & de Laat, W. (2002). Looping and interaction between hypersensitive sites in the active beta-globin locus. *Mol Cell* 10, 1453-1465.

Tonini, M.M., Passos-Bueno, M.R., Cerqueira, A., Matioli, S.R., Pavanello, R., & Zatz, M. (2004). Asymptomatic carriers and gender differences in facioscapulohumeral muscular dystrophy (FSHD). *Neuromuscul Disord* 14, 33-38.

Trevisan, C.P., Pastorello, E., Tomelleri, G., Vercelli, L., Bruno, C., Scapolan, S., Siciliano, G., & Comacchio, F. (2008). Facioscapulohumeral muscular dystrophy: hearing loss and other atypical features of patients with large 4q35 deletions. *Eur J Neurol 15*, 1353-1358.

Tsien, F., Sun, B., Hopkins, N.E., Vedanarayanan, V., Figlewicz, D., Winokur, S., & Ehrlich, M. (2001). Methylation of the FSHD syndrome-linked subtelomeric repeat in normal and FSHD cell cultures and tissues. *Mol Genet Metab* 74, 322-331.

Tsuji, M., Kinoshita, M., Imai, Y., Kawamoto, M., & Kohara, N. (2009). Facioscapulohumeral muscular dystrophy presenting with hypertrophic cardiomyopathy: a case study. *Neuromuscul Disord* 19, 140-142.

Tupler, R., Barbierato, L., Memmi, M., Sewry, C.A., De Grandis, D., Maraschio, P., Tiepolo, L., & Ferlini, A. (1998). Identical de novo mutation at the D4F104S1 locus in monozygotic male twins affected by facioscapulohumeral muscular dystrophy (FSHD) with different clinical expression. *J Med Genet* 35, 778-783.

Tupler, R., Berardinelli, A., Barbierato, L., Frants, R., Hewitt, J.E., Lanzi, G., Maraschio, P., & Tiepolo, L. (1996). Monosomy of distal 4q does not cause facioscapulohumeral muscular dystrophy. *J Med Genet* 33, 366-370.

Upadhyaya, M., Maynard, J., Osborn, M., Jardine, P., Harper, P.S., & Lunt, P. (1995). Germinal mosaicism in facioscapulohumeral muscular dystrophy (FSHD). *Muscle Nerve* 2, S45-49.

van der Maarel, S.M., Deidda, G., Lemmers, R.J., Bakker, E., van der Wielen, M.J., Sandkuijl, L., Hewitt, J.E., Padberg, G.W., & Frants, R.R. (1999). A new dosage test for subtelomeric 4;10 translocations improves conventional diagnosis of facioscapulohumeral muscular dystrophy (FSHD). *J Med Genet* 36, 823-828.

van der Maarel, S.M., Deidda, G., Lemmers, R.J., van Overveld, P.G., van der Wielen, M., Hewitt, J.E., Sandkuijl, L., Bakker, B., van Ommen, G.J., Padberg, G.W., *et al.* (2000). De novo facioscapulohumeral muscular dystrophy: frequent somatic mosaicism, sex-dependent phenotype, and the role of mitotic transchromosomal repeat interaction between chromosomes 4 and 10. *Am J Hum Genet* 66, 26-35.

van der Maarel, S.M., Frants, R.R., & Padberg, G.W. (2007). Facioscapulohumeral muscular dystrophy. *Biochim Biophys Acta* 1772, 186-194.

van Deutekom, J.C., Wijmenga, C., van Tienhoven, E.A., Gruter, A.M., Hewitt, J.E., Padberg, G.W., van Ommen, G.J., Hofker, M.H., & Frants, R.R. (1993). FSHD associated DNA rearrangements are due to deletions of integral copies of a 3.2 kb tandemly repeated unit. *Hum Mol Genet 2*, 2037-2042.

van Deutekom, J.C.(1996a) Toward the molecular mechanism of faciuscapulohumeral muscular dystrophy. *PhD Thesis,*Leiden University, Leiden van Deutekom, J.C., Bakker, E., Lemmers, R.J., van der Wielen, M.J., Bik, E., Hofker, M.H., Padberg, G.W., & Frants, R.R. (1996b). Evidence for subtelomeric exchange of 3.3 kb tandemly repeated units between chromosomes 4q35 and 10q26: implications for genetic counselling and etiology of FSHD1. *Hum Mol Genet* 5, 1997-2003.

van Deutekom, J.C., Lemmers, R.J., Grewal, P.K., van Geel, M., Romberg, S., Dauwerse, H.G., Wright, T.J., Padberg, G.W., Hofker, M.H., Hewitt, J.E., *et al.* (1996c). Identification of the first gene (FRG1) from the FSHD region on human chromosome 4q35. *Hum Mol Genet 5*, 581-590.

van Geel, M., Heather, L.J., Lyle, R., Hewitt, J.E., Frants, R.R., & de Jong, P.J. (1999). The FSHD region on human chromosome 4q35 contains potential coding regions among pseudogenes and a high density of repeat elements. *Genomics* 61, 55-65.

van Geel, M., Dickson, M.C., Beck, A.F., Bolland, D.J., Frants, R.R., van der Maarel, S.M., de Jong, P.J., & Hewitt, J.E. (2002). Genomic analysis of human chromosome 10q and 4q telomeres suggests a common origin. *Genomics* 79, 210-217.

van Koningsbruggen, S., Dirks, R.W., Mommaas, A.M., Onderwater, J.J., Deidda, G., Padberg, G.W., Frants, R.R., & van der Maarel, S.M. (2004). FRG1P is localised in the nucleolus, Cajal bodies, and speckles. *J Med Genet* 41, e46.

van Overveld, P.G., Lemmers, R.J., Deidda, G., Sandkuijl, L., Padberg, G.W., Frants, R.R., & van der Maarel, S.M. (2000). Interchromosomal repeat array interactions between chromosomes 4 and 10: a model for subtelomeric plasticity. *Hum Mol Genet* 9, 2879-2884.

van Overveld, P.G., Lemmers, R.J., Sandkuijl, L.A., Enthoven, L., Winokur, S.T., Bakels, F., Padberg, G.W., van Ommen, G.J., Frants, R.R., & van der Maarel, S.M. (2003). Hypomethylation of D4Z4 in 4q-linked and non-4q-linked facioscapulohumeral muscular dystrophy. *Nat Genet* 35, 315-317.

van Overveld, P.G., Enthoven, L., Ricci, E., Rossi, M., Felicetti, L., Jeanpierre, M., Winokur, S.T., Frants, R.R., Padberg, G.W., & van der Maarel, S.M. (2005). Variable hypomethylation of D4Z4 in facioscapulohumeral muscular dystrophy. *Ann Neurol 58*, 569-576.

Vitelli, F., Villanova, M., Malandrini, A., Bruttini, M., Piccini, M., Merlini, L., Guazzi, G., & Renieri, A. (1999). Inheritance of a 38-kb fragment in apparently sporadic facioscapulohumeral muscular dystrophy. *Muscle Nerve* 22, 1437-1441.

Wallace, L.M., Garwick, S.E., Mei, W., Belayew, A., Coppee, F., Ladner, K.J., Guttridge, D., Yang, J., & Harper, S.Q. (2011). DUX4, a candidate gene for facioscapulohumeral muscular dystrophy, causes p53-dependent myopathy in vivo. *Ann Neurol 69*, 540-552.

Weierich, C., Brero, A., Stein, S., von Hase, J., Cremer, C., Cremer, T., & Solovei, I. (2003). Three-dimensional arrangements of centromeres and telomeres in nuclei of human and murine lymphocytes. *Chromosome Res 11*, 485-502.

Weiffenbach, B., Dubois, J., Storvick, D., Tawil, R., Jacobsen, S.J., Gilbert, J., Wijmenga, C., Mendell, J.R., Winokur, S., Altherr, M.R., *et al.* (1993). Mapping the facioscapulohumeral muscular dystrophy gene is complicated by chromsome 4q35 recombination events. *Nat Genet* 4, 165-169.

Weiffenbach, B., bagley,R., Falls, K., Hyser, C. & Storvick, D., (1992). Linkage analyses of five chromosome 4 markers localizes the facioscapulohumeral muscular dystrophy (FSHD) gene to distal 4q35. *Am J Hum Genet* 51, 416-423.

Wijmenga, C., Frants, R.R., Brouwer, O.F., Moerer, P., Weber, J.L., & Padberg, G.W. (1990). Location of facioscapulohumeral muscular dystrophy gene on chromosome 4. *Lancet* 336, 651-653.

Wijmenga, C., Brouwer, O.F., Padberg, G.W., & Frants, R.R. (1992a). Transmission of de-novo mutation associated with facioscapulohumeral muscular dystrophy. *Lancet* 340, 985-986.

Wijmenga, C., Hewitt, J.E., Sandkuijl, L.A., Clark, L.N., Wright, T.J., Dauwerse, H.G., Gruter, A.M., Hofker, M.H., Moerer, P., Williamson, R., *et al.* (1992b). *Chromosome* 4q DNA rearrangements associated with facioscapulohumeral muscular dystrophy. Nat Genet 2, 26-30.

Winokur, S.T., Bengtsson, U., Feddersen, J., Mathews, K.D., Weiffenbach, B., Bailey, H., Markovich, R.P., Murray, J.C., Wasmuth, J.J., Altherr, M.R., *et al.* (1994). The DNA rearrangement associated with facioscapulohumeral muscular dystrophy involves a heterochromatin-associated repetitive element: implications for a role of chromatin structure in the pathogenesis of the disease. *Chromosome* Res 2, 225-234.

Winokur, S.T., Barrett, K., Martin, J.H., Forrester, J.R., Simon, M., Tawil, R., Chung, S.A., Masny, P.S., & Figlewicz, D.A. (2003a). Facioscapulohumeral muscular dystrophy (FSHD) myoblasts demonstrate increased susceptibility to oxidative stress. *Neuromuscul Disord* 13, 322-333.

Winokur, S.T., Chen, Y.W., Masny, P.S., Martin, J.H., Ehmsen, J.T., Tapscott, S.J., van der Maarel, S.M., Hayashi, Y., & Flanigan, K.M. (2003b). Expression profiling of FSHD muscle supports a defect in specific stages of myogenic differentiation. *Hum Mol Genet* 12, 2895-2907.

Wohlgemuth, M., Lemmers, R.J., van der Kooi, E.L., van der Wielen, M.J., van Overveld, P.G., Dauwerse, H., Bakker, E., Frants, R.R., Padberg, G.W., & van der Maarel, S.M. (2003). Possible phenotypic dosage effect in patients compound heterozygous for FSHD-sized 4q35 alleles. *Neurology* 61, 909-913.

Xu, G.L., Bestor, T.H., Bourc'his, D., Hsieh, C.L., Tommerup, N., Bugge, M., Hulten, M., Qu, X., Russo, J.J., & Viegas-Pequignot, E. (1999). Chromosome instability and immunodeficiency syndrome caused by mutations in a DNA methyltransferase gene. *Nature* 402, 187-191.

Yang, F., Shao, C., Vedanarayanan, V., & Ehrlich, M. (2004). Cytogenetic and immuno-FISH analysis of the 4q subtelomeric region, which is associated with facioscapulohumeral muscular dystrophy. *Chromosoma* 112, 350-359.

Yao, Y.L., Yang, W.M., & Seto, E. (2001). Regulation of transcription factor YY1 by acetylation and deacetylation. *Mol Cell Biol* 21, 5979-5991.

Zatz, M., Marie, S.K., Cerqueira, A., Vainzof, M., Pavanello, R.C., & Passos-Bueno, M.R. (1998). The facioscapulohumeral muscular dystrophy (FSHD1) gene affects males more severely and more frequently than females. *Am J Med Genet* 77, 155-161.

Zatz, M., Marie, S.K., Passos-Bueno, M.R., Vainzof, M., Campiotto, S., Cerqueira, A., Wijmenga, C., Padberg, G., & Frants, R. (1995). High proportion of new mutations and possible anticipation in Brazilian facioscapulohumeral muscular dystrophy families. *Am J Hum Genet* 56, 99-105.

Zeng, W., de Greef, J.C., Chen, Y.Y., Chien, R., Kong, X., Gregson, H.C., Winokur, S.T., Pyle, A., Robertson, K.D., Schmiesing, J.A., *et al.* (2009). Specific loss of histone H3 lysine 9 trimethylation and HP1gamma/cohesin binding at D4Z4 repeats is associated with facioscapulohumeral dystrophy (FSHD). *PLoS Genet* 5, e1000559.

Zouvelou, V., Manta, P., Kalfakis, N., Evdokimidis, I., & Vassilopoulos, D. (2009). Asymptomatic elevation of serum creatine kinase leading to the diagnosis of 4q35 facioscapulohumeral muscular dystrophy. *J Clin Neurosci* 16, 1218-1219.

3

AON-Mediated Exon Skipping for Duchenne Muscular Dystrophy

Ingrid E. C. Verhaart and Annemieke Aartsma-Rus
Department of Human Genetics,
Leiden University Medical Center
The Netherlands

1. Introduction

Duchenne muscular dystrophy (DMD) is a genetic, X-chromosome recessive, severe and progressive muscle wasting disorder, affecting around 1 in 3500 newborn boys. The onset of the disease is in early childhood and, nowadays, most children are diagnosed before the age of 5. The first signs of muscular weakness become apparent around the age of 2 or 3 years. In most patients the age at which the child starts to walk is delayed (retarded motor development). The children have less endurance and difficulties with running and climbing stairs (Moser, 1984). Gower's sign is a reflection of the weakness of the muscles of the lower extremities (knee and hip extensors): the child helps himself to get upright from sitting position by using his upper extremities: first by rising to stand on his arms and knees, and then "walking" his hands up his legs to stand upright (Gowers, 1895). Muscle wasting is often symmetrical, however not all muscles are affected to the same extent. A prominent feature of the disease is enlargement of the calve muscle, caused by replacement of muscle fibres by connective and adipose tissue. Furthermore, the pelvic girdle, trunk and abdomen are severely affected and to a lesser extent the shoulder girdle and proximal muscles of the upper extremities. Progressive weakness and contractures of the leg muscles lead to wheelchair-dependency around the age of 10. Thereafter the muscle contractions increase rapidly leading to spinal deformities and scoliosis, often with an asymmetric distribution pattern. Involvement of the intercostal muscles and distortion of the thorax lead to respiratory failure and patients often require assisted ventilation in the mid to late teens. Thereafter dilated cardiomyopathy becomes apparent and most patients die before the age of 30. Another common feature is mental retardation (IQ less than 70) in around 20-30% of the patients (Emery, 2002).

Becker Muscular Dystrophy (BMD) is a related, but much milder, form of muscular weakness, affecting around 1 in 20 000 men. The phenotype varies between individual patients, from very mild to moderately severe, but the course of the disease is more benign compared to DMD. On average, the age of onset is around 12 years; however some patients remain asymptomatic until much higher ages. The age of wheelchair-dependency also shows more variability, but in general is in their second or third decade of life. The most severely affected patients die between 40 and 50 years of age, whereas patients with a mild phenotype have (nearly) normal life expectancies. Around 50% of patients also develops cardiomyopathy (Emery, 1993).

The majority of female carriers shows no signs of disease. Only in 5 to 10% some degree of skeletal muscular weakness and enlarged calves are reported, but this is generally very mild and often does not affect daily activities. A small part of these carriers develops cardiomyopathy later in life; however most of the women with cardiac abnormalities on echocardiogram or ECG (left ventricular dilatation and decreased shortening fraction), are asymptomatic. There is no relation between the presence of skeletal muscle weakness and the development of cardiomyopathy (Grain et al., 2001).

At present there is no cure for DMD. However, during the past decades pharmacological interventions and improved care (e.g. physiotherapy and assisted ventilation) have led to increased function and quality of life and prolonged life expectancy for currently diagnosed patients into their forties. The current standard of care also consists of corticosteroids (mainly predniso(lo)ne or deflazacourt). These are anti-inflammatory/immunosuppressive drugs that have shown to improve muscle function, prolong ambulation for around 3 years and to have a positive effect on cardiac function (Bushby et al., 2010).

2. *DMD* gene and dystrophin protein

2.1 Genetic defect in DMD

DMD is caused by a genetic defect in the *DMD* gene. In approximately 33% of cases this is a de novo (new) mutation. The *DMD* gene is located on the short arm of the X-chromosome (at Xp21). It is the largest gene in the human genome consisting of 2 220 223 base pairs. The coding sequence spans around 0.5% (11 058 bases) of the gene, dispersed over 79 exons. Mutations in the gene causing a disruption of the open reading frame or introducing a premature stop codon lead to a complete absence of a functional dystrophin protein. Dystrophin consists of 3 685 amino acids and has a molecular weight of 427 kDa (Muntoni et al., 2003). The protein is located inside the muscle fibres and forms a bridge between the actin cytoskeleton and the extracellular matrix (ECM). Thereby it provides mechanical stability to the muscle fibres during each contraction. The protein consists of 4 domains: first an N-terminus, containing 2 actin-binding domains (ABD), both consisting of a CH1-and a CH2-domain, which are bound to contractile structures (F-actin) inside the muscle cells. This is followed by a central domain, so called central rod domain, consisting of 24 spectrin-like triple helical coiled repeat units, interrupted by 4 proline-rich hinge regions. A third actin-binding domain is present between repeat 11 and 17 (Amann et al., 1998), while repeat 16-17 contain a binding site for neuronal nitric oxide synthase (nNOS) (Lai et al., 2009). Subsequently the protein contains a cysteine-rich part and finally a C-terminal domain. The cysteine-rich domain binds to β-dystroglycan, which is part of a membrane bound dystrophin-associated glycoprotein complex (DGC) (fig. 1). Β-dystroglycan is a transmembrane protein that is bound to the extracellular α-dystroglycan, which in turn is bound to laminin-2, a part of the extracellular matrix (ECM). The central rod domain can absorb mechanical force. Hereby the protein transmits energy produced by the actin-myosin contraction machinery via the cell membranes to the connective tissue and tendons surrounding the muscles, to maintain the energy-balance and prevent overstressing of the muscle fibres (Ehmsen et al., 2002).

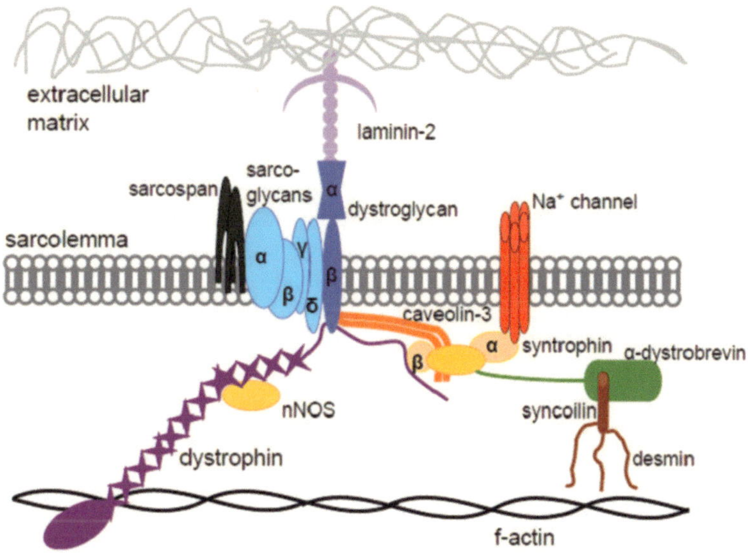

The dystrophin-associated glycoprotein complex (DGC) is composed of α- and β-dystroglycan, a sarcoglycan-sarcospan complex and the dystrophin containing cytoplasmic complex. Dystrophin (purple) forms the link between the actin cytoskeleton with its N-terminal domain and extracellular matrix component laminin-2 (lilac) via α- and β-dystroglycan (dark blue) with its C-terminal domain. B-dystroglycan is also bound to the sarcoglycan-sarcospan complex (light blue/black) and to caveolin-3 (orange), a scaffolding protein of skeletal muscle caveolae. Furthermore, the C-terminal domain of dystrophin is connected to α-dystrobrevin (green) and syntrophin (salmon pink), which recruits nNOS (yellow), a vasodilator, to the membrane. A-dystrobrevin, in turn, is linked to syncoilin (brown), forming a bridge between the DGC and the desmin intermediate filament protein network (brown).

Fig. 1. The dystrophin-associated glycoprotein complex

In addition to its mechanical linker function, dystrophin is involved in the organisation of the DGC as well as many other proteins, the maintenance of the calcium homeostasis and control of the growth of the muscle cells (Hoffman et al., 1987). In the DGC, β-dystroglycan is connected to a complex of α-, β-, γ- and δ-sarcoglycans and sarcospan. This complex functions in maintaining membrane stability (Miller et al., 2007). B-dystroglycan is also bound to caveolin-3, a structural protein of skeletal muscle caveolae, small invaginations of the plasma membrane playing a role in, among others, signal transduction. Caveolins act as scaffolding proteins to compartmentalise and functionally regulate signalling molecules (Hezel et al., 2010). Furthermore, the C-terminal domain of dystrophin is connected to α-dystrobrevin and syntrophin. nNOS is recruited to the membrane by binding to dystrophin and syntrophin. In contracting muscles, nNOS produces NO to induce vasodilatation in order to increase the local blood flow necessary for the increased mechanical load. The absence of nNOS in DMD causes abnormal vasoconstriction and ischemic stress, which contributes to the muscle degeneration (Brenman et al., 1995). Syntrophin is also connected to sodium channels, which are involved in regulating the Na+ distribution. In DMD, defects in cardiac conduction systems are thought to be caused by disturbances in Na+ distribution (Gee et al., 1998). A-dystrobrevin is linked to syncoilin too, thereby forming a bridge between the DGC and the desmin intermediate filament protein network at the neuromuscular junction (Newey et al., 2001).

Furthermore, in addition to the most common form of the dystrophin protein found in muscles, additional full-length and shorter isoforms of dystrophin exist. This is due to the presence of at least 7 different promoters and alternative splicing events. Three full-length variants exist (including the muscle isoform), which only differ in their first exon. In addition to the muscle promoter expressed in skeletal muscle and cardiomyocytes, a brain promoter drives expression in the cortical neurons and hippocampus of the brain and a Purkinje promoter in the cerebellar Purkinje cells. Four internal promoters lead to the production of shorter dystrophin proteins, lacking the actin-binding domains, expressed in specific tissues. In addition, alternative splicing facilitates the expression of many more dystrophins with a tissue-specific function (Muntoni et al., 2003).

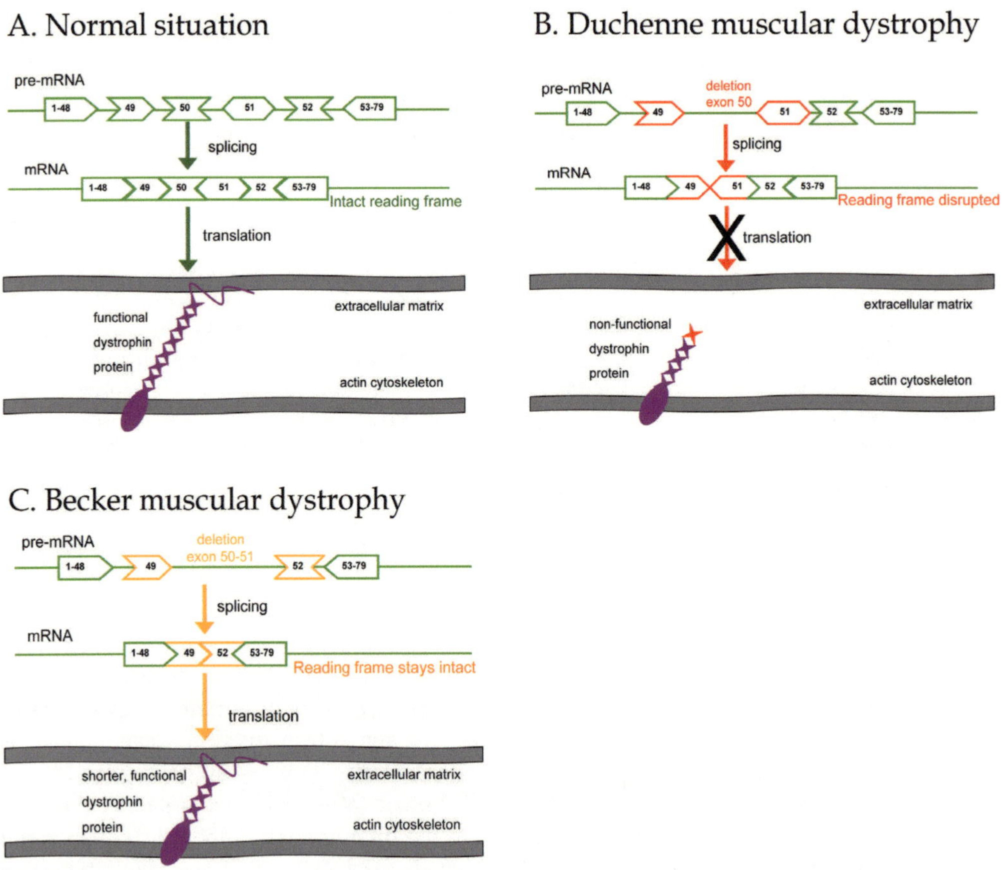

a.) In the normal situation pre-mRNA is spliced to produce mRNA, which in turn is translated into the dystrophin protein. This fully functional protein forms a bridge between the actin cytoskeleton and the extracellular matrix. b.) In DMD mutations lead to a disruption of the open reading frame and translation into protein stops prematurely. A truncated, non-functional dystrophin protein (which is degraded) is formed and the bridge function is lost. c.) In BMD mutations do not disrupt the open reading frame and translation into a shorter, but largely functional protein can occur. The bridge function is maintained.

Fig. 2. The reading frame rule

2.2 Genetic defect in BMD

In contrast to DMD, suffering from a complete absence dystrophin, in BMD a shorter, but partly functional, dystrophin protein is present. This discrepancy can be explained by the type of mutation that affects the *DMD* gene. In DMD mutations cause a disruption of the open reading frame or a premature stop codon, whereby the transcription of the gene stops prematurely and no functional protein is formed. In BMD the open reading frame stays intact (i.e. the size of the deletion in base pairs is divisible by 3), thereby translation can continue and a shorter protein is formed (fig. 2). This reading frame rule holds for over 90% of the cases (Aartsma-Rus et al., 2006b; Koenig et al., 1989). Only in-frame deletions that are very large (>36 exons) or deleting essential parts of the protein (the complete actin-binding domain or (part of) the cysteine-rich domain) lead to DMD. Furthermore, a small number of mutations that do disrupt the reading frame, lead to BMD instead of DMD (2%). This is probably due to correction of the reading frame at RNA level (Aartsma-Rus et al., 2006b).

2.3 Animal models for DMD

2.3.1 Mouse models for DMD

The most widely used model for DMD is the *mdx* mouse model (C57Bl/10ScSn-$DMD^{mdx/J}$). These mice have a single base substitution within exon 23, leading to a premature stop codon, so a truncated, non-functional dystrophin protein is formed (Sicinski et al., 1989). Despite the absence of dystrophin, the phenotype of the *mdx* mice is relatively mild compared to human DMD patients. However, compared to wild-type mice, their muscles are clearly dystrophic and functionally impaired (Chamberlain et al., 2007). Nevertheless, their life span is only slightly reduced and the muscular weakness is mild. This is probably due to compensatory mechanisms, like the upregulation of utrophin, a dystrophin homologue, which can partly take over its function. Mice that lack both dystrophin and utrophin (*mdx/utrn*$^{-/-}$, double knock-out mice) show a very severe, progressive muscular dystrophy. Their muscles display several signs of damage and are rapidly replaced by fibrotic and adipose tissue. Furthermore, these mice are functionally impaired, have an arched spine and a life span of 20 weeks at maximum (Deconinck et al., 1997). Due to the very severe phenotype and short life span, *mdx/utrn*$^{-/-}$ mice are not practical as experimental model. An intermediate model is the *mdx* mouse with haploinsufficiency for utrophin (*mdx/utrn*$^{+/-}$). Inflammation and fibrosis in both skeletal muscle and diaphragm are more severe than in the *mdx* mouse, but less than in the *mdx/utrn*$^{-/-}$ mouse. Their life span is significantly longer than that of *mdx/utrn*$^{-/-}$ mice (Zhou et al., 2008).

Next to the naturally occurring mutation in the *mdx* mouse, several DMD mutations have been induced in mice. For example, treatment of mice with the chemical *N*-ethylnitrosourea (ENU), a powerful mutagen in mice, resulted in several new *mdx*-like mouse models (B6Ros.Cg-Dmd$^{mdx\text{-}Cv}$/J). *Mdx*^{2Cv} has a mutation in a splice site in exon 43 (causing alternative splicing, resulting in out-of-frame transcripts), *mdx*^{3Cv} a mutation in intron 65 (inducing a new splice site, resulting in out-of-frame transcripts), *mdx*^{4Cv} a mutation in exon 53 (premature stop codon) and *mdx*^{5Cv} a mutation in exon 10 (frame-shift by introduction of a new splice site). All these mice have a phenotype comparable to the *mdx* mouse (Chapman et al., 1989). In addition, several mouse models have been generated that only affect 1 or a few of the different dystrophin isoforms.

2.3.2 Canine models for DMD

The Golden retriever muscular dystrophy (GRMD) dog is a spontaneously occurring canine model for Duchenne muscular dystrophy. These dogs have a single base substitution in the 3′ consensus splice site of intron 6, resulting in skipping of exon 7, thereby introducing a premature stop codon in exon 8. The course of the disease is more comparable to human patients than that of the *mdx* mouse. The dogs display rapid and fatal muscular dystrophy, characterised by muscle atrophy, myofibre degeneration, replacement by fibrotic and adipose tissue and cardiomyopathy (Sharp et al., 1992). Most affected animals die within a few years, mainly due to degeneration of the cardiac muscle (Howell et al., 1997). Although phenotypically the GRMD dog seems a better model for DMD, it shows a lot of interindividual variation in the severity of the pathology. Some animals die within days after birth, whereas others appear almost normal and live for years (Ambrosio et al., 2008). This makes the dogs less suitable for experimental use, due to standardisation problems.

Because of the large size of the golden retriever, the GRMD dog has been bred with a much smaller beagle to generate the canine X-linked muscular dystrophy ($CXMD_j$) model. These dogs have a milder phenotype compared to GRMD dogs and therefore have a longer life span (Shimatsu et al., 2003).

In addition to the above mentioned large phenotypical variation, experiments with dogs are very costly. Dogs have a long breeding time and the availability is low (a heterozygous breeding program is needed, due to the severity of the phenotype). Furthermore, for therapeutic studies the size of the dogs requires large amounts of compound.

3. Antisense oligonucleotide-mediated exon skipping

3.1 Introduction antisense oligonucleotides

Antisense oligonucleotides (AONs) are small synthetic pieces of DNA or RNA (15-30 bp), which are complementary to their target mRNA. Initially, DNA oligos were used for the specific knockdown of gene expression. These DNA oligos bind to the RNA to form DNA-RNA hybrids which activate RNase H. This enzyme cleaves the double-stranded mRNA, thereby preventing the translation into protein, thus decreasing protein expression. DNA oligos are fast degraded by endonucleases, therefore oligos with a phosphorothioate instead of a phosphodiester backbone (PS DNA oligos) were developed, which are more endonuclease-resistant. These led to very efficient expression knockdown of for example genes (UL36 or IL2) involved in CMV retinitis (85-95%) (Baker & Monia, 1999). In addition to activation of RNase H, AONs can also down regulate gene expression by inducing translational arrest through steric hindrance of ribosomal activity, interference with mRNA maturation by inhibiting splicing or destabilisation of pre-mRNA in the nucleus (Chan et al., 2006). Later, 2′O modified RNA oligos were developed, which have a higher affinity for mRNA and turned out not to induce RNase H-dependent cleavage (Sproat et al., 1989). The activation of RNase H is useful when down regulation of gene expression is required, but not when AONs are used for modulation of pre-mRNA splicing.

3.1.1 Antisense-mediated exon skipping for DMD

AON-mediated exon skipping for DMD is based on the reading frame rule (fig. 2), which underlies the phenotypic differences between DMD and BMD. Furthermore, in some DMD patients rare, dystrophin-positive (so-called "revertant" fibres) were found, which are the result of spontaneous exon skipping or secondary mutations restoring the reading frame in these fibres and allowing dystrophin production. Therefore it was hypothesised that using AONs to induces skipping of specific exons could lead to the restoration of the reading frame and thereby production of slightly shorter dystrophin proteins, as found in BMD and revertant fibres (fig. 3) (van Ommen et al., 2008). This approach is mutation-specific and a large variety in mutations exists among DMD patients. Fortunately, 2 "hotspots" (a major around exon 43 to 53 and a minor spanning exons 2 to 20) exist, comprising a large proportion of the mutations (Aartsma-Rus et al., 2006b). In this Chapter we will describe the development of this therapeutic approach. We are aware that many excellent papers about exon skipping for DMD exist. Due to space constraints it was not feasible to cover them all. For a recent overview see Aartsma-Rus, *RNA Biology* 2010 (Aartsma-Rus, 2010).

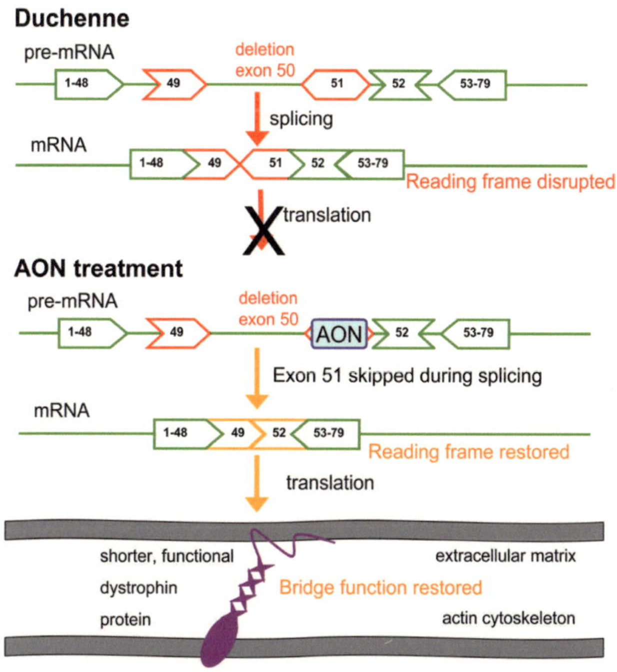

In DMD mutations in the *DMD* gene lead to a disruption of the open reading frame (in this example a deletion of exon 50), thereby preventing production of a functional dystrophin protein. Binding of an exon-specific AON (in this example against exon 51) hides the exon from the splicing machinery. The exon will be 'skipped' and not incorporated in the mRNA. Thereby the reading frame is restored and translation of a shorter, but still largely functional dystrophin protein can occur, which is similar to the proteins found in BMD.

Fig. 3. Antisense oligonucleotide-mediated exon skipping

3.2 Backbone chemistries

To prevent activation of RNase H the 2'-*O* position of the ribose was modified (2'-*O*-methyl (2OME) or 2'-*O*-methoxyethyl (2OMOE)). Furthermore, various chemical modifications (fig. 4) have been developed, which differ in sugar and backbone chemistry and have different biophysical, biochemical and biological properties. For a more detailed review see Chan et al., *Clin.Exp.Pharmacol.Physiol* 2006 (Chan et al., 2006). The 2OMePS chemistry has an increased affinity for RNA and nuclear uptake. Disadvantages are that the phosphorothioate backbone is toxic to some extent and some sequences elicit an immune response. This is partly counteracted by the 2OMe modification.

Peptide nucleic acids (PNA) contain a flexible, uncharged, achiral *N*-(2-aminoethyl)glycine backbone to which nucleobases are attached via methylenecarbonyl linkages in stead of the phosphodiester backbone of DNA oligos. PNAs have a high affinity for RNA, are not toxic even at high concentrations, are peptidase-and nuclease-resistant and have a high sequence-specificity. A disadvantage is the insolubility of PNAs, due to their hydrophobic nature, which makes transfection difficult. This can be solved by the attachment of carrier groups, which easily bind to the peptide backbone, or addition of cationic lysine residues to the C-terminus. Another disadvantage is the rapid clearance of PNAs *in vivo*. Their mechanism of action is mainly by steric hindrance (Larsen et al., 1999).

Locked nucleic acid (LNA) DNA oligos contain a 2′-*O*, 4′-*C*-methylene bridge in the β-D-ribofuranosyl configuration. They have a high hybridisation affinity towards target mRNA or DNA, thereby forming stable duplexes. This is an advantage, but also a disadvantage, since LNAs longer than 15 base pairs show self-annealing and are not very sequence-specific, which increases the chance of unwanted side effects (Aartsma-Rus et al., 2004b). However, currently mainly LNA/2'-O-methyl oligonucleotide mixmers are used, which show much more sequence-specificity (Fabani & Gait, 2008). LNAs have a good nuclear uptake and are nuclease-resistant.

Ethylene bridged nucleic acids (ENA) contain an ethylene bridge between the 2′-*O* and the 4′-*O*-C of the ribose. They have similar properties to LNAs, but have a higher affinity to RNA, are very stable and more nuclease-resistant (Morita et al., 2002; Yagi et al., 2004).

Phosphoroamidate morpholino oligomers (PMO) have a six-membered morpholino ring instead of the ribose sugar and the phosphodiester bond is replaced by a phosphoroamidate linkage. They do not activate RNase H, are very resistant to nucleases and are non-toxic. Furthermore, they are uncharged, which prevents undesired binding to proteins. However, this also results in limited nuclear uptake, where pre-mRNA splicing takes place. Their neutral charge also makes them hard to transfect in cell cultures, but *in vivo* PMOs can be taken up by tissues after local injection. This is probably due to the fact that the neutral nature does not form interactions with other cellular components. In general, PMOs are often a bit longer than 2OMePS AONs (25 nucleotides or more compared to around 20 nucleotides for 2OMePSs). They primarily act by steric prevention of ribosomal assembly (Aartsma-Rus et al., 2004b; Chan et al., 2006; Heemskerk et al., 2009b). PMOs have been linked to arginine-rich cell-penetrating peptides (pPMOs) to increase uptake and efficiency. These conjugates indeed have higher efficacy, but there are toxicity concerns and the peptide might evoke an immune response (Moulton & Moulton, 2010), though this has not yet been observed. Conjugation of PMOs with a dendrimeric octaguanidine polymer (vivo-morpholino) improves the delivery of the compound *in vivo*. Since this polymer is not a peptide, the risk of an immune response is small and has not been observed so far (Wu et al., 2009), though the polymer is toxic at higher concentrations as well.

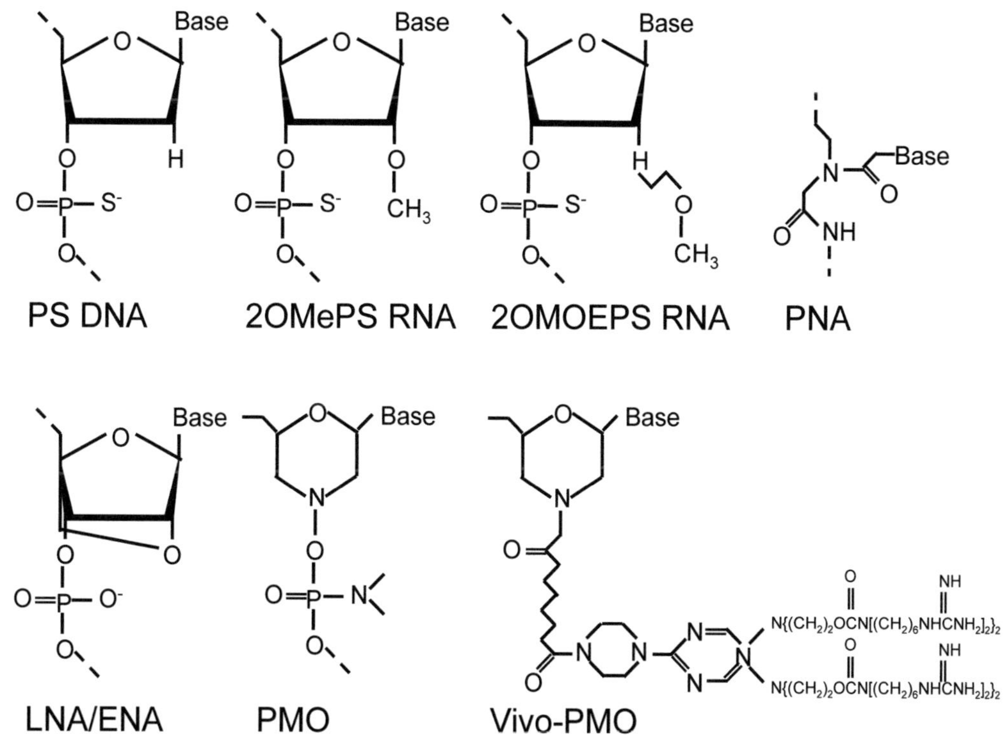

Phosphorothioate (PS) DNA, 2′-*O*-methyl phosphorothioate (2OMePS) RNA, 2′-*O*-methoxyethyl phosphorothioate (2OMOEPS) RNA, peptide nucleic acid (PNA), locked nucleic acid (LNA), ethylene bridged nucleic acid (ENA), phosphoroamidate morpholino (PMO) and dendrimeric octaguanidine conjugated phosphoroamidate morpholino (Vivo-PMO).

Fig. 4. Chemical structure of different antisense oligonucleotides

3.3 AON design and targets

Target sites for exon skipping AONs are splice sites (SS), exonic splicing enhancer (ESE) sites or exon inclusion sequences (EIS). Splice sites are required for the correct identification of exons by the spliceosome, a catalytic complex that coordinates the splicing process and consists of 5 small nuclear ribonucleoproteins (snRNP) and hundreds of other splicing factors. The 5′ (donor) splice site (beginning of an intron), the branch point (just upstream of the acceptor splice site) and the 3′ (acceptor) splice site (end of an intron) contain consensus sequences that are bound by snRNPs and splicing factors to bring about the removal of introns and ligation of exons. Blockage of splice sites or the branch point prevents incorporation of the exon in the mRNA. Exon recognition is further facilitated by ESE sites, which are exonic sequence motives to which certain splicing factors (Ser-Arg-rich (SR) proteins) can bind. AONs targeting ESEs have been proposed to sterically hinder the binding of SR proteins (Aartsma-Rus et al., 2005; Aartsma-Rus et al., 2009b; Kole et al., 2004; Tanaka et al., 1994).

4. Antisense-mediated exon skipping *in vitro*

4.1 Single exon skipping

First proofs-of-principle for the feasibility of restoring the reading frame by exon skipping have been shown *in vitro* in cultured primary human myoblasts, derived from DMD patients and in *mdx*-cell cultures.

In the early nineties, a DMD patient (named "DMD Kobe") was identified carrying a deletion of 52 base pairs within exon 19, which led to the skipping of the whole exon. The authors hypothesised that this sequence might be important for splicing. An AON targeting part of this exon induced exon skipping in human control lymphoblastoid cells (Pramono et al., 1996; Takeshima et al., 1995). In cells derived from a patient with a deletion of exon 20, PS AONs (able to activate RNase H) against the aforementioned sequence, resulted in exon 19 skipping and the restoration of dystrophin in ~20% of treated cells (Takeshima et al., 2001). By that time, exon skipping with 2OMePS AONs (unable to activate RNase H), had also been explored. In 2 patients with an out-of-frame exon 45 deletion treatment with AONs resulted in exon 46 skipping, which should restore the open reading frame. Exon skipping levels were ~15%, which restored the synthesis of functional dystrophin in more than 75% of the cells (van Deutekom et al., 2001). Subsequently, the skipping of different exons has been reported for patient-derived cells with other deletions, point mutations and duplications. For an overview see Aartsma-Rus, *RNA Biology* 2010 (Aartsma-Rus, 2010). Restoration of dystrophin synthesis was detectable at the membrane and the (at least partial) functionality of these BMD-like proteins was suggested by the reformation of the dystrophin-glycoprotein complex, shown by increased membrane expression of DGC-associated proteins. Another interesting finding were the higher exon skipping levels observed in these patient cell lines, than previously seen in control cell lines. This can be explained by nonsense-mediated decay (NMD) of the original out-of-frame transcripts, which are less stable than the newly formed in-frame transcripts (Aartsma-Rus et al., 2003).

4.2 Double and multiple exon skipping

In theory, skipping of a single exon would be beneficial for approximately 64% of the known mutations in DMD patients. However, there still is a large population which requires the skipping of 2 or more exons for reading frame restoration (Aartsma-Rus et al., 2009a). The theoretic applicability of exon skipping could be extended to 79% by double exon skipping and around 90% of patients by multiple exon skipping. Feasibility of double exon skipping was first shown in 2 different patient cell lines. One patient had a nonsense mutation in exon 43, for which dystrophin synthesis could be restored by skipping of exon 43 and 44. The second, carrying an exon 46-50 deletion, was successfully treated with a combination of AONs against exon 45 and 51. Dystrophin synthesis was found in 70% of the myotubes, which is almost as high as after single exon skipping (75-80%) (Aartsma-Rus et al., 2004a). Subsequently, successful double exon skipping has been proved by other groups (reviewed in Aartsma-Rus, *RNA Biology* 2010 (Aartsma-Rus, 2010)). The dog model for DMD needs double skipping to bypass the mutation and cells derived from these dogs have been used to show double exon skipping *in vitro* (see below) (McClorey et al., 2006).

A surprising finding in control myotubes was that combinational treatment with 45AON and 51AON caused the skipping of the entire stretch of exons from 45 through 51. This would largely increase its therapeutic applicability for a number of different mutations. Indeed the same result could be induced in patient cells with an exon 48-50 deletion (Aartsma-Rus et al., 2004a). Skipping of other large stretches of exons (multiple exon skipping) however turned out to be technically challenging and has had limited success so far (Aartsma-Rus et al., 2006a). The use of several ratios of 45AON and 55AON in both control as patient cell lines resulted in undetectable to very low exon 45-55 skipping frequencies (van Vliet L. et al., 2008).

Exon skipping is in theory useful for the majority of patients. Exceptions are mutations that involve regions in the gene that are essential for the function of the dystrophin protein: all actin-binding N-terminal parts, the cysteine-rich C-terminal part (binding to the DGC-complex), the promoter region or the first exon. Furthermore it is not applicable to translocations. Fortunately these kind of mutations make up only a small part (~8%) of all known mutations (Aartsma-Rus et al., 2009a). The largest part of mutations is made up by deletions and small mutations. A minor part consists of exon duplications (double or multiple). In the case of single duplications, skipping of one of these exons would in theory generate wild-type dystrophin transcripts. However, this turned out to be challenging. In cells with an exon 45 duplication this was indeed possible, but in other cases the skipping was so efficient that both exons were skipped, leading to an out-of-frame transcript (Aartsma-Rus et al., 2007). Skipping of an additional exon could restore the reading frame again. For example for an exon 18 duplication, successful skipping of exon 17 and both exon 18s resulted in restoration of the reading frame (Forrest et al., 2010). Successful skipping of multiple exon duplications has not yet been achieved (Aartsma-Rus et al., 2007). In total 6% of patients could benefit from single or multiple skipping of exon duplications.

5. Antisense-mediated exon skipping *in vivo* in animal models

5.1 AONs in mouse models for DMD

5.1.1 AONs in the *mdx* mouse model

After the promising *in vitro* results, AONs have been tested *in vivo* in animal models. As mentioned before, the *mdx* mouse is most widely used. The target site for exon 23 was first optimised in *mdx* myotube cell cultures. This resulted in a 5′ splice site targeting AON with a 2′-*O*-methoxyethyl phosphorothioate (2OMePS) backbone, which was tested locally in the *mdx* mouse. A single intramuscular injection of this compound in the tibialis anterior of both young (2 or 4 weeks old) and aged (6 months old) mice resulted in marked dystrophin expression 2 weeks after injection, which persisted up to 3 months after injection. The functionality of the dystrophin protein was suggested by the re-expression of dystroglycans, sarcoglycans and nNOS at the membrane. It also resulted in partial restoration of physiological function, maximum isometric titanic force, of the treated muscles. Importantly no auto-immune response against the newly formed dystrophin protein was observed (Lu et al., 2003). Of course, since DMD affects body-wide musculature, including heart and diaphragm, injection of every muscle separately is not feasible and systemic treatment is required. Three intravenous injections at weekly intervals resulted in dystrophin expression, highest in gastrocnemius, intercostal muscles and the diaphragm, without signs of toxicity or damage to other organs. However dystrophin could not be detected in the cardiac muscle (Lu et al., 2005). To optimise delivery and efficiency, different administration routes have been compared. Intravenous injection resulted rapidly in high plasma levels, which were quickly cleared. Peak plasma levels were twofold lower after subcutaneous and intraperitoneal injection, but clearance was much slower. Furthermore, intravenous injection resulted in very high AON levels in the kidney and liver, which might induce toxicity after long term treatment. Skipping levels were highest after intravenous injection and slightly lower for both subcutaneous and intraperitoneal injection. Dystrophin expression followed a similar pattern. Importantly, all 3 routes resulted in exon skipping and dystrophin expression in the heart, albeit at low levels. Due to the better pharmacokinetic profile of subcutaneous versus intravenous injection and slightly higher exon skipping compared to intraperitoneal administration, subcutaneous injection seemed to be the delivery method of choice. After subcutaneous treatment also a decrease in serum creatine kinase (CK) levels was observed. Creatine kinase is an enzyme that leaks out of the muscles into the blood stream when muscles are damaged, so a decrease indicates an improvement of muscle integrity (Heemskerk et al., 2010).

Morpholino (PMO) AONs have been shown to be effective *in vivo* as well. Intramuscular injection in the tibialis anterior elicited a dose-dependent increase in dystrophin expression in the majority of muscle fibres and dystrophin protein levels up to 60% of levels found in healthy muscle. Efficiency was comparable in both young (3 weeks old) and aged (6 months old) *mdx* mice. Repeated systemic (intravenous) injections induced exon skipping and expression of dystrophin protein body-wide, albeit with large variations between individual muscles. Highest levels were found in the quadriceps, abdominal and intercostal muscles. Lower levels were found in the tibialis anterior and diaphragm. CK levels were decreased and muscle function was improved as well. As with 2OMePS AONs, targeting of the cardiac muscle appeared difficult, since exon skipping and dystrophin expression were undetectable (Alter et al., 2006). Wu et al. showed that dystrophin restoration could be achieved (up to 30% of healthy levels) by systemic PMO treatment, although extremely high doses (up to 3 g/kg bodyweight) were required (Wu et al., 2010). Furthermore, a dosing regime of multiple low doses seems to be preferable above a few high doses to reduce the risk of toxicity and increase the efficiency, since both AONs and dystrophin protein show an accumulation over time (Malerba et al., 2009).

In the *mdx* mouse model PMOs appeared more effective and at lower doses compared to 2OMePS AONs. A direct comparison revealed that this was indeed the case for mouse exon 23 in the *mdx* mouse. Intramuscular injection of both AONs in the gastrocnemius, resulted in much higher skipping levels for PMOs than for 2OMePS AONs at the same molar amount. Systemic (intravenous) comparison in the *mdx* mouse showed, as had been noticed before, that most of the 2OMePS AONs are taken up by the liver and kidney. However the PMOs were almost exclusively taken up by the kidney. A possible explanation is that 2OMePS AONs bind to serum proteins, which prevents renal clearance (Geary et al., 2001), whereas PMOs do not, which explains their high renal clearance (Oberbauer et al., 1995). 2OMePS AON uptake was higher for all skeletal muscles, diaphragm and heart. In contrast to the biodistribution, exon skipping efficiency was much higher for the PMO AONs in skeletal muscle and diaphragm (approximately 40% versus 10%). Skipping levels in the heart were much lower and almost comparable between both compounds (2.5% for the PMOs versus 1.5% for the 2OMePS AONs). Protein levels followed the same pattern (Heemskerk et al., 2009b).

A PMO conjugated to a cell-penetrating peptide (pPMO) showed to be more effective than the naked PMO AON. Systemic (intravenous) treatment of *mdx* mice was very potent in both skeletal muscle, diaphragm and, importantly, heart. pPMOs lead to a decrease in CK levels (Jearawiriyapaisarn et al., 2008). Another study confirmed that the long term systemic treatment with pPMOs was effective in restoring dystrophin expression in skeletal muscle, improving muscle function and preventing heart failure (Wu et al., 2008). These pPMOs were also able to rescue the severe *mdx/utrn*$^{-/-}$ mouse model by systemic (intraperitoneal) treatment. Considerable improvement of muscle function was observed, combined with dystrophin expression in almost all muscles, except for the heart (Goyenvalle et al., 2010). Peptides might elicit an immune response, but no signs of such a response or toxicity were found in the mouse models so far. Unfortunately, when a pPMO compound was tested in primates, there were toxicity concerns. In cynomolgus monkeys pPMO doses equivalent to the ones used in mice, were not toxic, but also had little exon skipping effect. Higher doses were effective, but also caused tubular degeneration in the kidneys, a sign of renal toxicity (Moulton & Moulton, 2010). Yin et al. generated a chimeric fusion peptide consisting of a muscle-targeting heptapeptide (MSP) fused to an arginine-rich cell-penetrating peptide (B-peptide), which they conjugated to a PMO oligomer (B-MSP-PMO). These B-MSP-PMOs were already efficient at very low doses in restoring high levels of dystrophin expression body-wide (Yin et al., 2009). Novel cell-penetrating peptides have been discovered by inducing modifications to a *Drosophila melanogaster*-derived R6-Penetratin peptide. These peptides are called PNA or PMO internalisation peptides (Pips). A conjugate of Pip2b and a PNA AON (Pip2b-PNA) resulted in approximately threefold higher dystrophin-positive fibres compared to the naked AON after local injection in the tibialis anterior of *mdx* mice (Ivanova et al., 2008). More and improved Pips have been developed. Pip5e fused with a PMO (Pip5e-PMO) showed high exon skipping efficiency after a single intravenous injection in the *mdx* mouse. Most importantly it also efficiently targeted the heart, leading to dystrophin levels of more than 50% of wild-type levels (Yin et al., 2011).

Another modification of the PMO is conjugation to a dendrimeric octaguanidine polymer (vivo-morpholino). This modification also significantly improved the delivery and dystrophin production in *mdx* mice after intravenous injection. Repeated treatment resulted in dystrophin expression in almost 100% of the skeletal muscle fibres and levels of protein up to 50% of wild-type levels. Importantly, levels of ~10% of those found in healthy hearts were found in the cardiac muscle. In these mice no signs of an immune response or toxicity were observed (Wu et al., 2009).

5.1.2 AONs in the other mouse models

Both 2OMePS and PMO AONs have also been tested in the *mdx*^{4Cv} mouse. These mice require skipping of both exon 52 and 53 to remove the mutation and maintain the reading frame. Immortalised myoblast cell cultures from these mice were used to design the most effective AONs against exon 52 and 53, which were then tested *in vivo* in the *mdx*^{4Cv} mice. 2OMePS AONs induced exon skipping in these cell cultures, but no dystrophin protein was observed. Intramuscular injection of the cocktail of AONs in the tibialis anterior resulted in sporadic exon skipping in this muscle, but no detection of dystrophin protein. A combination of PMO AONs against both exons resulted both *in vitro* and *in vivo* (after injection in the tibialis anterior) in exon skipping and restoration of dystrophin expression (Mitrpant et al., 2009).

AONs are sequence-, and therefore species-, specific. So, to be able to test human-specific AONs, a mouse containing the full-length human *DMD* gene was generated (*hDMD*). These mice have a fully functional *hDMD* transgene integrated on mouse chromosome 5. The functionality of the transgene was proven by rescuing the severe dystrophic phenotype of the *mdx/utrn*$^{-/-}$ mouse after crossing of both models ('t Hoen et al., 2008). Intramuscular injection (gastrocnemius) of 2OMePS AONs against exon 44, 46 or 49, induced specific skipping of the targeted human exons. It also highlighted the sequence-specificity of the AONs, since in the corresponding mouse sequences, with only 2 or 3 mismatches, no detectable skipping was observed (Bremmer-Bout et al., 2004). As described before, PMOs were more efficient in the *mdx* mouse than 2OMePS AONs. However in the *hDMD* mouse, AONs targeting human exon 44, 45, 46 or 51 were comparably effective or only marginally different between both chemistries. This indicated that the differences between PMO and 2OMePS AONs are probably more due to sequence differences than to chemistry differences. Furthermore, it also suggested important differences in sequence-specificity. 2OMePS AONs with 2 mismatches had a greatly reduced efficiency, whereas PMO AONs remained equally effective. This can increase the risk of off-target side effects (Heemskerk et al., 2009b).

Studies in these *hDMD* mice revealed that the uptake of AON by the healthy *hDMD* muscle fibres is much lower than by dystrophic *mdx* fibres. This can probably be explained by the dystrophic nature of the *mdx* fibres: the lack of dystrophin results in damage to the muscle fibres, leading to leakage of the muscle enzyme creatine kinase into the bloodstream. It has been proposed that the AONs migrate into the muscle fibres through these same holes (Hoffman, 2007). In this way the disease is facilitating delivery of the potential therapeutic compound. Indeed AON uptake and skipping in the *hDMD* mouse is more difficult. The exon skipping levels observed after intramuscular injection with either 2OMePS or PMO AONs were lower than previously observed in the *mdx* mouse and in cell cultures (Heemskerk et al., 2009a). A pilot experiment with systemic (intravenous) injection of 2OMePS AONs targeting exon 51 in the *hDMD* mouse resulted in very low or undetectable exon skipping in the muscles (Heemskerk et al., 2010). Recently, vivo-morpholinos against exon 50 were shown to be able to achieve high levels of exon skipping after systemic (intravenous) injection in the healthy skeletal muscles of the *hDMD* mouse and even low levels in the cardiac muscle. There were no large signs of toxicity or adverse effects, only a small increase in serum CK levels, which could reflect a bit of membrane integrity disturbance (Wu et al., 2011). The influence of the nature of the muscle fibres on AON delivery efficiency might also explain why targeting of the heart is so difficult. The heart muscle is structurally and pathologically different from skeletal muscle, since it is made up of individual cardiomyocytes, which do not become 'leaky'.

5.2 AONs in the canine models

First AON experiments with the canine model have been performed *in vitro* in myoblast cell cultures of the GRMD dog. The nature of the mutation requires the skipping of 2 exons (exon 6 and exon 8) to restore the reading frame, thereby making it more challenging. *In vitro*, 2OMePS AONs induced higher exon skipping levels than the PMOs, but only for a short term and without induction of detectable dystrophin protein. PMOs could restore a low level of dystrophin production, but only at very high concentrations. pPMOs could induce slightly higher exon skipping levels and restored dystrophin expression (McClorey et al., 2006). Further testing of these AON cocktails *in vivo* by intramuscular injections, revealed that the AONs targeting exon 8 were effective, but the AONs targeting exon 6, which showed effectiveness *in vitro*, were not (Partridge, 2010). Another small experiment (in a 6 months old and a 5 years old dog) with cocktails of 2OMePS AONs or PMOs, resulted in high skipping levels of the desired exons and restoration of dystrophin protein to near normal levels after a single injection in the tibialis anterior with the highest test dose. The structure of the dystrophin-positive cells was reported to be improved. Furthermore, both backbone chemistries showed comparable results and results were better in the younger dog than in the older dog (Scheuerbrandt, 2009).

Systemic (intravenous) treatment of $CXMD_j$ dogs with a cocktail of 3 PMO AONs targeting exon 6 (2 PMOs) and exon 8 (1 PMO), generated body-wide production of functional dystrophin. In the heart there was only modest production of dystrophin, as observed in mice. Furthermore, an interindividual variation between dogs and intra-individual variation between different muscles of the same dog was seen. Functional improvement could be shown too and no signs of toxicity were observed (Yokota et al., 2009).

6. Clinical trials with antisense-mediated exon skipping

6.1 Local treatment with AONs

After the promising preclinical results *in vitro* and *in vivo*, the first clinical trials were initiated. These trials used local (intramuscular) injections to obtain proof-of-principle in humans and examine possible adverse effects. Normally, the first human trials are done in healthy volunteers (phase I). However, this is not possible in this case, since exon skipping in healthy persons would result in disruption of the reading frame. Therefore this phase was skipped and AONs were tested immediately in DMD patients (phase I). These first trials focused on skipping of exon 51 for both 2OMePS (in 2006) and PMO AONs (in 2008), since this would be applicable to the relatively largest group of known mutations (13%) (Aartsma-Rus et al., 2009a).

A single injection in the tibialis anterior with 0.8 mg of a 2OMePS AON (called PRO051) in 4 patients resulted in specific exon 51 skipping without adverse effects. It restored dystrophin expression at the sarcolemma in 64-97% of the myofibres and restored protein levels till 17-35% of control levels. However, it also clearly indicated the importance of muscle quality since the target of AONs, the dystrophin transcript, is only expressed in muscle fibres and not in adipose and fibrotic tissue, which replaces the muscle tissue when the disease progresses. The patient with the lowest dystrophin levels had the most advanced disease state and relatively little muscle tissue left (van Deutekom et al., 2007).

For PMO AONs a placebo-controlled, single-blinded study was performed. Seven patients received an injection with a PMO AON (called AVI-4658) into their extensor digitorum brevis (EDB) and saline into the contralateral muscle. In 2 patients receiving the lowest dose (0.09 mg) this resulted in low levels of exon 51 skipping, but no observed increase in dystrophin expression. However, a clear dystrophin restoration was observed in the higher dose (0.9 mg) group. As for the PRO051 study no adverse events, like an inflammatory response, were observed. Immunofluorescent staining for dystrophin indicated 11-21% higher intensity levels in the AON-treated muscle compared to the contralateral saline-treated muscle, and levels of 22-32% of control dystrophin levels (Kinali et al., 2009). Since both studies studied different muscles and used different techniques for quantifying immunocytochemistry the results are not directly comparable (Aartsma-Rus & van Ommen, 2009). However both studies showed unequivocal effectiveness of the used compound in the absence of side effects.

6.2 Systemic treatment with AONs

The next step towards clinical application of exon skipping are systemic clinical trials. The first pilot experiment has been conducted in Japan. Takeshima et al. treated 1 DMD patient intravenously with a weekly dose of 0.5 mg/kg bodyweight of a PS AON against exon 19 for 4 weeks. Only very low levels of exon skipping and dystrophin protein were observed in a muscle biopsy (Takeshima et al., 2006). This is not surprising, as the dose used was very low and the PS backbone chemistry is not ideal for exon skipping purposes (see above). Furthermore, this was only 1 single patient, so no real, reliable conclusions can be drawn from this experiment.

More extensive, open-label, dose-escalation, phase I/IIa studies have recently been completed for both 2OMePS and PMO AONs. The first was a study with abdominal subcutaneous injections of PRO051 (2OMePS AON, now called GSK2402968)) in 12 patients testing 5 weekly doses (0.5, 2, 4 and 6 mg/kg bodyweight) in groups of 3 patients. Doses of 2 mg/kg bodyweight or higher resulted in specific exon 51 skipping. In 10 out of 12 patients dystrophin expression in a tibialis anterior biopsy could be observed in 60-100% of the muscle fibres at levels up to 15.6% of healthy levels in a dose-dependent manner. After analysis of this first phase (6 to 15 months later), all patients entered an open-label extension study in which they received weekly injections of the highest dose. After 12 weeks, this resulted in functional improvement as measured by the 6-minute walk test. Since a placebo group is lacking, interpretation of this improvement must be done with caution. Nevertheless, the overall results are encouraging and only mild adverse events, like irritation at the injection side and mild proteinuria, were observed (Goemans et al., 2011).

AVI-4658 (PMO AON, also called eteplirsen) was tested by 12 weekly intravenous infusions of different doses (0.5, 1, 2, 4, 10 and 20 mg/kg bodyweight) in a total of 19 patients, without serious adverse events. In a biceps biopsy, exon 51 skipping and restoration of protein expression was observed starting at a dose of 2 mg/kg bodyweight, albeit variable between individual patients. The responding patients showed dystrophin levels of 8-16% of healthy controls by immunofluorescent staining. Notably, there were 3 patients who responded very well, with up to 55% of dystrophin-positive fibres by immunofluorescent staining and dystrophin levels up to 18% by western blot. In 4 other patients some improvement was observed. Furthermore, the functionality of the newly formed proteins was confirmed by the restoration of DGC-associated proteins at the sarcolemma. In addition, a reduction of inflammatory infiltrates was observed in the highest dose group, which probably indicates a reduction in necrosis and an increased resistance to mechanical load (Cirak et al., 2011). Not all patients responded equally well, which may be explained by the short serum half-life of PMOs. Since PMOs do not bind to plasma proteins (see above), they are rapidly filtered out by the kidney (accounting for 40-60% of total plasma clearance). Thus, the amount available for uptake by other tissues (e.g. muscles) is low. Therefore further optimisation (e.g. higher doses) is needed.

The next steps are larger randomised, placebo-controlled studies and targeting of other exons. For GSK2402968 a phase III study was initiated in January 2011. 180 ambulant patients will receive 6 mg/kg bodyweight AON once weekly for 1 year or placebo (http://clinicaltrials.gov/ct2/show/NCT01254019?term=GSK2402968&rank=1). This study will tell us whether long-term treatment is safe and leads to functional improvement or slowing down of disease progression (compared to placebo-treated patients). In parallel, a study in non-ambulant patients with different AON doses, primarily to determine the pharmacokinetical profile in older patients, and a study in ambulant patients where different treatment regimes are compared, are conducted (http://clinicaltrials.gov/ct2/show/NCT01128855?term=GSK2402968&rank=3 and http://clinicaltrials.gov/ct2/show/NCT01153932?term=GSK2402968&rank=2). In addition a clinical trial for AVI-4658 (eteplirsen) with higher doses (30 mg/kg and 50 mg/kg bodyweight) for 24 weeks has been initiated to assess its efficacy and safety (http://clinicaltrials.gov/ct2/show/NCT01396239?term=eteplirsen&rank=1). These trials focus on skipping of exon 51, applicable to the relative largest group of patients. Skipping of exon 44 would be useful for another large group of patients (6.2%) (Aartsma-Rus et al., 2006b). A phase I/IIa study with PRO044 (2OMePS AON against exon 44) with the same set-up as the phase I/IIa study for PRO051 is currently ongoing (http://clinicaltrials.gov/ct2/show/NCT01037309?term=PRO044&rank1). Furthermore, preclinical studies with other 2OMePS AONs (against exon 45, 52, 53 and 55) are performed by Prosensa Therapeutics. In addition to this, preclinical tests with AVI-5038 (pPMO AON against exon 50) are ongoing, although toxicity issues with this pPMO have been reported (http://investorrelations.avibio.com/phoenix.zhtml?c=64231%20&p=irol-newsArticle&ID=1406001&highlight=).

7. Improvement of AON delivery and efficiency

The efficacy of AONs depends partly on the amount of AON that reaches its target, i.e. the muscle fibre nuclei. Several strategies to improve muscle-specific uptake are under investigation, like muscle-homing peptides and cell-penetrating peptides (see above). Due to AON clearance and turnover, the effect of AONs is only temporarily, thus repeated, life-long, injections are required, should this approach prove to be efficacious. The first clinical trials showed that the average serum half-life was 29 days for 2OMePS AONs and around 1.5 hours for PMOs. A way to allow a more prolonged effect is the use of viral vectors stably expressing modified small nuclear ribonucleoprotein (snRNP) genes, in which the normal antisense sequence is replaced by an antisense sequence of choice. snRNPs are small protein-RNA hybrids that are amongst others involved in pre-mRNA splicing and histone processing. The U1 and U7 snRNPs have been used most in splicing modulation experiments (Brun et al., 2003). Exon 51 targeting U1 snRNPs induced effective skipping of exon 51 and rescue of dystrophin synthesis in a patient-derived cell line (De Angelis et al., 2002). Adeno-associated viruses (AAVs) are very efficient at transferring genes into skeletal muscles. Injection of AAV vectors expressing U7 or U1 snRNPs targeting mouse exon 23 resulted in sustained production of functional dystrophin in the *mdx* mouse after intramuscular injection and body-wide dystrophin expression and reduced muscle wasting after systemic treatment (Denti et al., 2008; Goyenvalle et al., 2004). However serious problems with the use of AAV vectors are the possibility of an immune response against the viral capsid and the difficulty to produce them on a large scale under good manufacturing practice (GMP), necessary for implementation in the clinic. Another problem is the translation from mice to larger animals or humans. In mice it is feasible to treat a whole muscle, but transfection of whole muscles body-wide is more challenging in larger animals and humans.

8. Conclusion

In summary, Duchenne muscular dystrophy is caused by genetic defects in the gene encoding the dystrophin protein. These mutations cause a premature stop codon or disrupt the reading frame, leading to a non-functional protein. In most cases this can be overcome by specific skipping of the mutated exon with AONs, to produce a slightly shorter, but largely functional dystrophin protein, as found in the related, but much milder Becker muscular dystrophy. Over the past years major steps have been made in development of this therapy. Proof-of-principle has first been shown *in vitro* in cultured muscle cell lines and *in vivo* in several animal models (e.g. *mdx* mice and GRMD dogs). Recently the first clinical trials with AONs of 2 different chemistries, targeting exon 51, applicable to the largest group of patients, have been completed with positive results. Larger trials are ongoing or planned for the near future. Although the results obtained in the past few years are very encouraging, precaution is needed and several problems still exist. First of all, this is not a cure, but a potential treatment that will hopefully lead to an improvement of the phenotype. Secondly, the approach is mutation-specific, i.e. requiring different AONs for different mutations. Luckily most mutations cluster in 2 hotspots (see above). However, development and application in the clinic of the therapy for rare mutations will be difficult, since at the moment each AON is considered as a new drug, therefore has to go through all (pre)clinical steps before it can be registered. For these rare mutations simply not enough patients are available for these studies. At the moment efforts to discuss this with the regulatory authorities are coordinated by the TREAT-NMD Network of Excellence. For example, it may be possible to reduce the toxicity trials for an AON with similar backbone chemistry, if 1 or 2 of this kind have been proven to be safe (Muntoni & Wood, 2011). Thirdly, the approach will not be useful for mutations affecting the essential parts (actin-or dystroglycan-binding domains) of the protein. Fortunately these make up only a small percentage of all known mutations. Furthermore, restoration of the reading frame is more challenging when double and especially multiple exon skipping is required. Finally, the preclinical studies and first clinical trials have shown that muscle quality is very important for the therapeutic success, since dystrophin transcripts are only produced in muscle cells and not in the fibrotic and adipose tissue that replaces the muscle cells when the disease progresses. Therefore early start of treatment will probably be required.

In conclusion, AONs are currently a promising therapeutic approach for DMD and major steps towards clinical implementation have been made over the past years, but further improvements are necessary for increasing therapeutic effectiveness and more research for broader clinical application of the technique.

9. References

't Hoen, P. A., de Meijer, E. J., Boer, J. M., Vossen, R. H., Turk, R., Maatman, R. G., Davies, K. E., van Ommen, G. J., van Deutekom, J. C., & Den Dunnen, J. T. (February 2008).

Generation and characterization of transgenic mice with the full-length human DMD gene. *J.Biol.Chem.*, Vol.283,No.9, (February 2008), pp. 5899-5907, ISSN

Aartsma-Rus, A. (July 2010). Antisense-mediated modulation of splicing: therapeutic implications for Duchenne muscular dystrophy. *RNA.Biol.*, Vol.7,No.4, (July 2010), pp. 453-461, ISSN

Aartsma-Rus, A., de Winter, C. L., Janson, A. A., Kaman, W. E., van Ommen, G. J., Den Dunnen, J. T., & van Deutekom, J. C. (December 2005). Functional analysis of 114 exon-internal AONs for targeted DMD exon skipping: indication for steric hindrance of SR protein binding sites. *Oligonucleotides.*, Vol.15,No.4, (December 2005), pp. 284-297, ISSN

Aartsma-Rus, A., Fokkema, I., Verschuuren, J., Ginjaar, I., van, D. J., van Ommen, G. J., & Den Dunnen, J. T. (March 2009a). Theoretic applicability of antisense-mediated exon skipping for Duchenne muscular dystrophy mutations. *Hum.Mutat.*, Vol.30,No.3, (March 2009a), pp. 293-299, ISSN

Aartsma-Rus, A., Janson, A. A., Kaman, W. E., Bremmer-Bout, M., Den Dunnen, J. T., Baas, F., van Ommen, G. J., & van Deutekom, J. C. (April 2003). Therapeutic antisense-induced exon skipping in cultured muscle cells from six different DMD patients. *Hum.Mol.Genet.*, Vol.12,No.8, (April 2003), pp. 907-914, ISSN

Aartsma-Rus, A., Janson, A. A., Kaman, W. E., Bremmer-Bout, M., van Ommen, G. J., Den Dunnen, J. T., & van Deutekom, J. C. (January 2004a). Antisense-induced multiexon skipping for Duchenne muscular dystrophy makes more sense. *Am.J.Hum.Genet.*, Vol.74,No.1, (January 2004a), pp. 83-92, ISSN

Aartsma-Rus, A., Janson, A. A., van Ommen, G. J., & van Deutekom, J. C. (2007). Antisense-induced exon skipping for duplications in Duchenne muscular dystrophy. *BMC.Med.Genet.*, Vol.8,No.2007), pp. 43-

Aartsma-Rus, A., Kaman, W. E., Bremmer-Bout, M., Janson, A. A., Den Dunnen, J. T., van Ommen, G. J., & van Deutekom, J. C. (September 2004b). Comparative analysis of antisense oligonucleotide analogs for targeted DMD exon 46 skipping in muscle cells. *Gene Ther.*, Vol.11,No.18, (September 2004b), pp. 1391-1398, ISSN

Aartsma-Rus, A., Kaman, W. E., Weij, R., Den Dunnen, J. T., van Ommen, G. J., & van Deutekom, J. C. (September 2006a). Exploring the frontiers of therapeutic exon skipping for Duchenne muscular dystrophy by double targeting within one or multiple exons. *Mol.Ther.*, Vol.14,No.3, (September 2006a), pp. 401-407, ISSN

Aartsma-Rus, A., van Deutekom, J. C., Fokkema, I. F., van Ommen, G. J., & Den Dunnen, J. T. (August 2006b). Entries in the Leiden Duchenne muscular dystrophy mutation database: an overview of mutation types and paradoxical cases that confirm the reading-frame rule. *Muscle Nerve.*, Vol.34,No.2, (August 2006b), pp. 135-144, ISSN

Aartsma-Rus, A. and van Ommen, G. J. (October 2009). Less is more: therapeutic exon skipping for Duchenne muscular dystrophy. *Lancet Neurol.*, Vol.8,No.10, (October 2009), pp. 873-875, ISSN

Aartsma-Rus, A., van, V. L., Hirschi, M., Janson, A. A., Heemskerk, H., de Winter, C. L., de, K. S., van Deutekom, J. C., 't Hoen, P. A., & van Ommen, G. J. (March 2009b). Guidelines for antisense oligonucleotide design and insight into splice-modulating mechanisms. *Mol.Ther.*, Vol.17,No.3, (March 2009b), pp. 548-553, ISSN

Alter, J., Lou, F., Rabinowitz, A., Yin, H., Rosenfeld, J., Wilton, S. D., Partridge, T. A., & Lu, Q. L. (February 2006). Systemic delivery of morpholino oligonucleotide restores dystrophin expression bodywide and improves dystrophic pathology. *Nat.Med.*, Vol.12,No.2, (February 2006), pp. 175-177, ISSN

Amann, K. J., Renley, B. A., & Ervasti, J. M. (October 1998). A cluster of basic repeats in the dystrophin rod domain binds F-actin through an electrostatic interaction. *J.Biol.Chem.*, Vol.273,No.43, (October 1998), pp. 28419-28423, ISSN

Ambrosio, C. E., Valadares, M. C., Zucconi, E., Cabral, R., Pearson, P. L., Gaiad, T. P., Canovas, M., Vainzof, M., Miglino, M. A., & Zatz, M. (November 2008). Ringo, a Golden Retriever Muscular Dystrophy (GRMD) dog with absent dystrophin but normal strength. *Neuromuscul.Disord.*, Vol.18,No.11, (November 2008), pp. 892-893, ISSN

Baker, B. F. and Monia, B. P. (December 1999). Novel mechanisms for antisense-mediated regulation of gene expression. *Biochim.Biophys.Acta*, Vol.1489,No.1, (December 1999), pp. 3-18, ISSN

Bremmer-Bout, M., Aartsma-Rus, A., de Meijer, E. J., Kaman, W. E., Janson, A. A., Vossen, R. H., van Ommen, G. J., Den Dunnen, J. T., & van Deutekom, J. C. (August 2004). Targeted exon skipping in transgenic hDMD mice: A model for direct preclinical screening of human-specific antisense oligonucleotides. *Mol.Ther.*, Vol.10,No.2, (August 2004), pp. 232-240, ISSN

Brenman, J. E., Chao, D. S., Xia, H., Aldape, K., & Bredt, D. S. (September 1995). Nitric oxide synthase complexed with dystrophin and absent from skeletal muscle sarcolemma in Duchenne muscular dystrophy. *Cell*, Vol.82,No.5, (September 1995), pp. 743-752, ISSN

Brun, C., Suter, D., Pauli, C., Dunant, P., Lochmuller, H., Burgunder, J. M., Schumperli, D., & Weis, J. (March 2003). U7 snRNAs induce correction of mutated dystrophin pre-mRNA by exon skipping. *Cell Mol.Life Sci.*, Vol.60,No.3, (March 2003), pp. 557-566, ISSN

Bushby, K., Finkel, R., Birnkrant, D. J., Case, L. E., Clemens, P. R., Cripe, L., Kaul, A., Kinnett, K., McDonald, C., Pandya, S., Poysky, J., Shapiro, F., Tomezsko, J., & Constantin, C. (January 2010). Diagnosis and management of Duchenne muscular dystrophy, part 1: diagnosis, and pharmacological and psychosocial management. *Lancet Neurol.*, Vol.9,No.1, (January 2010), pp. 77-93, ISSN

Chamberlain, J. S., Metzger, J., Reyes, M., Townsend, D., & Faulkner, J. A. (July 2007). Dystrophin-deficient mdx mice display a reduced life span and are susceptible to spontaneous rhabdomyosarcoma. *FASEB J.*, Vol.21,No.9, (July 2007), pp. 2195-2204, ISSN

Chan, J. H., Lim, S., & Wong, W. S. (May 2006). Antisense oligonucleotides: from design to therapeutic application. *Clin.Exp.Pharmacol.Physiol*, Vol.33,No.5-6, (May 2006), pp. 533-540, ISSN

Chapman, V. M., Miller, D. R., Armstrong, D., & Caskey, C. T. (February 1989). Recovery of induced mutations for X chromosome-linked muscular dystrophy in mice. *Proc.Natl.Acad.Sci.U.S.A*, Vol.86,No.4, (February 1989), pp. 1292-1296, ISSN

Cirak, S., Arechavala-Gomeza, V., Guglieri, M., Feng, L., Torelli, S., Anthony, K., Abbs, S., Garralda, M. E., Bourke, J., Wells, D. J., Dickson, G., Wood, M. J., Wilton, S. D., Straub, V., Kole, R., Shrewsbury, S. B., Sewry, C., Morgan, J. E., Bushby, K., & Muntoni, F. (July 2011). Exon skipping and dystrophin restoration in patients with Duchenne muscular dystrophy after systemic phosphorodiamidate morpholino oligomer treatment: an open-label, phase 2, dose-escalation study. *Lancet*, Vol.July 2011), pp.

De Angelis, F. G., Sthandier, O., Berarducci, B., Toso, S., Galluzzi, G., Ricci, E., Cossu, G., & Bozzoni, I. (July 2002). Chimeric snRNA molecules carrying antisense sequences against the splice junctions of exon 51 of the dystrophin pre-mRNA induce exon skipping and restoration of a dystrophin synthesis in Delta 48-50 DMD cells. *Proc.Natl.Acad.Sci.U.S.A.*, Vol.99,No.14, (July 2002), pp. 9456-9461, ISSN

Deconinck, A. E., Rafael, J. A., Skinner, J. A., Brown, S. C., Potter, A. C., Metzinger, L., Watt, D. J., Dickson, J. G., Tinsley, J. M., & Davies, K. E. (August 1997). Utrophin-dystrophin-deficient mice as a model for Duchenne muscular dystrophy. *Cell.*, Vol.90,No.4, (August 1997), pp. 717-727, ISSN

Denti, M. A., Incitti, T., Sthandier, O., Nicoletti, C., De Angelis, F. G., Rizzuto, E., Auricchio, A., Musaro, A., & Bozzoni, I. (June 2008). Long-term benefit of adeno-associated virus/antisense-mediated exon skipping in dystrophic mice. *Hum.Gene Ther.*, Vol.19,No.6, (June 2008), pp. 601-608, ISSN

Ehmsen, J., Poon, E., & Davies, K. (July 2002). The dystrophin-associated protein complex. *J.Cell Sci.*, Vol.115,No.Pt 14, (July 2002), pp. 2801-2803, ISSN

Emery, A. E. (1993). *Duchenne muscular dystrophy* (2nd), Oxford University Press, ISBN 9780192623706, Oxford

Emery, A. E. (February 2002). The muscular dystrophies. *Lancet*, Vol.359,No.9307, (February 2002), pp. 687-695, ISSN

Fabani, M. M. and Gait, M. J. (February 2008). miR-122 targeting with LNA/2'-O-methyl oligonucleotide mixmers, peptide nucleic acids (PNA), and PNA-peptide conjugates. *RNA.*, Vol.14,No.2, (February 2008), pp. 336-346, ISSN

Forrest, S., Meloni, P. L., Muntoni, F., Kim, J., Fletcher, S., & Wilton, S. D. (December 2010). Personalized exon skipping strategies to address clustered non-deletion dystrophin mutations. *Neuromuscul.Disord.*, Vol.20,No.12, (December 2010), pp. 810-816, ISSN

Geary, R. S., Watanabe, T. A., Truong, L., Freier, S., Lesnik, E. A., Sioufi, N. B., Sasmor, H., Manoharan, M., & Levin, A. A. (March 2001). Pharmacokinetic properties of 2'-O-(2-methoxyethyl)-modified oligonucleotide analogs in rats. *J.Pharmacol.Exp.Ther.*, Vol.296,No.3, (March 2001), pp. 890-897, ISSN

Gee, S. H., Madhavan, R., Levinson, S. R., Caldwell, J. H., Sealock, R., & Froehner, S. C. (January 1998). Interaction of muscle and brain sodium channels with multiple members of the syntrophin family of dystrophin-associated proteins. *J.Neurosci.*, Vol.18,No.1, (January 1998), pp. 128-137, ISSN

Goemans, N. M., Tulinius, M., van den Akker, J. T., Burm, B. E., Ekhart, P. F., Heuvelmans, N., Holling, T., Janson, A. A., Platenburg, G. J., Sipkens, J. A., Sitsen, J. M., Aartsma-Rus, A., van Ommen, G. J., Buyse, G., Darin, N., Verschuuren, J. J., Campion, G. V., de Kimpe, S. J., & van Deutekom, J. C. (March 2011). Systemic Administration of PRO051 in Duchenne's Muscular Dystrophy. *N.Engl.J.Med.*, Vol.March 2011), pp.

Gowers, W. R. (1895). *A manual of the nervous system.* (2nd), Philadelphia

Goyenvalle, A., Babbs, A., Powell, D., Kole, R., Fletcher, S., Wilton, S. D., & Davies, K. E. (January 2010). Prevention of dystrophic pathology in severely affected dystrophin/utrophin-deficient mice by morpholino-oligomer-mediated exon-skipping. *Mol.Ther.*, Vol.18,No.1, (January 2010), pp. 198-205, ISSN

Goyenvalle, A., Vulin, A., Fougerousse, F., Leturcq, F., Kaplan, J. C., Garcia, L., & Danos, O. (December 2004). Rescue of dystrophic muscle through U7 snRNA-mediated exon skipping. *Science.*, Vol.306,No.5702, (December 2004), pp. 1796-1799, ISSN

Grain, L., Cortina-Borja, M., Forfar, C., Hilton-Jones, D., Hopkin, J., & Burch, M. (March 2001). Cardiac abnormalities and skeletal muscle weakness in carriers of Duchenne and Becker muscular dystrophies and controls. *Neuromuscul.Disord.*, Vol.11,No.2, (March 2001), pp. 186-191, ISSN

Heemskerk, H., de Winter, C. L., van Ommen, G. J., van Deutekom, J. C., & Aartsma-Rus, A. (September 2009a). Development of antisense-mediated exon skipping as a treatment for duchenne muscular dystrophy. *Ann.N.Y.Acad.Sci.*, Vol.1175,No.September 2009a), pp. 71-79, ISSN

Heemskerk, H., de, W. C., van, K. P., Heuvelmans, N., Sabatelli, P., Rimessi, P., Braghetta, P., van Ommen, G. J., de, K. S., Ferlini, A., Aartsma-Rus, A., & van Deutekom, J. C. (June 2010). Preclinical PK and PD studies on 2'-O-methyl-phosphorothioate RNA antisense oligonucleotides in the mdx mouse model. *Mol.Ther.*, Vol.18,No.6, (June 2010), pp. 1210-1217, ISSN

Heemskerk, H. A., de Winter, C. L., de Kimpe, S. J., van Kuik-Romeijn, P., Heuvelmans, N., Platenburg, G. J., van Ommen, G. J., van Deutekom, J. C., & Aartsma-Rus, A. (March 2009b). In vivo comparison of 2'-O-methyl phosphorothioate and morpholino antisense oligonucleotides for Duchenne muscular dystrophy exon skipping. *J.Gene Med.*, Vol.11,No.3, (March 2009b), pp. 257-266, ISSN

Hezel, M., de Groat, W. C., & Galbiati, F. (January 2010). Caveolin-3 promotes nicotinic acetylcholine receptor clustering and regulates neuromuscular junction activity. *Mol.Biol.Cell*, Vol.21,No.2, (January 2010), pp. 302-310, ISSN

Hoffman, E. P. (December 2007). Skipping toward personalized molecular medicine. *N.Engl.J.Med.*, Vol.357,No.26, (December 2007), pp. 2719-2722, ISSN

Hoffman, E. P., Brown, R. H., Jr., & Kunkel, L. M. (December 1987). Dystrophin: the protein product of the Duchenne muscular dystrophy locus. *Cell*, Vol.51,No.6, (December 1987), pp. 919-928, ISSN

Howell, J. M., Fletcher, S., Kakulas, B. A., O'Hara, M., Lochmuller, H., & Karpati, G. (July 1997). Use of the dog model for Duchenne muscular dystrophy in gene therapy trials. *Neuromuscul.Disord.*, Vol.7,No.5, (July 1997), pp. 325-328, ISSN

Ivanova, G. D., Arzumanov, A., Abes, R., Yin, H., Wood, M. J., Lebleu, B., & Gait, M. J. (November 2008). Improved cell-penetrating peptide-PNA conjugates for splicing redirection in HeLa cells and exon skipping in mdx mouse muscle. *Nucleic Acids Res.*, Vol.36,No.20, (November 2008), pp. 6418-6428, ISSN

Jearawiriyapaisarn, N., Moulton, H. M., Buckley, B., Roberts, J., Sazani, P., Fucharoen, S., Iversen, P. L., & Kole, R. (September 2008). Sustained dystrophin expression induced by peptide-conjugated morpholino oligomers in the muscles of mdx mice. *Mol.Ther.*, Vol.16,No.9, (September 2008), pp. 1624-1629, ISSN

Kinali, M., Arechavala-Gomeza, V., Feng, L., Cirak, S., Hunt, D., Adkin, C., Guglieri, M., Ashton, E., Abbs, S., Nihoyannopoulos, P., Garralda, M. E., Rutherford, M., McCulley, C., Popplewell, L., Graham, I. R., Dickson, G., Wood, M. J., Wells, D. J., Wilton, S. D., Kole, R., Straub, V., Bushby, K., Sewry, C., Morgan, J. E., & Muntoni, F. (October 2009). Local restoration of dystrophin expression with the morpholino oligomer AVI-4658 in Duchenne muscular dystrophy: a single-blind, placebo-controlled, dose-escalation, proof-of-concept study. *Lancet Neurol.*, Vol.8,No.10, (October 2009), pp. 918-928, ISSN

Koenig, M., Beggs, A. H., Moyer, M., Scherpf, S., Heindrich, K., Bettecken, T., Meng, G., Muller, C. R., Lindlof, M., Kaariainen, H., & . (October 1989). The molecular basis for Duchenne versus Becker muscular dystrophy: correlation of severity with type of deletion. *Am.J.Hum.Genet.*, Vol.45,No.4, (October 1989), pp. 498-506, ISSN

Kole, R., Williams, T., & Cohen, L. (2004). RNA modulation, repair and remodeling by splice switching oligonucleotides. *Acta Biochim.Pol.*, Vol.51,No.2, (2004), pp. 373-378, ISSN

Lai, Y., Thomas, G. D., Yue, Y., Yang, H. T., Li, D., Long, C., Judge, L., Bostick, B., Chamberlain, J. S., Terjung, R. L., & Duan, D. (March 2009). Dystrophins carrying spectrin-like repeats 16 and 17 anchor nNOS to the sarcolemma and enhance exercise performance in a mouse model of muscular dystrophy. *J.Clin.Invest*, Vol.119,No.3, (March 2009), pp. 624-635, ISSN

Larsen, H. J., Bentin, T., & Nielsen, P. E. (December 1999). Antisense properties of peptide nucleic acid. *Biochim.Biophys.Acta*, Vol.1489,No.1, (December 1999), pp. 159-166, ISSN

Lu, Q. L., Mann, C. J., Lou, F., Bou-Gharios, G., Morris, G. E., Xue, S. A., Fletcher, S., Partridge, T. A., & Wilton, S. D. (August 2003). Functional amounts of dystrophin produced by skipping the mutated exon in the mdx dystrophic mouse. *Nat.Med.*, Vol.9,No.8, (August 2003), pp. 1009-1014, ISSN

Lu, Q. L., Rabinowitz, A., Chen, Y. C., Yokota, T., Yin, H., Alter, J., Jadoon, A., Bou-Gharios, G., & Partridge, T. (January 2005). Systemic delivery of antisense oligoribonucleotide restores dystrophin expression in body-wide skeletal muscles. *Proc.Natl.Acad.Sci.U.S.A.*, Vol.102,No.1, (January 2005), pp. 198-203, ISSN

Malerba, A., Thorogood, F. C., Dickson, G., & Graham, I. R. (September 2009). Dosing regimen has a significant impact on the efficiency of morpholino oligomer-induced exon skipping in mdx mice. *Hum.Gene Ther.*, Vol.20,No.9, (September 2009), pp. 955-965, ISSN

McClorey, G., Moulton, H. M., Iversen, P. L., Fletcher, S., & Wilton, S. D. (October 2006). Antisense oligonucleotide-induced exon skipping restores dystrophin expression in vitro in a canine model of DMD. *Gene Ther.*, Vol.13,No.19, (October 2006), pp. 1373-1381, ISSN

Miller, G., Wang, E. L., Nassar, K. L., Peter, A. K., & Crosbie, R. H. (February 2007). Structural and functional analysis of the sarcoglycan-sarcospan subcomplex. *Exp.Cell Res.*, Vol.313,No.4, (February 2007), pp. 639-651, ISSN

Mitrpant, C., Fletcher, S., Iversen, P. L., & Wilton, S. D. (January 2009). By-passing the nonsense mutation in the 4 CV mouse model of muscular dystrophy by induced exon skipping. *J.Gene Med.*, Vol.11,No.1, (January 2009), pp. 46-56, ISSN

Morita, K., Hasegawa, C., Kaneko, M., Tsutsumi, S., Sone, J., Ishikawa, T., Imanishi, T., & Koizumi, M. (January 2002). 2'-O,4'-C-ethylene-bridged nucleic acids (ENA): highly nuclease-resistant and thermodynamically stable oligonucleotides for antisense drug. *Bioorg.Med.Chem.Lett.*, Vol.12,No.1, (January 2002), pp. 73-76, ISSN

Moser, H. (1984). Duchenne muscular dystrophy: pathogenetic aspects and genetic prevention. *Hum.Genet.*, Vol.66,No.1, (1984), pp. 17-40, ISSN

Moulton, H. M. and Moulton, J. D. (December 2010). Morpholinos and their peptide conjugates: therapeutic promise and challenge for Duchenne muscular dystrophy. *Biochim.Biophys.Acta*, Vol.1798,No.12, (December 2010), pp. 2296-2303, ISSN

Muntoni, F., Torelli, S., & Ferlini, A. (December 2003). Dystrophin and mutations: one gene, several proteins, multiple phenotypes. *Lancet Neurol.*, Vol.2,No.12, (December 2003), pp. 731-740, ISSN

Muntoni, F. and Wood, M. J. (2011). Targeting RNA to treat neuromuscular disease. *Nat.Rev.Drug Discov.*, Vol.10,No.8, (2011), pp. 621-637, ISSN

Newey, S. E., Howman, E. V., Ponting, C. P., Benson, M. A., Nawrotzki, R., Loh, N. Y., Davies, K. E., & Blake, D. J. (March 2001). Syncoilin, a novel member of the intermediate filament superfamily that interacts with alpha-dystrobrevin in skeletal muscle. *J.Biol.Chem.*, Vol.276,No.9, (March 2001), pp. 6645-6655, ISSN

Oberbauer, R., Schreiner, G. F., & Meyer, T. W. (October 1995). Renal uptake of an 18-mer phosphorothioate oligonucleotide. *Kidney Int.*, Vol.48,No.4, (October 1995), pp. 1226-1232, ISSN

Partridge, T. (September 2010). The potential of exon skipping for treatment for Duchenne muscular dystrophy. *J.Child Neurol.*, Vol.25,No.9, (September 2010), pp. 1165-1170, ISSN

Pramono, Z. A., Takeshima, Y., Alimsardjono, H., Ishii, A., Takeda, S., & Matsuo, M. (September 1996). Induction of exon skipping of the dystrophin transcript in lymphoblastoid cells by transfecting an antisense oligodeoxynucleotide complementary to an exon recognition sequence. *Biochem.Biophys.Res.Commun.*, Vol.226,No.2, (September 1996), pp. 445-449, ISSN

Sharp, N. J., Kornegay, J. N., Van Camp, S. D., Herbstreith, M. H., Secore, S. L., Kettle, S., Hung, W. Y., Constantinou, C. D., Dykstra, M. J., Roses, A. D., & . (May 1992). An error in dystrophin mRNA processing in golden retriever muscular dystrophy, an animal homologue of Duchenne muscular dystrophy. *Genomics.*, Vol.13,No.1, (May 1992), pp. 115-121, ISSN

Shimatsu, Y., Katagiri, K., Furuta, T., Nakura, M., Tanioka, Y., Yuasa, K., Tomohiro, M., Kornegay, J. N., Nonaka, I., & Takeda, S. (April 2003). Canine X-linked muscular dystrophy in Japan (CXMDJ). *Exp.Anim.*, Vol.52,No.2, (April 2003), pp. 93-97, ISSN

Sicinski, P., Geng, Y., Ryder-Cook, A. S., Barnard, E. A., Darlison, M. G., & Barnard, P. J. (June 1989). The molecular basis of muscular dystrophy in the mdx mouse: a point mutation. *Science*, Vol.244,No.4912, (June 1989), pp. 1578-1580, ISSN

Sproat, B. S., Lamond, A. I., Beijer, B., Neuner, P., & Ryder, U. (May 1989). Highly efficient chemical synthesis of 2'-O-methyloligoribonucleotides and tetrabiotinylated derivatives; novel probes that are resistant to degradation by RNA or DNA specific nucleases. *Nucleic Acids Res.*, Vol.17,No.9, (May 1989), pp. 3373-3386, ISSN

Takeshima, Y., Nishio, H., Sakamoto, H., Nakamura, H., & Matsuo, M. (February 1995). Modulation of in vitro splicing of the upstream intron by modifying an intra-exon sequence which is deleted from the dystrophin gene in dystrophin Kobe. *J.Clin.Invest*, Vol.95,No.2, (February 1995), pp. 515-520, ISSN

Takeshima, Y., Wada, H., Yagi, M., Ishikawa, Y., Ishikawa, Y., Minami, R., Nakamura, H., & Matsuo, M. (December 2001). Oligonucleotides against a splicing enhancer sequence led to dystrophin production in muscle cells from a Duchenne muscular dystrophy patient. *Brain Dev.*, Vol.23,No.8, (December 2001), pp. 788-790, ISSN

Takeshima, Y., Yagi, M., Wada, H., Ishibashi, K., Nishiyama, A., Kakumoto, M., Sakaeda, T., Saura, R., Okumura, K., & Matsuo, M. (May 2006). Intravenous infusion of an antisense oligonucleotide results in exon skipping in muscle dystrophin mRNA of Duchenne muscular dystrophy. *Pediatr.Res.*, Vol.59,No.5, (May 2006), pp. 690-694, ISSN

Tanaka, K., Watakabe, A., & Shimura, Y. (February 1994). Polypurine sequences within a downstream exon function as a splicing enhancer. *Mol.Cell Biol.*, Vol.14,No.2, (February 1994), pp. 1347-1354, ISSN

van Deutekom, J. C., Bremmer-Bout, M., Janson, A. A., Ginjaar, I. B., Baas, F., Den Dunnen, J. T., & van Ommen, G. J. (July 2001). Antisense-induced exon skipping restores dystrophin expression in DMD patient derived muscle cells. *Hum.Mol.Genet.*, Vol.10,No.15, (July 2001), pp. 1547-1554, ISSN

van Deutekom, J. C., Janson, A. A., Ginjaar, I. B., Frankhuizen, W. S., Aartsma-Rus, A., Bremmer-Bout, M., Den Dunnen, J. T., Koop, K., van der Kooi, A. J., Goemans, N. M., de Kimpe, S. J., Ekhart, P. F., Venneker, E. H., Platenburg, G. J., Verschuuren, J. J., & van Ommen, G. J. (December 2007). Local dystrophin restoration with antisense oligonucleotide PRO051. *N.Engl.J.Med.*, Vol.357,No.26, (December 2007), pp. 2677-2686, ISSN

van Ommen, G. J., van, D. J., & Aartsma-Rus, A. (April 2008). The therapeutic potential of antisense-mediated exon skipping. *Curr.Opin.Mol.Ther.*, Vol.10,No.2, (April 2008), pp. 140-149, ISSN

van Vliet L., de Winter, C. L., van Deutekom, J. C., van Ommen, G. J., & Aartsma-Rus, A. (2008). Assessment of the feasibility of exon 45-55 multiexon skipping for Duchenne muscular dystrophy. *BMC.Med.Genet.*, Vol.9,No.2008), pp. 105-

Wu, B., Benrashid, E., Lu, P., Cloer, C., Zillmer, A., Shaban, M., & Lu, Q. L. (2011). Targeted skipping of human dystrophin exons in transgenic mouse model systemically for antisense drug development. *PLoS.One.*, Vol.6,No.5, (2011), pp. e19906-

Wu, B., Li, Y., Morcos, P. A., Doran, T. J., Lu, P., & Lu, Q. L. (May 2009). Octa-guanidine morpholino restores dystrophin expression in cardiac and skeletal muscles and ameliorates pathology in dystrophic mdx mice. *Mol.Ther.*, Vol.17,No.5, (May 2009), pp. 864-871, ISSN

Wu, B., Lu, P., Benrashid, E., Malik, S., Ashar, J., Doran, T. J., & Lu, Q. L. (January 2010). Dose-dependent restoration of dystrophin expression in cardiac muscle of dystrophic mice by systemically delivered morpholino. *Gene Ther.*, Vol.17,No.1, (January 2010), pp. 132-140, ISSN

Wu, B., Moulton, H. M., Iversen, P. L., Jiang, J., Li, J., Li, J., Spurney, C. F., Sali, A., Guerron, A. D., Nagaraju, K., Doran, T., Lu, P., Xiao, X., & Lu, Q. L. (September 2008). Effective rescue of dystrophin improves cardiac function in dystrophin-deficient mice by a modified morpholino oligomer. *Proc.Natl.Acad.Sci.U.S.A.*, Vol.105,No.39, (September 2008), pp. 14814-14819, ISSN

Yagi, M., Takeshima, Y., Surono, A., Takagi, M., Koizumi, M., & Matsuo, M. (2004). Chimeric RNA and 2'-O, 4'-C-ethylene-bridged nucleic acids have stronger activity than phosphorothioate oligodeoxynucleotides in induction of exon 19 skipping in dystrophin mRNA. *Oligonucleotides.*, Vol.14,No.1, (2004), pp. 33-40, ISSN

Yin, H., Moulton, H. M., Betts, C., Seow, Y., Boutilier, J., Iverson, P. L., & Wood, M. J. (November 2009). A fusion peptide directs enhanced systemic dystrophin exon skipping and functional restoration in dystrophin-deficient mdx mice. *Hum.Mol.Genet.*, Vol.18,No.22, (November 2009), pp. 4405-4414, ISSN

Yin, H., Saleh, A. F., Betts, C., Camelliti, P., Seow, Y., Ashraf, S., Arzumanov, A., Hammond, S., Merritt, T., Gait, M. J., & Wood, M. J. (July 2011). Pip5 transduction peptides direct high efficiency oligonucleotide-mediated dystrophin exon skipping in heart and phenotypic correction in mdx mice. *Mol.Ther.*, Vol.19,No.7, (July 2011), pp. 1295-1303, ISSN

Yokota, T., Lu, Q. L., Partridge, T., Kobayashi, M., Nakamura, A., Takeda, S., & Hoffman, E. (March 2009). Efficacy of systemic morpholino exon-skipping in duchenne dystrophy dogs. *Ann.Neurol.*, Vol.March 2009), pp.

Zhou, L., Rafael-Fortney, J. A., Huang, P., Zhao, X. S., Cheng, G., Zhou, X., Kaminski, H. J., Liu, L., & Ransohoff, R. M. (January 2008). Haploinsufficiency of utrophin gene worsens skeletal muscle inflammation and fibrosis in mdx mice. *J.Neurol.Sci.*, Vol.264,No.1-2, (January 2008), pp. 106-111, ISSN

4

Psychosocial Support Needs of Families of Boys with Duchenne Muscular Dystrophy

Jean K. Mah[1,*] and Doug Biggar[2]
[1]*Alberta Children's Hospital, University of Calgary, Calgary, Alberta,*
[2]*Bloorview Kids Rehab, University of Toronto, Ontario,*
Canada

1. Introduction

Duchenne muscular dystrophy (DMD, OMIM #310200) is the most common form of muscular dystrophy in childhood, with an incidence of approximately 1 per 3,500 live-born males [Emery, 1991]. It is caused by mutations of the *DMD* gene located on Xp21 which codes for dystrophin, a 427-kDa protein that is expressed at the sarcolemma of skeletal muscle. The *dystrophin* gene contains 79 exons, which includes an actin-binding domain at the N-terminus, 24 spectrin-like repeat units, a cysteine-rich dystroglycan binding site, and a C-terminal domain [Hoffman et al, 1987; Koenig et al, 1988]. The large size of the *dystrophin* gene results in a complex mutational spectrum (>4,700 different mutations) as well as a high spontaneous mutation rate [Aartsma-Rus et al, 2006]. Large deletions account for approximately 65% of DMD mutations while duplications occur in up to 10% of males with DMD. The remaining 25% include small deletions, insertions, point mutations, or splicing mutations. About two-thirds of DMD cases are inherited from mothers carrying the mutations, with the remaining one-third occurring as spontaneous mutations [Laing, 1993]. According to Monaco et al, DMD-causing mutations are typically associated with an out-of-frame mutation leading to a loss of functional gene product, whereas in-frame mutations that allow synthesis of an internally truncated but functional protein result in a milder Becker muscular dystrophy (BMD) phenotype [Monaco et al, 1988].

Dystrophin is an integral component of the dystrophin glycoprotein complex. It stabilizes the muscle membrane by bridging the basal lamina of the extracelluar matrix to the inner cytoskeleton of the contractile elements [Rybakova et al, 2000]. It also serve as a transmembrane signalling complex which is essential for cell survival [Chen et al, 2000]. Loss of dystrophin results in excessive membrane fragility, unregulated influx of calcium ions into the sarcoplasm, mitochondrial dysfunction, and increased oxidative stress, leading to progressive muscle degeneration, fibrosis, and fatty replacement [Wallace & McNally, 2009]. Early presenting features in DMD include developmental delay, proximal muscle weakness as evident by Gowers' sign and waddling gait, as well as varying degree of

* Corresponding Author

cognitive impairment and learning disability [Fitzpatrick et al, 1986; Leibowitz & Dubowitz, 1981]. Serum creatine kinase is usually markedly elevated due to on-going muscle damage and regenerative failure. Progressive muscle weakness leads to loss of independent ambulation by early teens, scoliosis, quadriplegia, respiratory insufficiency, cardiomyopathy, and death around the third decade of life.

Detection of *DMD* mutations include multiplex polymerase chain reaction (PCR) that examines the most commonly deleted regions of the gene, or other molecular genetic assays that interrogate all 79 exons, such as multiplex ligation-dependent probe amplification (MLPA) and comparative genomic hybridization (CGH) microarray. If the presence of a disease-causing deletion or duplication is not identified by a state-of-the-art DNA diagnostic technique, complete gene sequencing is needed to define the precise mutational event [Baskin et al, 2009; Takeshima et al, 2010]. A muscle biopsy can also be obtained for confirmation of dystrophin deficiency by immunostaining plus extraction of cDNA and RNA for further genetic testing [Mah et al, 2011].

Recent scientific advances have led to potentially new disease modifying treatments for many neuromuscular diseases including DMD [Wagner, 2008; Fairclough et al, 2011]. The main therapeutic strategies include: a) muscle membrane stabilization and up-regulation of compensatory cytoskeleton proteins such as biglycan and utrophin [Amenta et al, 2011; Tinsley et al, 2011]; b) enhancement of muscle regeneration via up-regulation of insulin growth factor (IGF-1) and modulation of members of transforming growth factor-beta such as myostatin [Schertzer et al, 2008; Morine et al, 2010]; c) reduction of the inflammatory cascade by selective nuclear factor-kappa B (NF-κB) inhibition [Tang et al, 2010]; and d) gene therapy including the use of adeno-associated virus microdystrophin [Trollet et al, 2009], nonsense suppression therapy [Welch et al, 2007; Malik et al, 2010], and exon-skipping to restore partial dystrophin protein production [Muntoni et al, 2005; van Deutekom et al, 2007]. Effective treatment of DMD will likely require multiple interventions targeting different disease processes, and updated information about DMD clinical trials is available at http://www.clinicaltrials.gov. The success of new and emerging therapeutic strategies depends on early diagnosis and precise mutational analysis for boys with DMD, the creation of a national or global disease-specific patient registries, plus on-going advocacy and interdisciplinary collaboration.

2. Current management strategies

Until there is a definitive cure for DMD, current treatment strategies focus on promoting well-balanced diet and physical activity as tolerated, delaying the onset of complications via pharmaceutical treatments, and optimizing health outcomes through appropriate medical and psychosocial support. Therapeutic interventions include the use of corticosteroids (such as prednisone or deflazacort) for skeletal muscle weakness and afterload reduction (such as angiotensin converting enzyme inhibitor or beta-blocker) for cardiomyopathy. Corticosteroid therapy offers benefit to DMD boys by improving muscle strength and function [Mendell et al, 1989; Griggs et al, 1991], prolonging independent ambulation [Biggar et al, 2001; Schara et al, 2001], plus slowing the progression of cardiomyopathy [Markham et al, 2008] and scoliosis [Kinali et al, 2007]. As well, the introduction of non-invasive positive pressure ventilation has prolonged the survival of individuals with DMD [Bach & Martinez, 2011].

A number of recent publications have provided comprehensive reviews on the diagnosis and multidisciplinary management of DMD, including the use of prednisone or deflazacort to preserve muscle strength [Bushby et al, 2004; Moxley et al, 2005], optimizing growth and development, surveillance for spinal deformities [Muntoni et al, 2006], managing respiratory complications [Finder et al, 2004; Birnkrant et al, 2010], and treating cardiomyopathy [American Academy of Pediatrics, 2005; Baxter, 2006]. As well, bone health, nutrition, learning disability, behaviour problems, access to wheelchair and other adaptive technology should be included as part of the comprehensive treatment plan [Bushby et al, 2010a; Bushby et al, 2010b]. As standard of care guidelines typically focus on medical management and there are no systematic strategies to meet the psychosocial needs of boys with DMD and their families, the remaining of this paper will present some of our results on pediatric HRQOL, parental experience, and family-centered care approach to DMD that may help to identify the needs and incorporate psychosocial support strategies into clinical practice. We propose the use of a modified Family Needs Survey for DMD (DMD-FNS) to help clinicians to address needs and tailor services for each family across the different stages of the disease.

3. DMD and health-related quality of life

Chronic neurological disorders such as DMD have a significant impact on pediatric health-related quality of life (HRQOL) and functional ability. Both medical services and community-based programs are often required to address their physical, emotional, social, and educational needs. A large prospective study led by Dr. Craig McDonald and his colleagues will provide valuable longitudinal data on the natural history of DMD, associated HRQOL, and health services utilization; this 5-year study includes more than three hundred boys with a confirmed diagnosis of DMD from 20 participating CINRG centers in the United States and other international sites (personal communication). Given the lack of information on the processes of care and health outcomes of children with chronic neurological disabilities in Canada, a brief 3-month cross-sectional pilot survey was performed at the Alberta Children's Hospital, a tertiary pediatric neurosciences center in Calgary, Alberta to explore the use of health services and HRQOL among DMD and other pediatric neurosciences patients. Specifically, parents of 278 children (165 male, mean age = 11 ± 4.5 years) were asked to describe their child's functional ability, health-related quality of life (HRQOL), and use of health services including access to medical professionals, rehabilitation programs, education, and social support in their communities. The children were followed because of chronic neurological diseases including brain tumour (n=33), traumatic brain injury (n=23), hydrocephalus (n=46), myelomeningocele (n=29), refractory epilepsy (n=89), or neuromuscular disease (n=58), including 14 boys with DMD. As part of the study procedure, the parents completed questionnaires regarding their socio-demographic status, their experience with rehabilitative and supportive services, their child's functional ability using the Functional Independence Measure (FIM™/WeeFIM®), and their child's HRQOL using the PedsQL™ (version 4.0) generic core.

The FIM and WeeFIM are designed to measure functional abilities and limitations in activities of daily living. The FIM is used for persons seven years of age or older, while the WeeFIM is designed for children between six months to seven years in age. Both versions measure independent performance in self-care, sphincter control, transfers, locomotion, communication, and social cognition. Response to each of the items ranges from 1 to 7, with higher scores indicating more independence. A total score is calculated by combining scores from all eighteen items, and ranges from 18 to 126. The psychometric properties of the FIM have been described in previous studies [Chau et al, 1994; Msall et al, 1994; Ottenbacher et al, 1997].

The PedsQL (version 4.0) generic core scale is a self-report multidimensional instrument designed by Varni et al to measure pediatric HRQOL [Varni et al, 1999]. The raw score for each item is transformed to a 0 to 100 scale, with a higher score indicating better quality of life. It has been validated for use in children [Varni et al, 2001]. The study was approved by the University of Calgary Conjoint Health Research and Ethics Board.

Among the 278 children, close to one-half (49%) had some limitations in daily activities, as reflected by their mean total FIM score of 90.6 (SD 34.4, max FIM score = 126). Approximately 25% were severely disabled and totally dependent on caregivers for self-care, sphincter control, and transfer. Nearly 40% of patients received regular (weekly to monthly) rehabilitation therapy. The majority of health services were financed by government health care program; 73 (27%) families reported additional out-of-pocket expenses. As anticipated, the use of supportive health services such as physiotherapy or occupational therapy was related to the child's diagnosis, degree of functional ability, and his/her HRQOL (**see Table 2**). On the other hand, socio-demographic variables such as parental age, marital status, education, employment, and place of residence were not significantly associated with health services utilization, except that parental income was associated with varying degree of funding support from the government. Only a small proportion (32%) of these families had access to regular respite, and the frequency of respite correlated with the severity of disability. Having a designated care coordinator was consistently associated with increased use of health services (OR 2.3 to 3.4).

Even though many pediatric neurosciences patients experienced significant functional limitations and required rehabilitative services, the majority (83%) of parents in this study felt that there was adequate medical, educational and financial support in their communities. However, almost half (49%) of the families indicated need for more psychosocial support, despite adequate medical, rehabilitative, and educational services. Parents from visible minority groups, those with English as a second language, and those who reported poor mental health were more likely to express need for more social support.

Overall, the physical and psychosocial HRQOL scores for this group of children were lower than published healthy controls; their mean PedsQL physical and psychosocial scores were 63.2 (SD 30.1) and 65.9 (SD 22.4) respectively (maximum PedsQL score = 100). Children with refractory epilepsy had the lowest mean psychosocial scores, while those with DMD and other neuromuscular diseases scored lowest on the physical scale (**see Table 1**). This suggests that despite their physical limitations, children with neuromuscular diseases enjoyed better HRQOL than those with refractory epilepsy. As seen in a subsequent study, children with DMD and other progressive neuromuscular diseases experienced further decline in their HRQOL, especially when they required the use of assisted mechanical ventilation at home [Mah et al, 2008].

	Mean	SD	Frequency
Physical functioning (/100)			
• Neuromuscular Disease	52.49	30.59	57
• Myelomeningocele	58.92	26.87	29
• Hydrocephalus	68.56	31.13	45
• Brain Injury	85.64	21.69	23
• Brain Tumour	83.09	20.26	33
• Refractory Epilepsy	53.99	30.81	88
Psychosocial functioning (/100)			
• Neuromuscular Disease	68.05	21.10	58
• Myelomeningocele	69.61	18.33	29
• Hydrocephalus	68.25	23.89	45
• Brain Injury	72.32	16.63	23
• Brain Tumour	80.96	17.90	33
• Refractory Epilepsy	54.10	21.36	89

Table 1. Comparison of Pediatric Health-Related Quality of Life Scores among children with chronic neurological disorders

Dependent variable	Independent variables	Odds Ratio	Wald's test	p value	95% CI
1. Utilization of Medical specialists	Child's age	0.911	-2.90	0.004	0.855 - 0.970
	Surgery	2.672	3.29	0.001	1.488 - 4.799
	Psychosocial HRQOL†	0.979	-3.13	0.002	0.965 - 0.992
	Care coordinator	3.407	4.03	0.000	1.877 - 6.184
2. Utilization of Allied Health Professionals	Diagnosis				
	Myelomeningocoele	0.295	-2.09	0.037	0.094 - 0.927
	Hydrocephalus	0.069	-3.92	0.000	0.018 - 0.263
	Brain injury	0.025	-3.13	0.002	0.002 - 0.251
	Brain tumor	0.261	-2.06	0.039	0.073 - 0.935
	Epilepsy	0.207	-3.13	0.002	0.077 - 0.555
	Child's age	0.851	-3.76	0.000	0.783 - 0.926
	FIM‡ score	0.969	-5.03	0.000	0.957 - 0.981
	Psychosocial HRQOL	0.978	-2.39	0.017	0.961 - 0.996
	Care coordinator	2.419	2.26	0.024	1.124 - 5.207
3. Utilization of Educational Services	FIM score	0.975	-3.64	0.000	0.961 - 0.988
	Psychosocial HRQOL	0.960	-3.69	0.000	0.939 - 0.980
	Parental education	2.521	2.09	0.037	1.060 - 5.998
	Care coordinator	3.359	2.97	0.003	1.509 - 7.477
4. Access to Social Support	FIM score	0.961	-6.96	0.000	0.950 - 0.972
	Care coordinator	2.294	2.62	0.009	1.232 - 4.272
5. Access to Funding Support	Psychosocial HRQOL	0.977	-2.46	0.014	0.959 - 0.995
	Family income	2.375	2.37	0.018	1.160 - 4.864

† Health-related quality of life
‡ Functional Independence Measure

Table 2. Multiple regression analysis of rehabilitation and supportive services utilization by children with chronic neurological disorders

4. Impact of home mechanical ventilation on HRQOL

The purpose of this study was to explore the impact of the use of life-sustaining assisted technologies such as home mechanical ventilation (HMV) on children and adolescents with NMD. We compared the HRQOL and parental stress among pediatric neuromuscular patients with or without home mechanical ventilation, and again boys with DMD (n = 24) were included as part of the study. Parents completed the Parenting Stress Index or the Stress Index for Parents of Adolescents, depending on their child's age. The Parenting Stress Index is a 120-item questionnaire that has been standardized for use with parents of children aged 1 month to 12 years [Abidin, 1993]. Each item is rated on a 5-point Likert-type scale that ranges from 1 (strongly agree) to 5 (strongly disagree). A Total Stress score, a Child Domain score, and a Parent Domain score are calculated from the responses. The 112-item Stress Index for Parents of Adolescents is an upward extension of the Parenting Stress Index for parents of adolescents aged 12 to 18 years [Sheras et al, 1998]. The Stress Index for Parents of Adolescents examines the relationship of parenting stress to adolescent characteristics, parent characteristics, the quality of adolescent-parent interactions, and stressful life circumstances. A Total Stress score, an Adolescent Domain score, a Parent Domain score, an Adolescent-Parent Relationship Domain score and a Life Stress score are calculated from the responses. Support for the content, convergent and discriminant validity of both versions of the Parental Stress Index is available. The PedsQL (version 4.0) generic core was again used to measure the HRQOL of children with neuromuscular disease.

109 families participated; 19 (17%) of them had a child with neuromuscular disease requiring HMV. Relative to healthy children and other chronically ill children, the pediatric neuromuscular patients in this study displayed poorer physical and psychosocial HRQOL. In addition, children on HMV had significantly lower mean total PedsQL scores than non-ventilated children (47.9 vs. 61.5 respectively, p=0.013) (**see Table 3**); the difference was likely the consequence of a more severe disease process in children requiring assisted ventilation. Furthermore, the opportunities that these children have to be involved in social activities outside of home and at school may be limited by the lack of portability of the assisted ventilation devices and/or availability of trained caregivers. However, no significant difference in mean total stress scores was found between parents of pediatric neuromuscular patients with or without HMV. We postulated that these parents had been living with the constant demands of caring for their child with neuromuscular disease requiring home mechanical ventilation and that over time, these caretaking demands had become part of "normal" life and were not identified as creating additional stress.

Mean PedsQL* Scores	HMV† Status	Number	Mean	Standard deviation	p value
Physical	Non-HMV	92	54.85	27.53	0.001
	HMV user	14	28.82	22.38	
Psychosocial	Non-HMV	87	63.22	18.89	0.028
	HMV user	13	51.06	13.87	
Total	Non-HMV	91	61.54	18.91	0.013
	HMV user	13	47.93	12.01	

* PedsQL refers to Pediatric Quality of Life Inventory; † HMV refers to Home Mechanical Ventilation

Table 3. Comparison of Mean Pediatric Quality of Life Inventory scores between Mechanically Ventilated and Non-Ventilated Pediatric Neuromuscular Subgroups [Mah et al, 2008a]. Reproduced with permission.

5. Understanding the parental experience

In order to further understand parental stress and psychosocial support needs of families caring for children with DMD and other neuromuscular diseases (NMD), a qualitative research study based on phenomenology was used to describe the experience of parents caring for children affected by NMD requiring HMV [Mah et al, 2008]. Data was collected from interviews in parents' homes. The interviews were subsequently modified based on an iterative approach to identify the core of the parents' caregiving experience (**see Figure 1**).

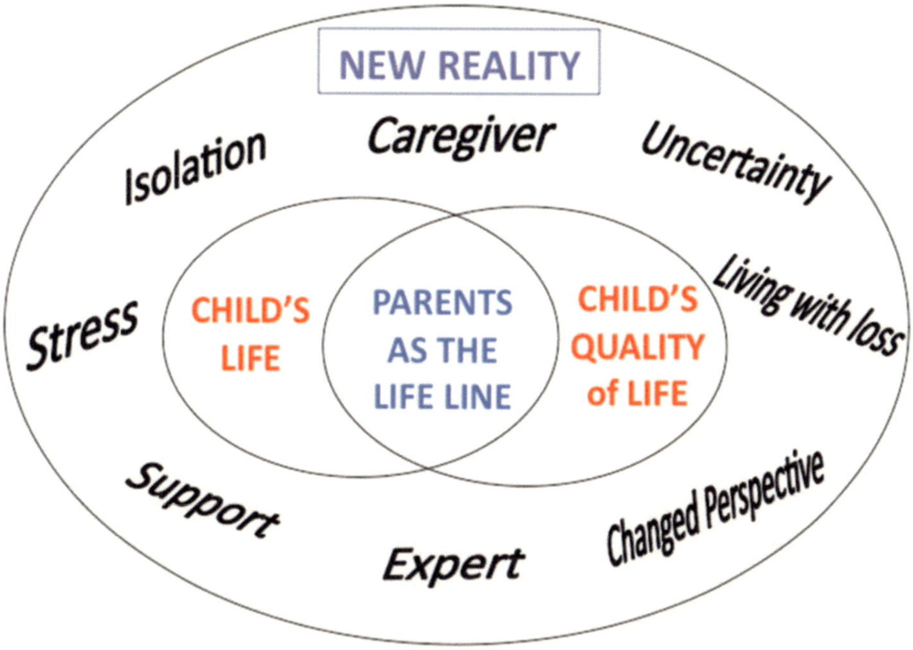

Fig. 1. Parental experience in caring for a child with neuromuscular disease [Mah et al, 2008b]. Reproduced with permission.

Given the emphasis by parents on providing the best possible care and ensuring optimal HRQOL for their child with NMD, the rest of the family unit's needs including those of the siblings, the spouse, and the primary caregiver tended to become secondary priorities. In addition being their child's primary caregivers, parents also took on the various functions of health care professionals (HCP) such as nursing and respiratory therapy. Given sufficient practice, they soon became experts on their child's care and the child's NMD. For most parents, the demand of caring for their child with NMD was disruptive to family life; they found it hard to spend quality time together. Over time, these demands became part of their normal daily routine. One parent summed up major losses such as friendship, income, privacy, and personal identity. The loss was not solely related to the child's NMD and declining health, but also due the impact of the parents' decision to give up their careers, passions, and personal desires to meet their child's needs. Parents lived with uncertainty in anticipation of future losses and limitations that their children might experience, as well as anxiety as to how their children would react to those losses.

Despite a recurring sense of loss, many parents opted to look beyond the negatives and focused on the positive aspects of their lives. Most families accepted the reality of caring for their child with NMD, and worked through the experience in order to move forward to live their lives as best they could. Living for the present helped parents to accept their changed lives and to live with the uncertainty that became their "new" normal. Most families also lived with the hope that there would be some improvement, a new treatment, or a cure around the corner that could benefit their children with NMD.

The core of the parental experience can be summarized as "being the lifeline" for their child with NMD Being the "lifeline" symbolized the vital role and the weight of the responsibility that parents had assumed to ensure the survival and well-being of their child with NMD. The core experience conveyed the love and devotion of parents for their child, and their desire for their child to live and to enjoy good quality of life despite the physical and sometimes cognitive limitations. The lifeline also embodied the mutually dependent and nurturing relationship that existed between the parents and their child with NMD. Most parents in this study acknowledged that they were receiving as much or more from their child than what they were giving to their child. Despite the many challenges and hardships these parents dealt with on a daily basis, they could not imagine life without their child, as he/she was also their "lifeline." Therefore, the "lifeline" theme serves as an important reminder to HCP in regards to to the parents' key role in safe guarding their child's life and ensuring their child's quality of life. Awareness of this reciprocal "lifeline" relationship between the parents and the child with NMD should also facilitate the recognition of parents as experts and key partners in decisions related to the child's medical management.

This study also highlights the importance of support from HCP, extended family, and community agencies. As consistent with results by van Kesteren and his colleagues [van Kesteren et al, 2001], families with NMD children requiring continuous assisted ventilation in our study were more likely to experience increased stress, particularly when support was inadequate. Potential gaps in the health care system that were identified by these parents included insufficient funding for essential supportive equipment, lack of appreciation for the "whole" child and the entire family unit, and unavailability of respite workers due to suboptimal wages and manpower shortages in our health regions. Families who perceived a lack of support were burdened with the responsibility of being the sole caregivers for their child, and might therefore be at higher risk for stress-related illnesses and adverse psychological outcomes. Specific strategies to improve support for these families will require greater coordination of services, reliable access to respite personnel, and an individualized approach to address each family's needs and priorities.

6. Family-centered care approach to DMD

The management of boys with DMD may benefit from a family centered model of care that promotes communication and consensus-building among HCP, administrative staff, and community agencies, with each family being an integral part of the interdisciplinary team [Ivey et al, 1988]. Accordingly, family-centered practice perceives "the entire family as the unit of attention" and provides services in a collaborative fashion based on informed choice, in accordance with each individual family's strengths, needs, and goals. Family centered care (FCC) acknowledges the importance of the family in meeting the physical, psychosocial, and developmental needs of children [Bissell et al, 2004; American Academy of Pediatrics, 2004]. The premise for a family-centered model of service delivery is based on the assumption that "parents know their children best and they want the best for their children"[Bamm & Rosenbaum, 2008]. An essential element of this model of care is to align the clinical practice with the needs of patients and families, as each family may not want the same degree of participation in their health care due to social and cultural factors [Boon et al, 2004; Deber, 1994a; Deber, 1994b; Deber et al, 1996]. As needs may change over time, it is also important to identify the support needs of individuals and families at different stages of the illness [Trivette et al, 1993]. In addition, children thrive within a supportive family and community environment. Thus, the purpose of FCC is to empower the caregivers and to enhance their well-being in order to maximize positive health and developmental outcomes for their children. This model of care reflects a paradigm shift away from the traditional paternalistic model of physician-patient relationship towards an equal partnership between families and HCP in order to arrive at mutually agreed goals. Early anticipatory guidance may help families cope with disease progression (see Table 4) [Dawson & Kristjanson, 2003].

The main guiding principle of FCC is to align the clinical practice with the needs of the families and to enable each family to be involved in making decisions for their child's health care. In order to accomplish this goal, special attention should be paid to the service providers' interactions with the families as well as the organizational approach to service delivery. From an interpersonal level, the practice of FCC will require the service providers to: a) show respect for the family's perspective, values, and cultural diversity; b) identify family strengths, needs, and priorities on an on-going basis; c) provide information about their child's condition in a way that matches the family's needs; d) involve families in decision-making; and e) develop services that are flexible to the needs of individual families. From an organizational or institutional level, the delivery of family centered services will require the managers and policy-makers to provide: a) service coordination and integration within and between sectors; b) expedients for family-to-family support; c) family-friendly physical environments; d) high quality general and illness-specific information; and e) opportunities for family involvement in decision-making at all levels of the organization.

Previous studies of FCC effectiveness have focused primarily on the impact on FCC practices on parental outcomes, such as a reduction in caregivers' stress, an improvement in their overall well-being, or an increase in satisfaction with care [Dunst et al, 2007]. In 2008, Dempsey and Keen summarized the findings of 35 studies published during 1993 to 2004 pertaining to the processes and outcomes of family centered services for children with disabilities [Dempsey et al, 2009]. Most of these studies examined health care providers' interpersonal strategies such as the provision of help-giving practices or other processes of care. The impact on parent outcomes included: a) a mild to moderate increase in psychological well-being; b) an increase sense of empowerment; and c) a greater degree of satisfaction with services. The effects on child outcomes were less evident, and included some (albeit inconsistent) degree of improvement in child development or health. Recently, Moore et al examined the relationship of processes of care to children's HRQOL [Moore et al, 2009]. The study included 187 caregivers of children from the pediatric neurosciences clinics at the Alberta Children's Hospital; 44 (24%) of these children suffered from a neuromuscular disease. FCC was found to be a significant predictor of parent-reported children's physical, psychosocial, and total HRQOL, independent of the illness severity. The provision of family-centred care practices by service providers had a positive impact on the quality of life of children with neurological disorders.

Key Stages & FCC Strategies	Early to late ambulatory stage (4 to 10 years old)	Early non-ambulatory stage (10 to 16 years old)	Late non-ambulatory stage (>16 years old)
Family knowledge: *Show respect for the family's perspective & expertise* *Identify family's needs, strengths, & priorities on an on-going basis* *Provide information that matches the family's needs* *Facilitate family-to-family support*	<u>Discuss</u>: DMD natural history & genetics Role of corticosteroids Research studies Genetic counselling referral Carrier testing if indicated Provide written material, websites &peer support information Muscular Dystrophy Association (MDA) & Parent Project contact information	<u>Discuss</u>: Nutrition Complications of DMD (scoliosis, cardiac, and respiratory) Complications of corticosteroids Symptoms of nocturnal hypoventilation Options for long-term ventilation assistance (i.e. BiPAP, CPAP) Medical management of cardiomyopathy if present School & social support Respite & financial issues Adolescent needs & quality of life Review previous topics	<u>Discuss</u>: Transition to adult care Options for long-term ventilation support Nutritional support (i.e. gastrostromy tube) End-of-life counseling and advance medical directive Review previous topics
Professional Support *Involve families in decision-making* *Develop services that are flexible to the needs of individual families* *Provide service coordination and integration within and between sectors*	**<u>Medical consultations:</u>** Genetics Respirology Orthopaedics (night splints, scoliosis) Cardiology Neurology / Physiatry Ophthalmology (cataracts) **<u>Allied health support:</u>** Clinic Nurse - Dietician Physiotherapist - Psychologist Occupational therapy Social worker MDA community liaison	**<u>Medical consultations (as before, plus)</u>** Endocrinology (osteoporosis, bisphosphonate therapy) **<u>Teach:</u>** Chest physiotherapy to family Breath stacking, cough assist Seating for wheelchair Passive & active exercises	**<u>Medical consultations (as before)</u>**
Medical Therapy: *Provide high quality general and illness-specific information* *Establish opportunities for family involvement in decision-making at all levels of the organization*	**<u>Immunizations</u>**: Varicella vaccine Pneumococcal vaccine Influenza vaccine **<u>Corticosteroids</u>** Deflazacort (0.9 mg/kg/d) or Prednisone (0.75 mg/kg/d) **<u>Physiotherapy</u>**: Passive stretching, night splints **<u>Bone health:</u>** Calcium supplementation Vitamin D supplementation **<u>Other:</u>** Behavioral intervention Weight management	**<u>Review previous topics</u>** **<u>Interventions</u>** (as required): Angiotensin converting enzyme inhibitor and/ or beta-blocker (cardiomyopathy) Diuretics (congestive heart failure) Antibiotics (respiratory tract infections) Sitting ankle-foot orthosis Scoliosis surgery (pre-op Cardiology, Respirology & Anaesthesiology consults)	**<u>Review previous topics</u>**

Key Stages & FCC Strategies	Early to late ambulatory stage (4 to 10 years old)	Early non-ambulatory stage (10 to 16 years old)	Late non-ambulatory stage (>16 years old)
Clinical / Laboratory Monitoring: *Create family-friendly physical environments*	Weight, height, & blood pressure Formal muscle function & strength test ECG, echocardiogram (every 2 year) Pulmonary function testing Wrist x-ray for bone age Bone densitometry scan	**Same as before, except:** ECG, echocardiogram (yearly)	**Same as before**
	25-hydroxyvitamin D level	**Same as before, plus:** PCO_2 measurement as needed	**Same as before**
Clinical review:	**6 to 12 months**	**3 to 6 months**	**1 to 3 months**

Table 4. Summary of Family Centred Care (FCC) Strategies for Duchenne Muscular Dystrophy [McMillan et al, 2010]. Reproduced with permission.

Thus, currently available evidence suggests that interpersonal strategies of FCC are positively associated with parental well-being, satisfaction, and empowerment. There is limited evidence of positive impact of family centered services on children's health and development. Further studies are needed to determine the key outcome variables as well as the longer-term effects of FCC strategies on parent and child outcomes. Subsequent studies should also examine if family centered services affect pediatric health outcomes directly or indirectly through improving parent outcomes, and how the practice can be incorporated as standard of care for children with severe neuromuscular disorders such as DMD.

7. Challenges related to unmet support needs

Similar to the reports from caregivers of children with other neuromuscular diseases, parents of DMD boys may experience frustration due to poor communication and fragmentation of care within the health care system. It is therefore important for clinicians to understand the priority support needs of individuals with DMD and their families across different stages of the disease. Accordingly, the natural history of DMD can be summarized into five main stages, including: a) the pre-symptomatic phase; b) the early ambulatory phase; c) the late ambulatory phase; d) the early non-ambulatory phase; and e) the late non-ambulatory phase [Weidner, 2005]. The purpose of this next study was to explore the unmet support needs of families of boys with DMD at different stages of the disease. We adapted the Family Needs Survey [Bailey 1990] by adding items specific to DMD, and administered it to a representative sample of parents of boys with DMD from two tertiary pediatric neuromuscular clinics in Canada, a country where health care is publicly funded. We hypothesized that the number of unmet needs might increase over time due to progression of the disease and vary by parental sociodemographic characteristics such as ethnicity or education.

7.1 Methods

This was a mixed method study with participation from parents of children and youth with DMD. For the purpose of this study, individuals were considered to have DMD if they fulfilled all of the following criteria: a) onset of weakness before age 5; b) male gender; c) evidence of proximal muscle weakness; d) increased serum creatine kinase; and e) confirmed mutation in the *dystrophin* gene or dystrophic muscle biopsy with marked deficiency in dystrophin immunostaining consistent with a diagnosis of DMD. Families with limited English comprehension or those who were unable to provide informed consent were excluded. Written informed consent from caregivers and assent from children was obtained prior to enrolment. The study was approved by the institutional review boards from the two participating centers.

The Family Needs Survey (FNS) was developed by Bailey and Simeonsson as a parsimonious approach to identify specific family needs and to elicit parents' priorities for services in children with disabilities [Bailey & Simeonsson, 1990], and it has been adapted for use across different cultures [Chen et al; 1994; Hendriks et al, 2000]. The original version contained 35 self-report items grouped into seven general categories, including the need for: 1) information; 2) family and social support; 3) financial support; 4) explaining to others; 5) child care; 6) professional support; and 7) community services. Parents who indicate "yes," to each item are given a score of 1, and other responses (no, or not sure) are scored as 0 [Bailey et al, 2004]. Previous studies have indicated strong inter-item reliability, with a reported Cronbach's alpha coefficient of 0.91 for the total score [Sexton et al, 1992]. Good agreement was found between mothers and fathers, and the responses were stable within a six-month period [Bailey & Simeonsson, 1988]. Permission from the authors was obtained to modify the Family Needs Survey for this study. The DMD Family Needs Survey (DMD-FNS) contained an additional 31 items exploring disease specific information and support needs of families caring for individuals with DMD, reflecting current clinical practice guidelines. The maximum score of the DMD Family Needs Survey was 66, with higher scores indicating more unmet needs. In addition, families were asked to rate the importance of each unmet need on a 5-point Likert scale, with a score of 1 indicating a "somewhat important" need, and a score of 5 indicating a "very important" need. The questionnaire also included items on the caregivers' socio-demographic characteristics and their child's current health status.

The DMD-FNS was reviewed by six paediatric neuromuscular clinic staff (including physicians and allied professionals) for content validity, and then piloted with five parents of boys with DMD for input regarding the area of needs, the appropriateness of items on the scale, the wording, and other content issues. Upon completion of the pilot, a cover letter and the revised DMD Family Needs Survey were distributed to the rest of the parents of DMD boys followed at the Alberta Children's Hospital in Calgary, Alberta and the Bloorview Kids Rehab in Toronto, Ontario. Both centers provide care for individuals with DMD in a similar multidisciplinary team setting, including assessments by paediatrics, social work, nursing, occupational therapy, physiotherapy, orthopaedic surgery, dietician, respirology and/or cardiology on the same clinic day [McMillan et al, 2010].

Parents who consented to participating in the study completed the questionnaire on their own and then returned it by mail or in person in a self-addressed and stamped envelope. A minimum sample size of 60 responses from the DMD Family Needs Survey was planned, with at least 10 to 15 families representing each of the four stages of DMD, including: a) at diagnosis (< 8 years); b) near cessation of ambulation (8 - 12 years); c) during adolescence (13 - 18 years); d) at advanced stage of the disease (> 18 years). Descriptive statistics were used to summarize the characteristics of the study participants and their priority support needs. Categorical variables were expressed as frequencies and percentages, and bivariate comparisons were made using Pearson's chi-square or Fisher's exact test. Continuous variables were reported as means with standard deviations or as medians with interquartile ranges if the data was skewed, and comparisons were made using unpaired Student's t-tests or one-way analyses of variance. All tests were two-tailed, and p values less than 0.05 were considered to be statistically significant.

In addition, parents who completed the DMD-FNS at the Bloorview Kids Rehab were invited to participate in a focus group meeting. The focus group was an ideal setting to verify the survey results, to explore ideas on how to address the identified priority needs, and to provide mutual support for the participants based on shared experiences [Kitzinger, 1995]. Written consent was obtained prior to the start of the meeting. Discussion from the focus group was audio-recorded and then transcribed verbatim. The analysis was performed in accordance with the phenomenological method of inquiry, by engaging in repeated immersions in the data prior to descriptive coding, and then using topic and analytic codes to identify themes that were central to the parents' experience and needs in caring for their child with DMD [Coffey & Atkinson, 1996].

7.2 Results

A total of 61 (59.8%) out of 102 eligible families participated in the DMD-FNS. Forty-five (74%) of the respondents were mothers, and the mean age was 45.3 (standard deviation 7.5, range 32-59) years. Fifty-four (89%) respondents were married; 49 (80%) respondents had post-secondary education, and the majority (46 families, 75%) were from Bloorview Kids Rehab program. The mean age of the boys with DMD was 11.8 (standard deviation 6.4, range 1 - 25) years; they were diagnosed at a mean age of 4.2 (standard deviation 2.3, range 0 to 12) years. Thirty-four (66%) boys were walking independently, 10 (16%) required the use of bi-level positive airway pressure ventilatory support, and the majority (51 boys, 84%) were on deflazacort as disease modifying treatment for DMD. There was no significant difference between the study participants and study non-responders in regards to the child's age, ambulatory status, need for assisted ventilation, or use of corticosteroids.

7.2.1 Unmet family support needs

The mean DMD-FNS total score was 25.1 (standard deviation 15.0), reflecting a large number of unmet family support needs. Cronbach alpha for the total score was 0.95, which suggested a high level of inter-item reliability. We found no significant differences between the mean number of needs and the stage of the disease by age group (see **Table 5**). The categories with the largest numbers of unmet needs overall, and for which a majority of parents expressed unmet needs were related to information, financial, and psychosocial supports. All items that the majority of families (i.e., >50%) indicated were unmet needs are listed in **Table 6**. Each of these items had mean Likert rating scores greater than 4, confirming that these were "important" or "very important" needs for the parents. There were no significant differences between the mean number of needs and the child's characteristics such as age, ambulatory status, need for ventilation support, and other co-morbidities such as learning disability, behavioural problems, or scoliosis. Similarly, socio-demographic factors including the parent's age, ethnicity, marital status, education, and place of residence (Ontario versus Alberta) were not associated with significant differences in the mean number of identified needs.

Unmet Needs	All ages (n = 57*)	< 8 yrs (n = 19)	8 – 12 yrs (n = 14)	13 – 18 yrs (n = 8)	>18 yrs (n = 16)	p value
Information						
Mean (SD†)	11.5 (6.4)	11.8 (6.8)	10.8 (6.2)	14.6 (5.1)	10.2 (6.6)	0.44
Family and social support						
Mean (SD)	4.1 (3.8)	3.3 (4.0)	4.6 (3.2)	4.6 (3.4)	4.4 (4.3)	0.75
Financial support						
Mean (SD)	3.5 (3.0)	2.8 (3.5)	3.9 (2.2)	3.7 (3.0)	4.0 (3.2)	0.63
Explaining to others						
Mean (SD)	1.4 (1.5)	1.9 (1.7)	1.3 (1.3)	1.2 (0.7)	0.8 (1.6)	0.17
Child care						
Mean (SD)	1.1 (0.9)	0.9 (1.1)	1.4 (0.6)	1.0 (0.8)	1.0 (0.9)	0.56
Professional support						
Mean (SD)	1.3 (1.8)	1.3 (2.4)	1.1 (1.1)	1.2 (1.4)	1.7 (1.8)	0.82
Community services						
Mean (SD)	2.0 (1.3)	2.2 (1.5)	1.6 (1.1)	2.0 (1.2)	2.2 (1.4)	0.51
Total						
Mean (SD)	24.9 (15.2)	24.2 (18.3)	24.6 (13.2)	28.5 (10.7)	24.4 (15.8)	0.92

* Four had incomplete responses and were removed from the analyses of variance
† SD referred to standard deviation of the mean

Table 5. Comparison of total mean number of unmet needs by different age categories of boys with DMD

	Percent	Number of Respondents
General Information Needs		
Information about services presently available for my child	74†	61
Information about services for parents and siblings*	74†	61
How my child will grow and develop	64†	59
Information about services my child might receive in the future	62	61
Reading materials or websites about other families who have a child like mine	59	61
DMD Specific Information Needs		
Improving my child's bone health*	66†	60
Issues related to spinal deformity or scoliosis*	62	61
Helping my child to be more physically active*	61	61
The diagnosis of DMD and what it means for my child and my family*	54	60
Stretching exercises, night splints or orthotics*	54	61
Issues related to my child's lung function*	54	60
Use of corticosteroids and/or other treatment*	51	61
Use of bi-level positive airway pressure or other assisted breathing devices*	51	60

	Percent	Number of Respondents
Financial Support Needs		
Paying for medications, treatment or equipment that my child needs	56	61
Paying for complementary or alternative therapies for my child*	54	61
Paying for expenses related to modifications in our home and or vehicle*	51	61
Psychosocial Support Needs		
Meeting and talking with other parents who have a child like mine	67†	61
Helping my child to make new friends*	56	61
Locating babysitters or respite care providers who are willing and able to care for my child	53	61

* New items specific for DMD are marked with an asterix
† Indicated the top five most frequently expressed needs in the DMD Family Needs Survey

Table 6. Unmet information, financial and psychosocial support needs identified by the majority of the parents of boys with DMD

7.2.2 Needs across stages of the illness

Participants of the 3-hour DMD focus group meeting included eight (3 dads, 5 moms) parents of boys (aged 6 to 21 years) with DMD. The main interview questions were: 1) When you first learned your son had DMD, what did you need? 2) How did your needs change over time? The responses of participants confirmed that information, financial support, and psychosocial supports were important needs across the course of the illness. However, the types and intensity of supports needed varied according to the stage of the illness, and according to each family situation. Themes emerged for the different stages of the illness, and these are described below.

7.2.2.1 Needs at diagnosis

Parents described their needs for information and emotional support at the time of diagnosis. They emphasized that the diagnosis should be given by a knowledgeable and empathetic physician, and immediate psychosocial support should be available, preferably by connecting with other parents who had gone through the same experience. However, some families were not ready to discuss their information needs soon after the diagnosis, due to the overwhelming sense of grief. One parent expressed it as a need to "*take the time to grieve over it first.*" The ideal time for discussion might occur much later for these families.

7.2.2.2 Needs during adolescence

This period is marked by progressive loss of mobility for boys with DMD. Therefore it is not surprising that a dominant need during this time is financial assistance for equipment, transportation, and modifications to the family home. Parents identified their struggles with bureaucracy and the lack of financial support from public and private sources. They indicated that there was a lack of coordination and information about services and financial support, as articulated by one parent: "*There isn't a single body that can sort of bring all of these things together and say, 'okay look, this is where you need to go; this is what you need to do, and these are the people you need to get money from … All those agencies, none of them talked to each other."* Parents talked about how this forced them into an advocacy role in order to get necessary supports and services. They reported that lack of coordination and the subsequent need for them to act as advocates resulted in much wasted time, time that could be spent caring for their family.

7.2.2.3 Needs at advanced stage of the disease

At this point, parents' needs for information and psychosocial supports seemed to decrease. Parents of young adults with DMD described how they had accepted the reality that their child could die soon. Despite the relentless progression of the disease, these parents were able to offer meaningful support, encouragement, and practical advice to younger families, as summed up by one parent: *"I think it really teaches you that … the moment is the most important; this day is wonderful, … you learn a lot from your child actually, because they have this sort of innate strength that is quite remarkable."*

Across all the stages parents indicated that they were very interested in participating in research, particularly if it would eventually lead to a cure. Those that had been actively involved in research activities or fundraising indicated that it gave them hope for the future, and helped them feel as if they were helping others.

8. Discussion

Consistent with previous research, our study found that parents of boys with DMD have many unmet needs, despite living in a country like Canada where health care is publically funded [Abresch et al, 1998; Buchanan et al, 1979; Firth et al, 1983]. Their needs may be unmet due to a lack of awareness or inability of available resources to adequately target their children needs. In this study we did not find a significant difference in the mean number of unmet needs across key stages of the illness, which suggests that families have needs throughout the course of the illness. As well, there was no significant difference in the mean number of needs by disease severity or parental socio-demographic characteristics.

Although the number of needs did not vary, the results of the group interview indicated that types of needs within the categories of information, financial, and psychosocial supports varied according to the stage of the illness and family situation. By using the DMD-FNS during clinic visits, health care professionals may be in a better position to understand each family's unique priority needs and strengths, instead of having to second guess what they might be or be influenced by clinician's personal bias [Gibson, 2001; Kinali et al, 2007]. The revised DMD-FNS that was used in this study incorporates topics specific to the care of individuals with DMD, and therefore may serve as an ideal prompt for parents to discuss these issues during their child's regular clinic visits. For example, it is important to acknowledge the frequent use of complementary or alternative therapies and the resultant financial burden on families of children with severe neurological disorders such as DMD [Soo et al, 2005]. The parents rated each identified need as very important, so the Likert scale did not provide additional information and we recommend it be removed from subsequent needs surveys for this population.

As the families' ability to cope during the course of the illness may be modified by their interaction with HCP, a major implication of our results is that HCP should make it a priority to provide information to families about DMD that is accessible and customized to their situation [Fitzpatrick & Barry, 1986; Steele, 2002]. A second priority pertains to the coordination of community based services to assist families to access financial supports for equipment and housing modifications in a timely fashion. A third priority is the provision of ongoing psychosocial supports, which may include individual counselling or family peer support programs.

A limitation of the DMD-FNS study relates to the small sample size. The mixed methodology compensated for the low numbers by using a group interview to verify and extend the results of the mailed survey. Future studies could recruit a larger sample to further explore differences across stages of the illness and across family demographics. A second limitation was that we relied on parent report and did not directly survey older children and youth for their perceived needs. During the pilot we found that most boys in the initial pilot phase of the study did not have the ability to work independently through a lengthy questionnaire like the DMD Family Needs Survey. However, previous research indicates that the needs of adolescents may vary significantly from their parents, and it is important to give the youth a voice [Mah et al, 2006]. Future studies could use an abbreviated DMD youth survey to clarify the changing needs of adolescents and young adults with DMD over time. Lastly, our survey was limited to families of boys who were currently living with DMD and may not provide a complete picture of family needs at the final stage of the illness. It may be helpful to interview families after their child has passed away.

Parents who participated in the group interview reflected that they appreciated the opportunity to share and to meet each other and were glad to participate in a research project. They indicated that participation in research projects gave them hope for the future. Based on this experience we recommend that parents of boys with DMD be included in future research initiatives as they have an important perspective and stake in the outcomes of such research.

9. Implications for clinical practice

Individuals with DMD and their families have to adjust to many challenges because of the progressive nature of the disease. The family resilience framework developed by Dr. Froma Walsh, Co-Founder and Co-Director of the Chicago Center of Family Health, can be applied to the neuromuscular population to serve as a guide to target and strengthen key processes that will encourage optimal adaptation of children and adolescents with DMD [Walsh, 2003]. Resilience involves a dynamic process that enables individuals "to withstand and rebound from disruptive life challenges, becoming strengthened, and more resourceful" [Rolland & Walsh, 2006]. Resilience is not innate or restricted to certain people only, and it can be learned over time. A resilience framework for supporting boys with DMD targets on strengths rather than problems, partnership instead of paternalism, and families (rather than the clinicians) as the center of attention. It acknowledges the family as the unit of operation, with tremendous potentials for growth and transformation. Each family in turn has unique perspectives, resources, strengths, and challenges.

According to Walsh, the key processes in family resilience focus on: 1) beliefs system, including making meaning of adversity, contextualizing distress, having a positive outlook, and developing transcendence and spirituality; 2) organization pattern (in partnership with community agencies, schools, healthcare, workplace and other larger systems) that provides flexibility, connectedness, social and economic resources; 3) communication strategy, with emphasis on clarity, open emotional expression, and collaborative problem-solving. Relational attributes of this framework include peers, extended family members, and other mentors. The goal of the resilience framework is to promote strong and enduring relationships, to help shape and sustain them to meet life challenges.

In practice, integration of the beliefs system should include: a) assessing family network and their prior experience; b) providing peers and extended family support; c) establishing routines for young children and their siblings; and d) offering genetic counselling to alleviate parental guilt. Positive outlook can be fostered by a) presenting research and current available supporting treatment as opportunities for hope; b) affirming the child's potentials and encouraging the family to look forward to college and beyond; and c) celebrating successes, initiatives, and perseverance, using life examples such as Jesse's Journey and other parent support organizations. In regards to transcendence and spirituality, it is helpful for family to: a) see the bigger picture and purpose, as one family said that they were "chosen to live a better life"; b) embrace spiritual domain of being human, which includes suffering and injustice; c) learn to living with paradox, to make the best out of the worst of times; and d) offer spiritual and inspirational support as necessary.

Using Walsh's conceptual approach, clinicians may be in a better position to help adolescents and their families to gain insight about their illness experience, to appreciate the strengths and vulnerabilities of each family member and the emerging adolescent developmental needs, and to recognize key family beliefs that explain their illness narratives and relationships with healthcare professionals. Clinicians can also foster the development of resilience through their direct interactions with DMD patients and their families. The discussion regarding the diagnosis and management of DMD should take place with both the child/adolescent and parents present, and they should be encouraged to participate in all treatment decisions. The treating physician should provide written information about the illness and realistic expectations regarding potential benefits of potentially new disease-modifying therapies. Financial resources including funding for adaptive equipments should be offered regardless of parental employment status or family income.

Parents should encourage their teenagers to meet age-appropriate developmental goals, including gradual transfer of decision-making authority over time. A resilience-oriented approach also draws upon extended family and peer resources as potential mentors and positive role models in mediating adolescent adjustment to DMD. Clinicians can help families resolve conflicts, identify coping strategies, develop realistic goals, and seek help when needed. Periodic family meetings and multidisciplinary consultations for anticipated transitions, including going away for college and/or transfer to adult services, can facilitate proactive planning and alleviate unnecessary anxiety.

10. Conclusion

DMD is a challenging chronic disease that requires multidisciplinary collaboration of healthcare professionals and individualized treatment approach for the adolescent patients and their families. The modified Family Needs Survey for DMD is a useful tool for needs assessment, continuing dialogue with families, and tailoring services to address individual families' needs. It may be used as part of a family-centered approach to the care of boys with DMD, in order to promote family resilience and their increase their capacity to deal with the challenges related to this devastating disease.

11. Acknowledgements

The authors would like to thank the families who participated in the research studies, the contribution of Dr. Melanie Moore, other collaborators, research assistants, and the paediatric neuromuscular clinic staff in Calgary and Toronto for their on-going support. Funding was provided in part by the Alberta Center for Child, Family, and Community Research, the Stichting Porticus Foundation, the Cooperative International Neuromuscular Research Group, and the Alberta Children's Hospital Foundation. The Duchenne muscular dystrophy Family Needs Survey (DMD-FNS) is available by request.

12. References

Aartsma-Rus, A., Van Deutekom, J. C., Fokkema, I. F., Van Ommen, G. J., & Den Dunnen, J. T. (2006). Entries in the Leiden Duchenne muscular dystrophy mutation database: An overview of mutation types and paradoxical cases that confirm the reading-frame rule. *Muscle & Nerve, 34*(2), 135-44.

Abidin, R. R. (1983). Parenting stress and the utilization of pediatric services. *Children's Health Care: Journal of the Association for the Care of Children's Health, 11*(2), 70-3.

Abresch, R. T., Seyden, N. K., & Wineinger, M. A. (1998). Quality of life. Issues for persons with neuromuscular diseases. *Physical Medicine and Rehabilitation Clinics of North America, 9*(1), 233-48.

Amenta, A. R., Yilmaz, A., Bogdanovich, S., McKechnie, B. A., Abedi, M., Khurana, T. S., & Fallon, J. R. (2011). Biglycan recruits utrophin to the sarcolemma and counters dystrophic pathology in mdx mice. *Proceedings of the National Academy of Sciences of the United States of America, 108*(2), 762-7.

American Academy of Pediatrics Committee on Hospital Care (2003). Family-Centered care and the pediatrician's role. *Pediatrics, 112*(3 Pt 1), 691-7.

American Academy of Pediatrics Section on Cardiology and Cardiac Surgery. (2005). Cardiovascular health supervision for individuals affected by Duchenne or Becker muscular dystrophy. *Pediatrics, 116*(6), 1569-73.

Bach, J. R., & Martinez, D. (2011). Duchenne muscular dystrophy: Continuous noninvasive ventilatory support prolongs survival. *Respiratory Care, 56*(6), 744-50.

Bailey, D. B., Hebbeler, K., Scarborough, A., Spiker, D., & Mallik, S. (2004). First experiences with early intervention: A national perspective. *Pediatrics, 113*(4), 887-96.

Bailey, D B., & Simeonsson, R. J. (1988). Assessing needs of families with handicapped infants. *Journal of Special Education,* 22(1), 117-127.

Bailey, D. B., & Simeonsson, R. J. (1990). Family Needs Survey. Frank Porter Graham Child Development Center Chapel Hill, NC: University of North Carolina; Available from URL: http://www.fpg.unc.edu/~publicationsoffice/pdfs/familyneedssurvey.pdf.

Bamm, E. L., & Rosenbaum, P. (2008). Family-Centered theory: Origins, development, barriers, and supports to implementation in rehabilitation medicine. *Archives of Physical Medicine and Rehabilitation, 89*(8), 1618-24.

Baskin, B., Banwell, B., Khater, R. A., Hawkins, C., & Ray, P. N. (2009). Becker muscular dystrophy caused by an intronic mutation reducing the efficiency of the splice donor site of intron 26 of the dystrophin gene. *Neuromuscular Disorders: NMD, 19*(3), 189-92.

Baxter, P. (2006). Treatment of the heart in Duchenne muscular dystrophy. *Developmental Medicine and Child Neurology, 48*(3), 163.

Biggar, W. D., Gingras, M., Fehlings, D. L., Harris, V. A., & Steele, C. A. (2001). Deflazacort treatment of Duchenne muscular dystrophy. *The Journal of Pediatrics, 138*(1), 45-50.

Birnkrant, D. J., Bushby, K. M., Amin, R. S., Bach, J. R., Benditt, J. O., Eagle, M., . . . Kravitz, R. M. (2010). The respiratory management of patients with Duchenne muscular dystrophy: A DMD care considerations working group specialty article. *Pediatric Pulmonology, 45*(8), 739-48.

Bissell, P., May, C. R., & Noyce, P. R. (2004). From compliance to concordance: Barriers to accomplishing a re-framed model of health care interactions. *Social Science & Medicine (1982), 58*(4), 851-62.

Boon, H., Verhoef, M., O'Hara, D., & Findlay, B. (2004). From parallel practice to integrative health care: A conceptual framework. *BMC Health Services Research, 4*(1), 15.

Buchanan, D. C., LaBarbera, C. J., Roelofs, R., & Olson, W. (1979). Reactions of families to children with Duchenne muscular dystrophy. *General Hospital Psychiatry, 1*(3), 262-9.

Bushby, K., Muntoni, F., Urtizberea, A., Hughes, R., & Griggs, R. (2004). Report on the 124th ENMC international workshop. Treatment of Duchenne muscular dystrophy; defining the gold standards of management in the use of corticosteroids. 2-4 April 2004, Naarden, the Netherlands. *Neuromuscular Disorders: NMD, 14*(8-9), 526-34.

Bushby, K., Finkel, R., Birnkrant, D. J., Case, L. E., Clemens, P. R., Cripe, L., . . . DMD Care Considerations Working Group. (2010). Diagnosis and management of Duchenne muscular dystrophy, part 1: Diagnosis, and pharmacological and psychosocial management. *Lancet Neurology, 9*(1), 77-93.

Bushby, K., Finkel, R., Birnkrant, D. J., Case, L. E., Clemens, P. R., Cripe, L., . . . DMD Care Considerations Working Group. (2010). Diagnosis and management of Duchenne muscular dystrophy, part 2: Implementation of multidisciplinary care. *Lancet Neurology, 9*(2), 177-89.

Chau, N., Daler, S., Andre, J. M., & Patris, A. (1994). Inter-rater agreement of two functional independence scales: The functional independence measure (FIM) and a subjective uniform continuous scale. *Disability and Rehabilitation, 16*(2), 63-71.

Chen, J., & Simeonsson, R. J. (1994). Child disability and family needs in the People's Republic of China. *International Journal of Rehabilitation Research. Internationale Zeitschrift Für Rehabilitationsforschung. Revue Internationale De Recherches De Réadaptation, 17*(1), 25-37.

Chen, Y. W., Zhao, P., Borup, R., & Hoffman, E. P. (2000). Expression profiling in the muscular dystrophies: Identification of novel aspects of molecular pathophysiology. *The Journal of Cell Biology, 151*(6), 1321-36.

Coffey, A., Atkinson, P (1996). *Making sense of qualitative data: Complementary Strategies.* Thousand Oaks, CA: Sage.

Dawson, S., & Kristjanson, L. J. (2003). Mapping the journey: Family carers' perceptions of issues related to end-stage care of individuals with muscular dystrophy or motor neurone disease. *Journal of Palliative Care, 19*(1), 36-42.

Deber, R. B. (1994). Physicians in health care management: 7. The patient-physician partnership: Changing roles and the desire for information. *CMAJ : Canadian Medical Association Journal = Journal De L'association Medicale Canadienne, 151*(2), 171-6.

Deber, R. B. (1994). Physicians in health care management: 8. The patient-physician partnership: Decision making, problem solving and the desire to participate. *CMAJ: Canadian Medical Association Journal = Journal De L'association Medicale Canadienne, 151*(4), 423-7.

Deber, R. B., Kraetschmer, N., & Irvine, J. (1996). What role do patients wish to play in treatment decision making? *Archives of Internal Medicine, 156*(13), 1414-20.

Dempsey, I., Keen, D., Pennell, D., O'Reilly, J., & Neilands, J. (2009). Parent stress, parenting competence and family-centered support to young children with an intellectual or developmental disability. *Research in Developmental Disabilities, 30*(3), 558-66.

Dunst, C. J., Trivette, C. M., & Hamby, D. W. (2007). Meta-Analysis of family-centered helpgiving practices research. *Mental Retardation and Developmental Disabilities Research Reviews, 13*(4), 370-8.

Emery, A. E. (1991). Population frequencies of inherited neuromuscular diseases--a world survey. *Neuromuscular Disorders : NMD, 1*(1), 19-29.

Fairclough, R. J., Bareja, A., & Davies, K. E. (2011). 2010 Joan Mott prize lecture: Progress in therapy for Duchenne muscular dystrophy. *Experimental Physiology.*, 96(11), 1101-13.

Finder, J. D., Birnkrant, D., Carl, J., Farber, H. J., Gozal, D., Iannaccone, S. T., . . . American Thoracic Society. (2004). Respiratory care of the patient with Duchenne muscular dystrophy: ATS consensus statement. *American Journal of Respiratory and Critical Care Medicine, 170*(4), 456-65.

Firth, M., Gardner-Medwin, D., Hosking, G., & Wilkinson, E. (1983). Interviews with parents of boys suffering from Duchenne muscular dystrophy. *Developmental Medicine and Child Neurology, 25*(4), 466-71.

Fitzpatrick, C., Barry, C., & Garvey, C. (1986). Psychiatric disorder among boys with Duchenne muscular dystrophy. *Developmental Medicine and Child Neurology, 28*(5), 589-95.

Fitzpatrick, C., & Barry, C. (1986). Communication within families about Duchenne muscular dystrophy. *Developmental Medicine and Child Neurology, 28*(5), 596-9.

Gibson, B. (2001). Long-Term ventilation for patients with Duchenne muscular dystrophy: Physicians' beliefs and practices. *Chest, 119*(3), 940-6.

Griggs, R. C., Moxley, R. T., Mendell, J. R., Fenichel, G. M., Brooke, M. H., Pestronk, A., & Miller, J. P. (1991). Prednisone in Duchenne dystrophy. A randomized, controlled trial defining the time course and dose response. Clinical investigation of Duchenne dystrophy group. *Archives of Neurology, 48*(4), 383-8.

Hendriks, A. H., De Moor, J. M., Oud, J. H., & Franken, W. M. (2000). Service needs of parents with motor or multiply disabled children in Dutch therapeutic toddler classes. *Clinical Rehabilitation, 14*(5), 506-17.

Hoffman, E. P., Brown, R. H., & Kunkel, L. M. (1987). Dystrophin: The protein product of the Duchenne muscular dystrophy locus. *Cell, 51*(6), 919-28.

Ivey, S. L., Brown, K. S., Teske, Y., & Silverman, D. (1988). A model for teaching about interdisciplinary practice in health care settings. *Journal of Allied Health, 17*(3), 189-95.

Kinali, M., Main, M., Eliahoo, J., Messina, S., Knight, R. K., Lehovsky, J., . . . Muntoni, F. (2007). Predictive factors for the development of scoliosis in Duchenne muscular dystrophy. *European Journal of Paediatric Neurology: EJPN : Official Journal of the European Paediatric Neurology Society, 11*(3), 160-6.

Kinali, M., Manzur, A. Y., Mercuri, E., Gibson, B. E., Hartley, L., Simonds, A. K., & Muntoni, F. (2006). UK physicians' attitudes and practices in long-term non-invasive ventilation of Duchenne muscular dystrophy. *Pediatric Rehabilitation, 9*(4), 351-64.

Kitzinger, J. (1995). Qualitative research. Introducing focus groups. *BMJ (Clinical Research Ed.), 311*(7000), 299-302.

Koenig, M., Monaco, A. P., & Kunkel, L. M. (1988). The complete sequence of dystrophin predicts a rod-shaped cytoskeletal protein. *Cell, 53*(2), 219-28.

Laing, N. G. (1993). Molecular genetics and genetic counselling for Duchenne/Becker muscular dystrophy. *In: Partridge TA, editor. Molecular and cell biology of muscular dystrophy.* (pp. p. 37-84). London: Chapman & Hall.

Leibowitz, D., & Dubowitz, V. (1981). Intellect and behaviour in Duchenne muscular dystrophy. *Developmental Medicine and Child Neurology, 23*(5), 577-90.

Mah, J. K., Tough, S., Fung, T., Douglas-England, K., & Verhoef, M. (2006). Adolescent quality of life and satisfaction with care. *The Journal of Adolescent Health : Official Publication of the Society for Adolescent Medicine, 38*(5), 607.e1-7.

Mah, J. K., Thannhauser, J. E., Kolski, H., & Dewey, D. (2008). Parental stress and quality of life in children with neuromuscular disease. *Pediatric Neurology, 39*(2), 102-7.

Mah, J. K., Thannhauser, J. E., McNeil, D. A., & Dewey, D. (2008). Being the lifeline: The parent experience of caring for a child with neuromuscular disease on home mechanical ventilation. *Neuromuscular Disorders: NMD, 18*(12), 983-8.

Mah, J. K., Selby, K., Campbell, C., Nadeau, A., Tarnopolsky, M., McCormick, A., . . . Yoon, G. (2011). A population-based study of dystrophin mutations in Canada. *The Canadian Journal of Neurological Sciences. Le Journal Canadien Des Sciences Neurologiques, 38*(3), 465-74.

Malik, V., Rodino-Klapac, L. R., Viollet, L., Wall, C., King, W., Al-Dahhak, R., . . . Mendell, J. R. (2010). Gentamicin-Induced readthrough of stop codons in Duchenne muscular dystrophy. *Annals of Neurology, 67*(6), 771-80.

Markham, L. W., Kinnett, K., Wong, B. L., Woodrow Benson, D., & Cripe, L. H. (2008). Corticosteroid treatment retards development of ventricular dysfunction in Duchenne muscular dystrophy. *Neuromuscular Disorders: NMD, 18*(5), 365-70.

McMillan, H. J., Campbell, C., Mah, J. K., & Canadian Paediatric Neuromuscular Group. (2010). Duchenne muscular dystrophy: Canadian paediatric neuromuscular physicians survey. *The Canadian Journal of Neurological Sciences. Le Journal Canadien Des Sciences Neurologiques, 37*(2), 195-205.

Mendell, J. R., Moxley, R. T., Griggs, R. C., Brooke, M. H., Fenichel, G. M., Miller, J. P., . . . Florence, J. (1989). Randomized, double-blind six-month trial of prednisone in Duchenne's muscular dystrophy. *The New England Journal of Medicine, 320*(24), 1592-7.

Moore, M. H., Mah, J. K., & Trute, B. (2009). Family-Centred care and health-related quality of life of patients in paediatric neurosciences. *Child: Care, Health and Development, 35*(4), 454-61.

Morine, K. J., Bish, L. T., Selsby, J. T., Gazzara, J. A., Pendrak, K., Sleeper, M. M., . . . Sweeney, H. L. (2010). Activin IIB receptor blockade attenuates dystrophic pathology in a mouse model of Duchenne muscular dystrophy. *Muscle & Nerve, 42*(5), 722-30.

Moxley, R. T., Ashwal, S., Pandya, S., Connolly, A., Florence, J., Mathews, K., . . . Practice Committee of the Child Neurology Society. (2005). Practice parameter: Corticosteroid treatment of Duchenne dystrophy: Report of the quality standards subcommittee of the American Academy of Neurology and the practice committee of the child neurology society. *Neurology, 64*(1), 13-20.

Msall, M. E., DiGaudio, K., Rogers, B. T., LaForest, S., Catanzaro, N. L., Campbell, J., . . . Duffy, L. C. (1994). The functional independence measure for children (WeeFIM). Conceptual basis and pilot use in children with developmental disabilities. *Clinical Pediatrics, 33*(7), 421-30.

Muntoni, F., Bushby, K., & van Ommen, G. (2005). 128Th ENMC international workshop on 'preclinical optimization and phase I/II clinical trials using antisense oligonucleotides in Duchenne muscular dystrophy' 22-24 October 2004, Naarden, the Netherlands. *Neuromuscular Disorders : NMD, 15*(6), 450-7.

Muntoni, F., Bushby, K., & Manzur, A. Y. (2006). Muscular dystrophy campaign funded workshop on management of scoliosis in Duchenne muscular dystrophy 24 January 2005, London, UK. *Neuromuscular Disorders: NMD, 16*(3), 210-9.

Ottenbacher, K. J., Msall, M. E., Lyon, N. R., Duffy, L. C., Granger, C. V., & Braun, S. (1997). Interrater agreement and stability of the functional independence measure for children (WeeFIM): Use in children with developmental disabilities. *Archives of Physical Medicine and Rehabilitation, 78*(12), 1309-15.

Rolland, J. S., & Walsh, F. (2006). Facilitating family resilience with childhood illness and disability. *Current Opinion in Pediatrics, 18*(5), 527-38.

Rybakova, I. N., Patel, J. R., & Ervasti, J. M. (2000). The dystrophin complex forms a mechanically strong link between the sarcolemma and costameric actin. *The Journal of Cell Biology, 150*(5), 1209-14.

Schara, U., Mortier, & Mortier, W. (2001). Long-Term steroid therapy in Duchenne muscular dystrophy-positive results versus side effects. *Journal of Clinical Neuromuscular Disease, 2*(4), 179-83.

Sheras PL, Abidin RR, Konold TR (1998). *Stress Index for Parents of Adolescents: Professional manual.* Odessa, FL: Psychological Assessment Resources, 7-49.

Schertzer, J. D., van der Poel, C., Shavlakadze, T., Grounds, M. D., & Lynch, G. S. (2008). Muscle-Specific overexpression of IGF-I improves E-C coupling in skeletal muscle fibers from dystrophic mdx mice. *American Journal of Physiology. Cell Physiology, 294*(1), C161-8.

Sexton, D., Burrell, B., Thompson, B (1992). Measurement integrity of the Family Needs Survey. *Journal of Early Intervention, 16(4),* 343-352.

Soo, I., Mah, J. K., Barlow, K., Hamiwka, L., & Wirrell, E. (2005). Use of complementary and alternative medical therapies in a pediatric neurology clinic. *The Canadian Journal of Neurological Sciences. Le Journal Canadien Des Sciences Neurologiques, 32*(4), 524-8.

Steele, R. G. (2002). Experiences of families in which a child has a prolonged terminal illness: Modifying factors. *International Journal of Palliative Nursing, 8*(9), 418-34.

Takeshima, Y., Yagi, M., Okizuka, Y., Awano, H., Zhang, Z., Yamauchi, Y., . . . Matsuo, M. (2010). Mutation spectrum of the dystrophin gene in 442 Duchenne/Becker muscular dystrophy cases from one Japanese referral center. *Journal of Human Genetics, 55*(6), 379-88.

Tang, Y., Reay, D. P., Salay, M. N., Mi, M. Y., Clemens, P. R., Guttridge, D. C., . . . Wang, B. (2010). Inhibition of the IKK/NF-κb pathway by AAV gene transfer improves muscle regeneration in older mdx mice. *Gene Therapy, 17*(12), 1476-83.

Tinsley, J. M., Fairclough, R. J., Storer, R., Wilkes, F. J., Potter, A. C., Squire, S. E., . . . Davies, K. E. (2011). Daily treatment with SMTC1100, a novel small molecule utrophin upregulator, dramatically reduces the dystrophic symptoms in the mdx mouse. *Plos ONE, 6*(5), e19189.

Trivette, C. M., Dunst, C. J., Allen, S., & Wall, L. (1993). Family-Centeredness of the children's health care journal. *Children's Health Care: Journal of the Association for the Care of Children's Health, 22*(4), 241-56.

Trollet, C., Athanasopoulos, T., Popplewell, L., Malerba, A., & Dickson, G. (2009). Gene therapy for muscular dystrophy: Current progress and future prospects. *Expert Opinion on Biological Therapy, 9*(7), 849-66.

van Deutekom, J. C., Janson, A. A., Ginjaar, I. B., Frankhuizen, W. S., Aartsma-Rus, A., Bremmer-Bout, M., . . . van Ommen, G. J. (2007). Local dystrophin restoration with antisense oligonucleotide PRO051. *The New England Journal of Medicine, 357*(26), 2677-86.

van Kesteren, R. G., Velthuis, B., & van Leyden, L. W. (2001). Psychosocial problems arising from home ventilation. *American Journal of Physical Medicine & Rehabilitation / Association of Academic Physiatrists, 80*(6), 439-46.

Varni, J. W., Seid, M., & Rode, C. A. (1999). The PedsQL: Measurement model for the pediatric quality of life inventory. *Medical Care, 37*(2), 126-39.

Varni, J. W., Seid, M., & Kurtin, P. S. (2001). PedsQL 4.0: Reliability and validity of the pediatric quality of life inventory version 4.0 generic core scales in healthy and patient populations. *Medical Care, 39*(8), 800-12.

Wagner, K. R. (2008). Approaching a new age in Duchenne muscular dystrophy treatment. *Neurotherapeutics : The Journal of the American Society for Experimental Neurotherapeutics, 5*(4), 583-91.

Wallace, G. Q., & McNally, E. M. (2009). Mechanisms of muscle degeneration, regeneration, and repair in the muscular dystrophies. *Annual Review of Physiology, 71*, 37-57.

Walsh, F. (2003). Family resilience: A framework for clinical practice. *Family Process, 42*(1), 1-18.

Weidner, N. J. (2005). Developing an interdisciplinary palliative care plan for the patient with muscular dystrophy. *Pediatric Annals, 34*(7), 546-52.

Welch, E. M., Barton, E. R., Zhuo, J., Tomizawa, Y., Friesen, W. J., Trifillis, P., . . . Sweeney, H. L. (2007). PTC124 targets genetic disorders caused by nonsense mutations. *Nature, 447*(7140), 87-91.

5

Comparison Between Courses of Home and Inpatients Mechanical Ventilation in Patients with Muscular Dystrophy in Japan

Toshio Saito[1] and Katsunori Tatara[2]
[1]*Division of Neurology, National Hospital Organization Toneyama National Hospital*
[2]*Division of Pediatrics, National Hospital Organization Tokushima National Hospital*
Japan

1. Introduction

In Japan, 27 hospitals specialize in treatment of muscular dystrophy patients, including inpatient care, of which 26 belong to the National Hospital Organization, and the other is the National Center of Neurology and Psychiatry. Since 1999, Japanese muscular dystrophy research groups investigating nervous and mental disorder have been developing a database of cases treated at these 27 institutions. In that regard, we conducted a survey of inpatients and home-mechanical ventilation patients (HMV patients) with muscular dystrophy and other neuromuscular disorders based on data collected by the National Hospital Organization and National Center of Neurology and Psychiatry.

Herein, we examined data obtained in order to evaluate efficacy of mechanical ventilation therapy for HMV patients and mechanical ventilation-dependent inpatients (MV inpatients) with those wards.

2. Subjects and methods

The database includes numbers of inpatients, gender, age, diagnosis, respiratory condition, nutritional state, number of death cases, causes of death, and other relevant findings from data collected annually on October 1 every year since 1999. Additionally we collected the data of HMV patients from 27 institutes for this study.

By using the database and newly collected HMV data, we analyzed the courses of HMV patients group and those of MV inpatients of wards. We compared data of these two groups. Examination points are mechanical ventilation periods, outcome of these two groups, and caregiver for HMV patients.

2.1 Objective diseases

Objective diseases of this study were muscular dystrophy and spinal muscular atrophy, in particular Duchenne muscular dystrophy and myotonic dystrophy. Amyotrophic lateral sclerosis was not included.

2.2 Patients introduced HMV after 1999

The data which we requested 27 institutes specializing muscular dystrophy care was as follows; the number of patients introduced HMV after 1999, diagnosis of disease, gender, age at being introduced HMV, type of mechanical ventilation, such as non-invasive positive pressure ventilation (NPPV) or tracheostomy intermittent ventilation (TIV), present status, death cause for death case, main caregiver, and so on.

2.3 Patients introduced MV in muscular dystrophy wards after 1999

We selected data of newly MV introduced inpatients after 1999 from the database of the muscular dystrophy wards.

3. Results

3.1 Demographic features of HMV patients group and MV inpatients

3.1.1 HMV patients group

HMV patients group included 434 patients from 14 institutes. Gender was male: 356, female: 78. The number of representative disease were as follows; 262 patients with Duchenne muscular dystrophy, 60 myotonic dystrophy, 17 Becker muscular dystrophy, 16 limb-girdle muscular dystrophy, 14 spinal muscular atrophy, and so on (Table 1-1).

Diagnosis	HMV	Inpatient	Total	Death cases
BMD	17	35	52	10
CMD	12	6	18	2
DMD	262	476	738	96
EDMD	2	0	2	
FCMD	16	43	59	13
FSHD	6	33	39	7
LGMD	16	42	58	12
MD	60	222	282	62
MG	1	0	1	
SMA	13	19	32	6
SPMA	0	11	11	4
UCMD	9	1	10	
Mitochondrila disease	0	5	5	1
Distal myopathy	2	3	5	2
Congenital myopathy	8	12	20	
Glycogen storage disease	2	1	3	
Other myopathies	3	1	4	
Other dystrophies	4	5	9	
Unknown	1	0	1	
total	434	915	1349	215

BMD, Becker muscular dystrophy; CMD, congenital muscular dystrophy; DMD, Duchenne muscular dystrophy; EDMD, Emery-Dreifuss muscular dystrophy; FCMD, Fukuyama congenital muscular dystrophy; FSHD, facio-scapulo-humeral muscular dystrophy; LGMD, limb-girdle muscular dystrophy; MD, Myotonic dystrophy; MG, myasthenia gravis; SMA, spinal muscular atrophy; SPMA, spinal progressive muscular atrophy, UCMD, Ullrich congenital muscular dystrophy

Table 1-1. Details of disease (HMV: from 14 institutes)

3.1.2 MV inpatients group

MV inpatients group included 915 inpatients. Gender was male: 718, female: 197. The number of representative disease were as follows; 476 Duchenne muscular dystrophy, 222 myotonic dystrophy, 35 Becker muscular dystrophy, 58 limb-girdle muscular dystrophy, 19 spinal muscular atrophy, and so on (Table 1-1).

3.1.3 Mean age at starting mechanical ventilation and type of ventilation

The range of mechanical ventilation introduction age for HMV patients was 6.3~72.8 years old (mean 25.9), and that of MV inpatients was 0.0~78.0 years old (mean 33.2). The number of NPPV introduction cases of HMV patients was 420, and that of MV inpatients was 517 (Table 1-2). Fifty of NPPV cases of HMV group were switched to tracheostomy during the course.

	HMV	Inpatient	
Age at starting mechanical ventilation (years old)	25.9	33.2	$p<0.05$
NPPV introduced case	420	517	

Table 1-2. Mean age at starting mechanical ventilation and type of ventilation

3.2 Survival analysis of HMV patients group and MV inpatients

We performed survival analysis of those two groups. The endpoint for HMV patients was death or transition to hospitalization, and that for MV inpatient was death. Kaplan-Meier analysis showed that 75% life time of HMV patients was 1,689 days, while that of inpatients was 2,988 days (Log Rank (Mantel-Cox) $p<0.01$) (Fig. 1).

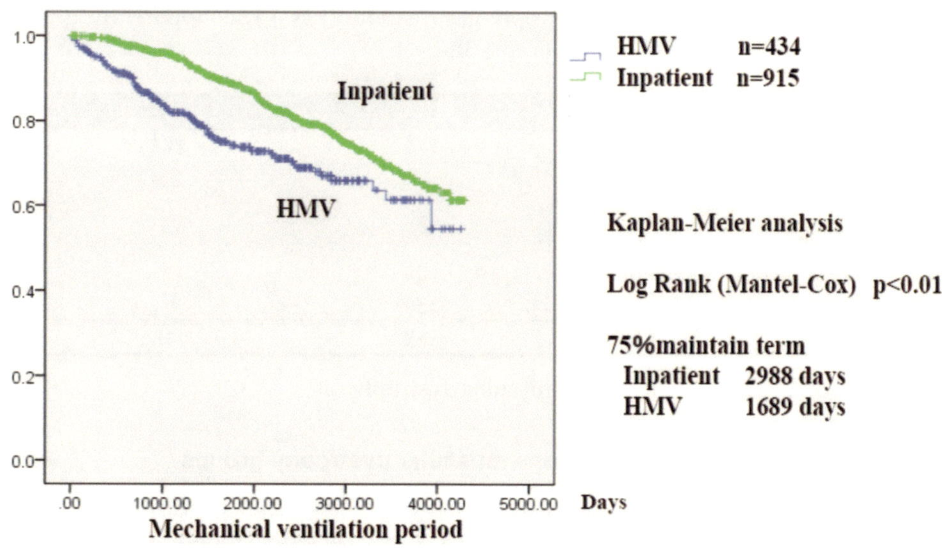

Fig. 1. Comparison between HMV Patients and Mechanical Ventilation Inpatients (Total)
Endpoint for HMV patient: death or transition to hospitalization
Endpoint for MV inpatient: death

3.3 Analysis data of Duchenne muscular dystrophy and myotonic dystrophy

As the number of patients with Duchenne muscular dystrophy and myotonic dystrophy was great in these two groups, we analyzed the data of Duchenne muscular dystrophy and myotonic dystrophy separately.

3.3.1 Mean age at starting mechanical ventilation and type of ventilation of patients with Duchenne muscular dystrophy

Mean age at starting mechanical ventilation of Duchenne muscular dystrophy was 19.8 years old, ranged from 11.5 to 39.9 years old. While that of inpatient with Duchenne muscular dystrophy was 21.5 years old, ranged from 10.0 to 42.0 years old. There was no significant difference. The number of NPPV introduction cases of HMV patients with Duchenne muscular dystrophy was 220, and that of MV inpatients was 338 (Table 2).

	HMV	Inpatient	
Age at starting mechanical ventilation (years old)	19.8	21.5	NS
NPPV	220	338	
TIV	42	138	
total	262	476	

Table 2. Mean age at starting mechanical ventilation and type of mechanical ventilation (Duchenne muscular dystrophy)

3.3.2 Type of nutrition of patients with Duchenne muscular dystrophy

The number of patients who required tube feeding, including a nasal or oral nutrition tube, and undergoing a percutaneous endoscopic gastrostomy (PEG) was apparently greater in MV inpatients group than HMV group (Table 3).

	HMV	Inpatient
Oral nutritional supply	118	314
PEG	11	78
Tube feeding (per nasal or per oral)	3	71
Intravenous hyperamelitaion	0	13
unknown	130	0
total	262	476

Table 3. Type of nutrition (Duchenne muscular dystrophy)

3.3.3 Survival analysis of two Duchenne muscular dystrophy groups

We performed survival analysis of those two Duchenne muscular dystrophy groups. The endpoint for HMV patients was death or transition to hospitalization, and that for MV inpatient was death. Kaplan-Meier analysis showed that 75% life time of HMV patients was 1,562 days, while that of inpatients was 3,739 days (Log Rank (Mantel-Cox) $p<0.01$) (Fig. 2).

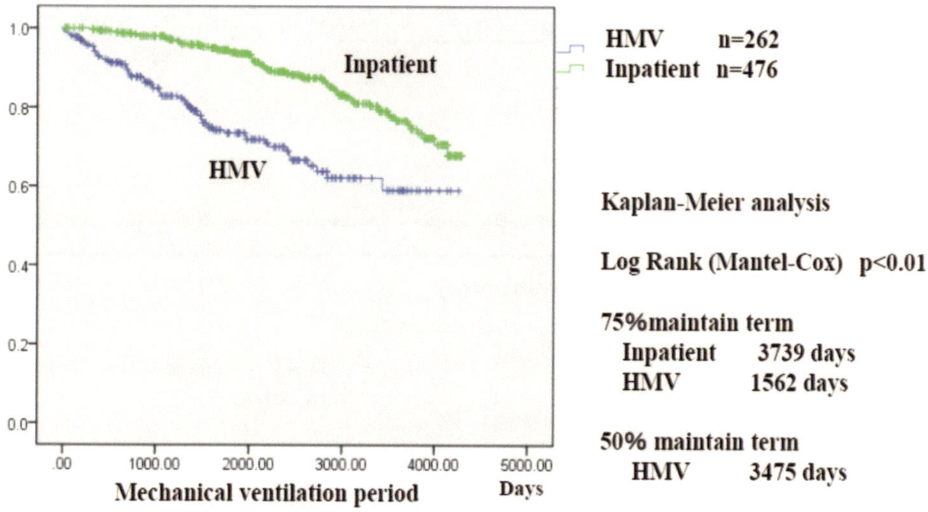

Fig. 2. Comparison between HMV Patients and Mechanical Ventilation Inpatients (Duchenne muscular dystrophy)
Endpoint for HMVpatient: death or transition to hospitalization
Endpoint for MV inpatient: death

3.3.4 Mean age at starting mechanical ventilation and type of ventilation of patients with myotonic dystrophy

Mean age at starting mechanical ventilation of myotonic dystrophy was 46.8 years old, ranged from 15.8 to 72.8 years old. While that of inpatient with myotonic dystrophy was 50.6 years old, ranged from 12.0 to 76.0 years old. There was no significant difference between two groups. The number of NPPV introduction cases of HMV patients with myotonic dystrophy was 55, and that of TIV was 5. The number of NPPV case was greater than TIV. While the number of NPPV introduction cases of MV patients with myotonic dystrophy was 108, and that of TIV was 114. In MV patients with myotonic dystrophy, the number and proportion of NPPV and TIV were almost equal (Table 4).

	HMV	Inpatient	
Age at starting mechanical ventilation (years old)	46.8	50.6	NS
NPPV	55	108	
TIV	5	114	
total	60	222	

Table 4. Mean age at starting mechanical ventilation and type of mechanical ventilation (myotonic dystrophy)

3.3.5 Type of nutrition of patients with myotonic dystrophy

The trend of nutrition was similar to Duchenne muscular dystrophy. The number who required tube feeding in MV inpatients group was apparently greater than HMV group (Table 5).

	HMV	Inpatient
Oral nutritional supply	18	93
PEG	1	69
Tube feeding (per nasal or per oral)	0	50
Intravenous hyperamelitaion	0	10
unknown	41	0
total	60	222

Table 5. Type of nutrition (myotonic dystrophy)

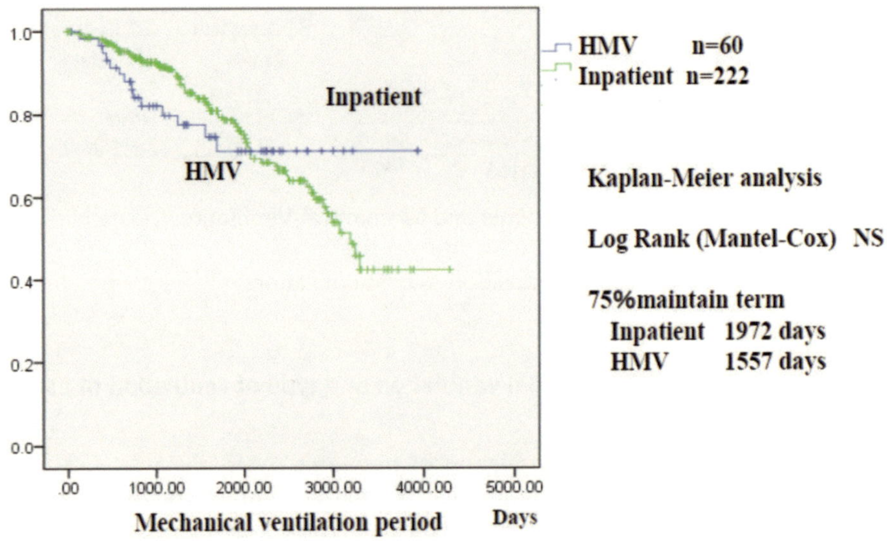

Fig. 3. Comparison between HMV Patients and Mechanical Ventilation Inpatients (myotonic dystrophy)
Endpoint for HMVpatient: death or transition to hospitalization
Endpoint for MV inpatient: death

3.3.6 Survival analysis of two myotonic dystrophy groups

Similarly, we performed survival analysis of those two myotonic dystrophy groups. The endpoint for HMV patients was death or transition to hospitalization, and that for MV inpatient was death. Kaplan-Meier analysis showed that 75% life time of HMV patients was 1,557 days, while that of inpatients was 1,972 days. There was no significance (Fig. 3).

3.4 Death case

The total number of death cases was 215 (Table 1-1). As the number of death case of Duchenne muscular dystrophy and myotonic dystrophy was the majority, we analyzed the data of Duchenne muscular dystrophy and myotonic dystrophy separately.

3.4.1 Cause of death of Duchenne muscular dystrophy

The number of death cases of HMV patients was 29, and that of MV inpatients was 67.

The most frequent cause of death was heart related disorders, such as heart failure and arrhythmia, accounting for 16/29 for HMV group and 33/67 for MV inpatient group. Frequency was not significantly different between two groups. In MV inpatient group, respiratory related disorders, such as respiratory failure and respiratory infection, accounted for 23/67. HMV group included more sudden death cases than MV inpatient, and had an accidental case (Table 6).

	HMV	Inpatient	Total
Heart failure	13	27	40
Arrhythmia	3	6	9
Respiratory failure	2	11	13
Respiratory infection	1	12	13
Tracheal bleeding	1	0	1
Pneumothorax	0	1	1
Renal failure	0	1	1
Infectious disease	2	0	2
Malignancy	1	0	1
Ileus	1	0	1
Sudden death	4	2	6
Power supply accident	1	0	1
Others	0	7	7
total	29	67	96

Table 6. Cause of death (Duchenne muscular dystrophy)

3.4.2 Cause of death of myotonic dystrophy

The majority of death case of myotonic dystrophy was reported from MV inpatient group. The most frequent cause was respiratory related disorders, such as respiratory tract infection and respiratory failure, which accounted for 29/56. Sudden death case was conspicuous in HMV group, accounting for 3/6(Table 7).

	HMV	Inpatient	Total
Respiratory infection	1	19	20
Respiratory failure	2	10	12
Heart failure	0	8	8
DIC	0	1	1
MOF	0	2	2
Cholangitis	0	2	2
Ileus	0	1	1
Choking	0	1	1
Malignancy	0	2	2
Intestinal bleeding	0	1	1
Hepatic failure	0	1	1
Sudden death	3	2	5
Others	0	6	6
total	6	56	62

Table 7. Cause of death (myotonic dystrophy)

3.5 Outcome of HMV patients and MV inpatients with Duchenne muscular dystrophy and myotonic dystrophy

One hundred ninty four cases with Duchenne muscular dystrophy among 262 cases continued HMV, while 46 cases with myotonic dystrophy among 60 cases continued HMV (Table 8). Twenty two cases with Duchenne muscular dystrophy were switched to hospitalization.

	DMD		MD	
	HMV	Inpatient	HMV	Inpatient
Continuing HMV	194	-	46	-
Continuing hospitalization	-	407	-	151
Death	29	67	6	56
Transition to hospitalization	22	-	3	-
Introduction to other institution	10	-	-	-
Withdrawing MV	-	-	3	-
Unknown	7	2	-	-
Others	-	-	2	15
total	262	476	60	222

Table 8. Outcome (Duchenne muscular dystrophy and myotonic dystrophy)

3.6 Caregivers for HMV patients

Caregivers for most of HMV patients with Duchenne muscular dystrophy were patients' families (Table 9). In particular, patients' mothers were playing important role in continuing HMV. Similarly, caregivers for HMV patients with myotonic dystrophy were patients' families. On reflecting their age, some caregivers were patient' spouse (Table 9).

Caregiver	DMD	MD
Mother	94	6
Parents	22	
Father	3	2
Family	3	
Mother/sibling	1	
Mother/uncle	1	
Mother/grandmother	1	
Grandmother	1	
Husband		2
Wife		1
Sister		1
daughter		1
foundation		2
Helper	2	2
(Response)	(134/262)	(17/60)

Table 9. HMV-continuing cases main caregiver (Duchenne muscular dystrophy and myotonic dystrophy)

3.7 Summary of results of Duchenne muscular dystrophy and myotonic dystrophy

Proportion of TIV was higher in MV inpatients group than HMV group. And proportion of tube feeding was also higher in MV inpatients group than HMV group. Namely, respiratory condition and nutritional status were more severe in MV inpatients group than HMV group (both Duchenne muscular dystrophy and myotonic dystrophy).

In Survival analysis, outcome of patients with Duchenne muscular dystrophy of MV inpatients group was better than HMV group. Meanwhile in that of myotonic dystrophy, HMV group was better than inpatient group.

In MV inpatient group of Duchenne muscular dystrophy, respiratory related death was remarkable.

In HMV group, some sudden death cases and accidental death case were conspicuous.

Caregivers of HMV group were constructed by patients' families, centrally mother.

4. Conclusion

Approximate 2500 beds for patients with muscular dystrophy and related disorders are now provided among 27 institutions in Japan. In accordance with progress in therapeutic strategies for respiratory failure (American Thoracic Society Documents, 2004) and heart failure (Ishikawa, 1999; Matsumura, 2010), the life span of patients with muscular dystrophy prolonged (Bushby 2010a, b). Now, most inpatients admitted to muscular dystrophy wards have severe general conditions and many are assisted by mechanical ventilation (Tatara, 2006; 2008), which is accordance with our data of MV patients in this study.

In recent two decades, social welfare systems and home medical care systems in Japan have been changing gradually. HMV has been penetrating into home medical care (Joseph, 2007). The number of HMV patients has been increasing (Tatara, 2006). Stable mechanical ventilated patients have been getting back home.

Our study demonstrated that the course of HMV patients was fairly good, although there was difference between Duchenne muscular dystrophy and myotonic dystrophy in long term outcome. However, the support system for patients and caregivers is not perfect. Our study also showed that burden of caregivers was supposed to be severe. The system for patients and caregivers should be adjusted (Dybwik, 2011). And safety net systems also should be adjusted to avoid accidental event leading to patient's death.

The muscular dystrophy wards may be requested to offer the circumstances for those who have difficulties in continuing HMV. There is necessarily needs for hospitalization of HMV patients (Windisch, 2008).

Study limitation: This study has limitation on bias of collecting patients' information. Specifically, information of HMV patients were reported from 14 institutes among 27 institutes, and MV inpatient information is the result of extraction from muscular dystrophy wards database. Extracted data from database has some ambiguous points in connection with obscure time-sequential analysis.

On analysis of institutes-restricted HMV patients group and MV inpatients group, differences in regard to therapeutic conditions among institutions may be problem.

5. Acknowledgments

This study was supported by a Research Grant for Nervous and Mental Disorders from the Ministry of Health, Labour and Welfare of Japan.

We are grateful to the members of the FUKUNAGA (1999-2005) and SHINNO (2006-2011) muscular dystrophy research groups of the National Hospital Organization for the data collection.

Institutions specializing in muscular dystrophy treatment in Japan (Fig.4)

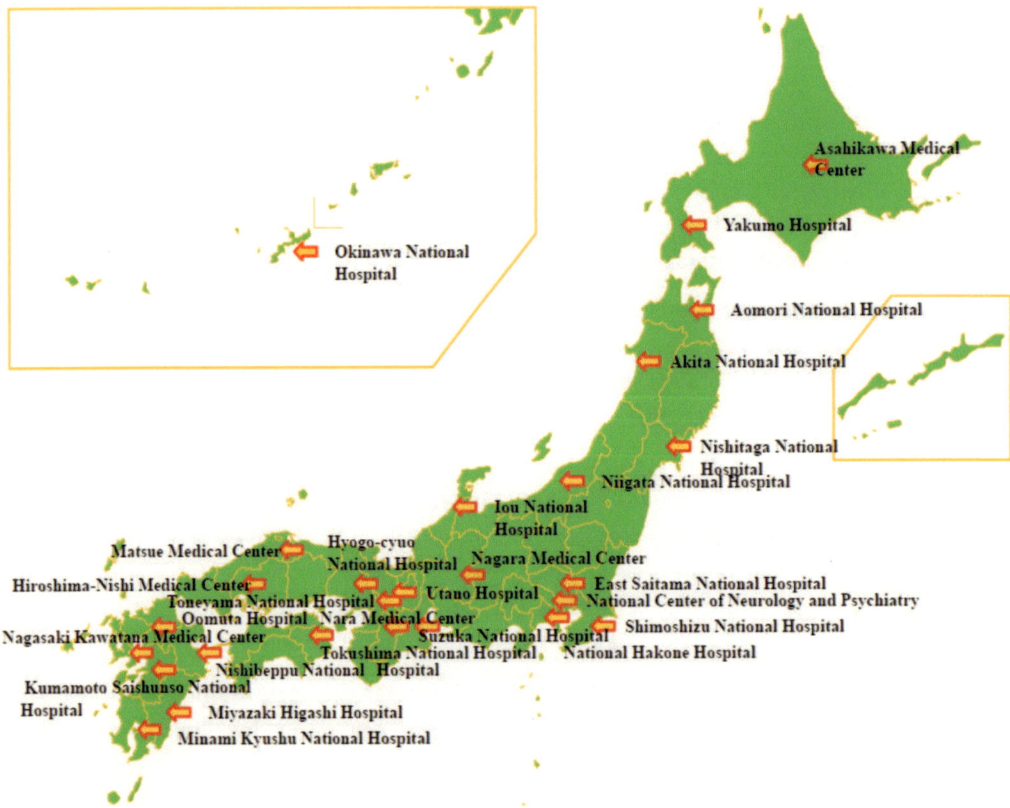

Fig. 4. Institutions specializing in muscular dystrophy treatment in Japan

National Hospital Organization:

Asahikawa Medical Center, Yakumo Hospital, Aomori National Hospital,

Akita National Hospital, Nishitaga National Hospital, East Saitama National Hospital,

Shimoshizu National Hospital, National Hakone Hospital, Niigata National Hospital,

Iou National Hospital, Nagara Medical Center, Suzuka National Hospital,

Nara Medical Center, Utano Hospital, Toneyama National Hospital,

Hyogo-cyuo National Hospital, Hiroshima-Nishi Medical Center, Matsue Medical Center,

Tokushima National Hospital, Oomuta Hospital, Nagasaki Kawatana Medical Center,

Kumamoto Saishunso National Hospital, Nishibeppu National Hospital,

Miyazaki Higashi Hospital, Minami Kyushu National Hospital, Okinawa National Hospital

National Center of Neurology and Psychiatry

6. References

American Thoracic Society Documents (2004). Respiratory Care of the Patient with Duchenne Muscular Dystrophy. ATS Consensus Statement *American Journal of Respiratory and Critical Care Medicine*, Vol 170, pp 456–465.

Bushby K, Finkel R, Birnkrant DJ, Case LE, Clemens PR, Cripe L, Kaul A, Kinnett K, McDonald C, Pandya S, Poysky J, Shapiro F, Tomezsko J, Constantin C, for the DMD care considerations working group (2010a). Diagnosis and management of Duchenne muscular dystrophy, part 1: diagnosis, and pharmacological and psychosocial management. *The Lancet Neurology*, Vol.9, pp 77-93.

Bushby K, Finkel R, Birnkrant DJ, Case LE, Clemens PR, Cripe L, Kaul A, Kinnett K, McDonald C, Pandya S, Poysky J, Shapiro F, Tomezsko J, Constantin C, for the DMD care considerations working group (2010b). Diagnosis and management of Duchenne muscular dystrophy, part 2: implementation of multidisciplinary care. *The Lancet Neurology*, Vol.9, pp 177–189.

Dybwik.K, Nielsen.E.W,Brinchmann. B. S (2011).Home mechanical ventilation and specialized health care in the community: Between a rock and a hard place. *BMC Health Services Research*, Vol. 11, pp 115-123.

Ishikawa Y, Bach JR, Minami R (1999). Cardioprotection for Duchenne's muscular dystrophy.*American Heart Journal* Vol.137, pp 895–902.

Joseph S. L, Peter C. G (2007). Current Issues in Home Mechanical Ventilation. *Chest*, Vol. 132, pp 671-676.

Matsumura T, Tamura T, Kuru S, Kikuchi Y, Kawai M (2010) · Carvedilol can prevent cardiac events in Duchenne muscular dystrophy. *Internal Medicine* Vol. 49, pp 1357-1363.

Tatara K, Fukunaga H, Kawai M (2006). Clinical survey of muscular dystrophyin hospitals of National Hospital Organization. *IRYO*, Vol. 60, pp 112-118.

Tatara K, Shinno S (2008). Management of mechanical ventilation and prognosis in Duchenne muscular dystrophy. *IRYO*, Vol. 62, pp 566–571.

Windisch W; Quality of life in home mechanical ventilation study group (2008). Impact of home mechanical ventilation on health-related quality of life. *Eur Respir J*. Vol. 32, pp 1328-1336.

6

Myopathy in Autoimmune Diseases – Primary Sjögren's Syndrome and Dermatomyositis

Fumio Kaneko[1,2,*], Ari Togashi[2], Erika Nomura[2],
Teiji Yamamoto[3] and Hideo Sakuma[4]
[1]*Institute of Dermat-Immunology and Allergy,*
Southern TOHOKU Research Institute for Neuroscience
[2]*Dermatology, Southern TOHOKU General Hospital,*
[3]*Neurological Institute, Southern TOHOKU Research Institute for Neuroscience*
[4]*Pathology Department, Southern TOHOKU Research Institute for Neuroscience*
Japan

1. Introduction

Myopathy, which clinically shows muscular pain (myalgia), weakness, cramps, stiffness and spasm, is one of neuromuscular disorders due to inflammation and/or dysfunction of muscle fibers. "Myositis", which is a general term for inflammation of the muscle, is pathologically an inflammatory myopathy seen seen mainly in autoimmune disorders including dermatomyositis (DM). The myopathy is classified by National Institute of Neurological Disorders and Stroke (NINDS) as indicated in Table 1 (1). We here focus myopathy on primary Sjögren's syndrome (pSjS) associated with myalgia "mimicking DM", as previously reported (2), and the inflammatory myopathy of DM (Table 2). Most of SjS is a secondary disorder to systemic autoimmune diseases including systemic lupus erythematosus (SLE), systemic sclerosis, DM, and so on. However, SjS, which is not associated with other autoimmune diseases, is considered to be an idiopathic primary disorder characterized by sicca symptoms. It is known that pSjS may be associated with fever, fatigue, myalgia, arthralgia, cutaneous vasculitis, etc. in addition to sicca symptoms (4-8).

DM is also characterized by myalgia, muscular weakness and fatigue due to inflammatory myopathy that ultimately progresses to muscle degeneration and the cutaneous involvements. The skin manifestations include helio-trope-like colored erythema and swelling on the eye-lids, cheeks, neck and upper extremities of the sun-exposed areas and Gottron's papules on the dorsa of the hand fingers (3). Although the etiology of DM remains unknown, internal maligmant disorders including lung and/or other organ cancers are frequently associated. Generally DM is classified as shown in Table 3 (9).

---

* Corresponding Author

Congenital myopathies: characterized by developmental delays in motor skills; skeletal and facial abnormalities are occationally evident at birth
Muscular dystrophies: caused by progressive weakness in voluntary muscles; sometimes evident at birth
Mitochondrial myopathies: caused by genetic abnormalities in mitochondria, cellular structures that control energy; include Kearns-Sayre syndrome,
Glycogen storage diseases of muscle: caused by mutations in genes controlling enzymes that metabolize glycogen and glucose (blood sugar); include Pompe's, Anderson's and Cori's disease
Myoglobulinurias: caused by disorders in the metabolisum of a fuel (myoglobulin) necessary for muscle work; include McArdle, Tarui and DiMauro diseases
Dermatomyositis: an inflammatory myopathy and skin lesions
Myositis ossificans: characterized by bone growing in muscle tissue
Familiar periodic paralysis: characterized by episodes of weakness in arms and legs
Polymyositis inclusion body myositis and related myopathies: inflammatory myopathies of skeletal muscles
Neuromyotonia: characterized by alternating episodes of twiching and stiffness
Stiff-man syndrome: characterized by episodes of rigidity and reflex spasms
Common muscular cramps and stiffness and tetany: characterized by prologed spasms of the arms and legs

(National Institute of Neurological Disorders and Stroke, National Institutes of Health, USA[1])

Table 1. Classification of myopathy

Patient	Gender	Age years	Disease	Enzyme	Muscle biopsy	Auto-antibody	Observation term	Compli-cation	Outcome
1.	F	37	pSjS	No abnormatities	myopathy	ANA nv SSA 61.4 SSB 21.6	3.0 y	no	remission
2.	M	32	pSjS	CK 147 ALD 5.8	myopathy	ANA 20 SSB 15.7	8 m	no	remission
3.	F	29	DM	CK 883 ALD 11.2	myositis	nv	2.6 y	no	remission
4.	F	42	DM	CK 212 KL-6 2485	nd	nv	4.3 y	intestinal peumonia	remission
5.	M	45	DM	CK 302 ALD 8.4	myositis	nv	3.8 y	no	remission
6.	F	55	DM	SLD 5.7	nd	nv	3.11 y	no	remission
7.	F	60	DM	CK 364	nd	nv	2.0 y	no	remission
8.	M	66	DM	CK 1706 ALD 8.2 KL-6 1876 myoglobin 29.7	myositis	ANA 20	2.0 y	pneumonia and cancer	death

ALD: aldolase, ANA: anti-nuclear antibody, CK: creatine kinase, DM: dermatomyositis,
F: female, M: male, nd: not done, Nv: negative, pSjS: primary Sjögren's syndrome,
SSA: anti-SjS A antibody, SSB: anti-SjS B antibody
Myopathy: non-inflammatory myopathy, Myositis: inflammatory myopathy

Table 2. Myopathy and myositis in primary Sjögren's syndrome (pSjS) and dermatomyositis (DM)

- **Dermatomyosistis**
- Without muscle weakness (amyopathic dermatomyositis or dermatomyositis sine myositis)
- With muscle weakness
- Adult
- associated with cancer
- not associated with cancer
- Pediatric
- **Polymyositis**
- Adult
- Pediatric
- Inclusion-body myositis
- Overlap (myositis associated with a connective tissue disease)

Drake LA, et al[9].: Guidelines of care of dermatomyositis. J Am Acard Dermatol 1996; 34: 824

Table 3. Classification of Dermatomyositis/ Polymyositis

2. Cases

pSjS: A 37-year-old woman (Case 1 in Table 2) was suffered from fever around 37.5℃, fatigue, proximal muscle pain and weakness in her limbs and arthralgia since a week before her visiting our hospital. She presented herself with swelling and helio-trope-like colored erythema on the eye-lids (Fig. 1a,b), purpurish erythema-spots on the elbows, thin-reddish erythema patches on the legs (Fig.1c) and red palms. On the dorsa of the hand-fingers, the eruption looked like Gottron's papules was seen and thin purpuric spots were also noted on the paronychial areas. The electromyography showed low amplitude motor units (less than 1 mV) from muscles of the upper extremities that were suggestive myopathy. We suspected the patient had DM and the skin biopsy was taken from the erythematous patches on the left leg. The histology revealed so-called "lymphocytic vasculitis" which showed swollen

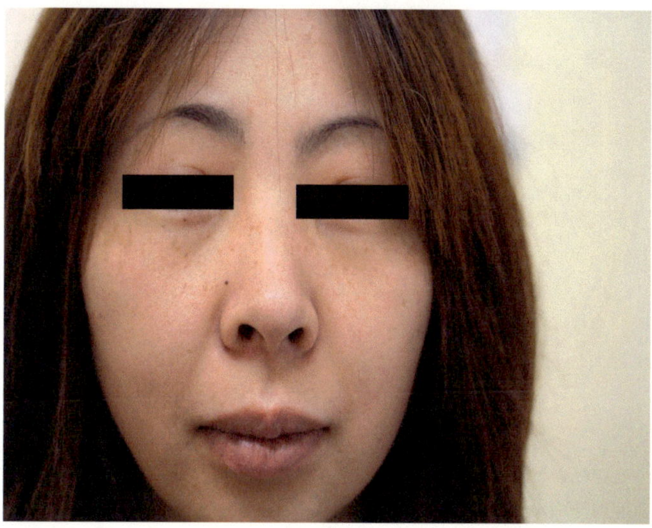

a)

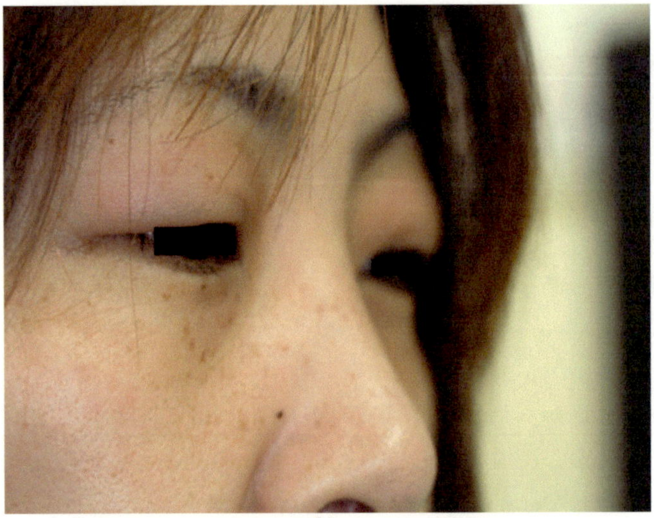

b)

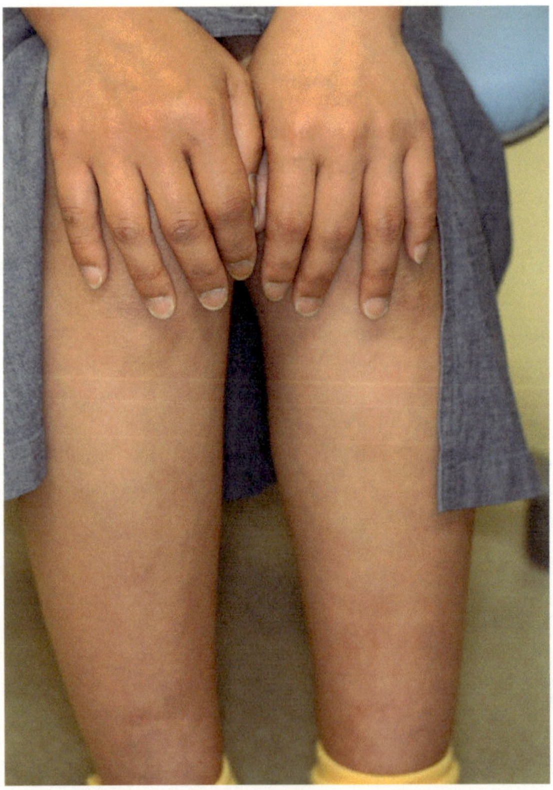

c)

Fig. 1. a,b) Close-up view of the right upper eye-lid showing slightly swollen and heliotrope-like colored erythema (Case 1 in Table 2). c) Gottron's nodule-like eruption on the dorsa of the fingers and thin-reddish erythematous patches on the lower legs.

vascular walls surrounded by mainly monocytes and a few of neutrophils in the middle and deep dermis (Fig. 2a,b). No deposit of IgG, IgA, IgM and C3 was seen at the dermo-epidermal (D-E) junction and vascular walls in the dermis by immunofluorescent microscopy. The immunochemical histology revealed $CD4^{+}>CD8^{+}>CD56^{+}$ cells distributed around vessels in the deep dermis. A muscle biopsy was performed from the biceps muscle of the left-upper arm where the patient was complaining of pain. No features of inflammation associated the "muscle fiber degeneration" could be found though slight vascular infiltration was seen in the interstitial tissue.

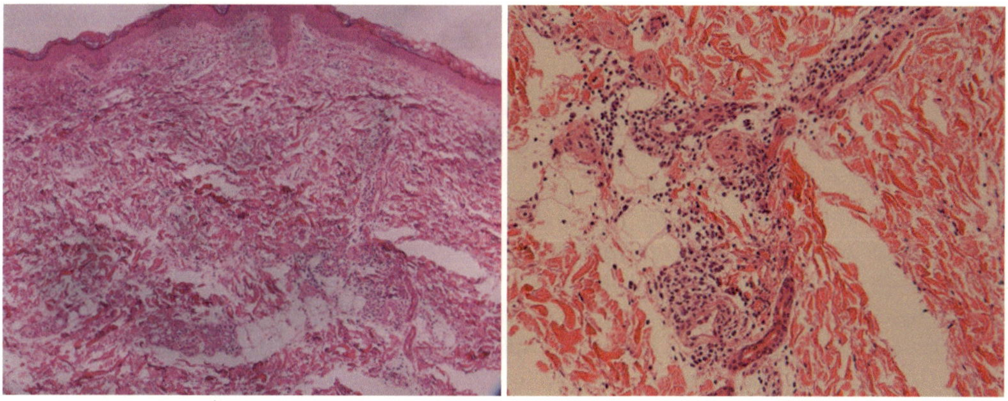

a) b)

Fig. 2. a) A skin biopsy from the left side of the lower leg revealed, a. vascular infiltration with lymphoid cells and a few neutrophils in the middle and deep dermis (H&E stain, x40). b) The magnified view showed swelling of the vascular endothelial cells with slight degeneration infiltrated by lymphoid cells, suggesting so-called "lymphocytic vasculitis" (x 200)

Laboratory examinations revealed within normal-limit (WNL) ranges of white blood cells (WBC), red blood cells (RBC) and serum AST (aspartate aminotransferase), ALT (alanine aminotransferase), and CK (creatine kinase) (28 IU/L, WNL: 48~259) and aldolase (ALD) (2.2 IU/L, WNL: 2.5~5.6) were rather lower than WNL. The serum levels of complement were high in CH50 (58.4 u/ml, WNL: 31.0~48.0) but levels of C3 and C4 were WNL. Although auto-antibodies (auto-Abs) including anti-nuclear Ab (ANA), anti-Jo-1, anti-DNA and anti-acetylcholine receptor Abs and RA factor were negative, anti-Sjögren's syndrome A (anti-SSA) and anti-SSB Abs showed the titers of 61.4 and 21.6 (WNL: less than 1.0), respectively, which were highly positive in detection by ELISA. Serum carcinoembryonic antigen (CEA) was not detected. Urinalysis revealed no abnormalities except detection of acetone body. The chest X-ray and positron emission tomography (PET) with ^{18}FDG (2-deoxy-2-fluoro-D-glucose) were performed but no abnormal uptakes were detected except for an enlarged lymphnode at the right-side neck and slight enlargement of the liver and spleen. Ophthalmological examinations revealed positive Schirmer's test (10mm/6mm) and fluorescein test which showed dry-eyes, although the amount of saliva was 3.5 ml/10 min which seemed to be low But WNL. The pain of visual analog scale (VAS) score was 75 mm when she initially visited our clinic.

The patient was diagnosed as having pSjS with myalgia mimicking DM, which may be classified as the extraglandular type. She was treated with prednisolone (PSL) 20mg/day and non-steroidal anti-inflammatory drugs (NSAIDs). The symptoms including the cutaneous manifestations completely disappeared and pain VAS score also gradually decreased to 55 mm in a week. The patient was quickly recovered from fatigue, subfebrile state, myalgia and arthralgia two weeks after treatment by oral steroid. However, PSL administration of within 10 mg/day was needed to keep her well condition, although more than two years have been passed since her first visit.

Although the other 32 year-old male patient (Case 2) complained of dry eyes, mild fever, myalgia and muscle weakness of the upper extremities for more than one year, we initially suspected DM and examined for possibility of his having SjS regardless of absence of a DM-like eruption. Ophthalmologically he was suggested to have SjS. The blood examination revealed ALT 40 U/L (WNL: 6-36), ALD 5.8 IU/L, titers of ANA 20x (speckled type) and anti-SSA Ab 15.7 which were relatively high. However, a biopsy from the biceps muscle of the left upper arm was free from inflammation, and no internal malignancy was associated through examinations including PET with ^{18}FDG. He has been followed as pSjS similarly to the Case 1 for the duration of more than half a year.

DM: A 29 year-old female (Case 3) visited our clinic for helio-trope-like eruptions on the sun-exposed areas including upper eye-lids, cheeks and V-neck area (Fig. 3a), swollen fingers with periungual hemorrhage of the hands (Fig. 3b) and myalgia of the upper extremities. The examination revealed a rise of AST and ALT (65 and 46 U/L; WNL: 35-11 and 39-6, respectively), CK 883 U/L and ADL 11.2 IU/L, but no auto-Abs including ANA, anti- SSA and SSB Abs were found. No internal malignancies were found. However, a biopsy from left biceps muscle revealed the typical myositis with intersititial vascular infiltration (Fig. 4a). The immunochemistry of infiltrated cells around the interstitial vessels of the muscle tissue revealed $CD4^{+}$> $CD8^{+}$> $CD68^{+}$ cells and little of $CD20^{+}$ cells as similarly seen in the cutaneous findings of Case 1 (Fig.4b). We made a diagnosis of early stage of DM.

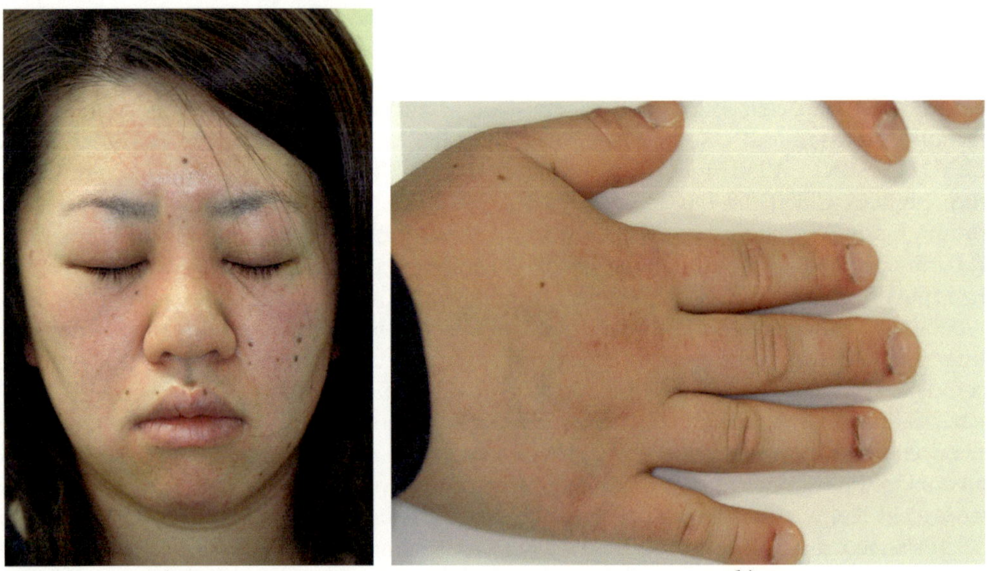

a) b)

Fig. 3. a) A 29 year-old female with dermatomyositis (DM) (Case 3). Swollen helio-trope-like erthema on the upper eye-lids and cheeks. b) Swollen erythema on the dorsa of the hands and periungual hamorrhage of the fingers.

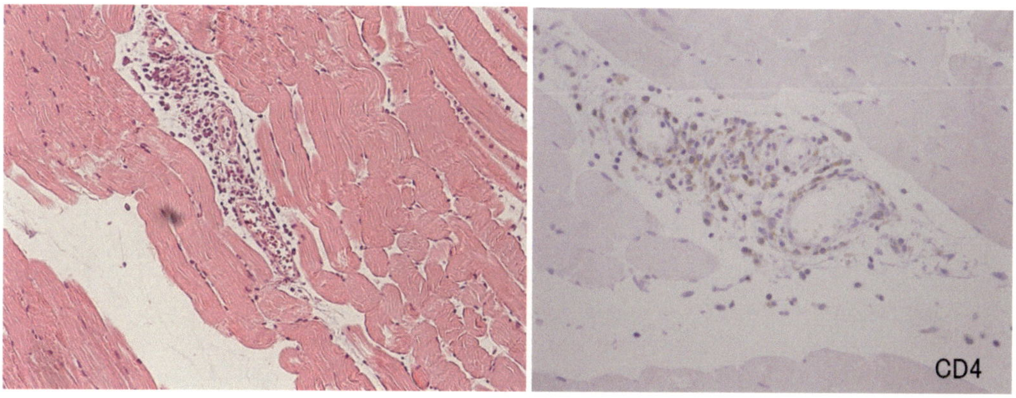

a) b)

Fig. 4. a) A biopsy specimen of muscle tissue from the left biceps muscle of patient with dermatomyositis (DM) (Case 3). Lymphoid cell infiltration around the vessels was found in the interstitial tissue (HE, 200x). b) Immunohistology of $CD4^{+}$T cells in the interstitial perivascular infiltration of the biceps muscle (Avidin-biotin stain, 20x). The infiltrated cells are $CD4^{+}$>$CD8^{+}$>$CD56^{+}$ mononuclear cells.

A 66 years old man (Case 8) was referred to our clinic for sudden episode of helio-trope-like colored erythematous eruption on the sun-exposed areas including the face, V-neck area, upper back and upper extremities associated with "myopathy" exhibiting muscle weakness and myalgia (Fig. 5). The patient had heavily smoked cigarettes a pack or more a day. He was initially suspected to have photosensitive dermatitis due to some photosensitizer and/ or DM and the examinations including skin and muscle biopsy from left-upper arm were performed. Laboratory examinations revealed WBC 11,070 / μl, RBC 327 x 10^4 / μl , CRP 14.28 mg/dL (WNL: 0.30), WNL of serum transaminases (AST and ALT), high levels of CK 1,706 U/L (WNL: 259-2.5) , ALD 8.2 IU/L (WNL: 5.6-2.5), myoglobulin-U 29.7 ng/mg (WNL: 10~0) and KL-6 1876 U/mL (WNL: 499-0). The titers of auto-Abs showed WNL as to anti-DNA, anti-Jo-1, anti-RNP, Sm, and anti-SSA and anti-SSB Abs except for ANA 20x (speckled type). Although CEA, CA15-3, AFP-L3, -L2,-L2, 3 and CA602 were negative, we suspected the patient might have an association with lung carcinoma after the chest X-ray and CT examination. The skin histology of the helio-trope-like erythema revealed as SLE-like findings exhibiting liquefaction degeneration of the D-E junction and edema of the upper dermis with a little lymphoid cell infiltration (Fig. 6) and immunohistologically, IgG, IgM and complement C3 were linearly deposited at the D-E junction. The muscle biopsy from the biceps of the left arm exhibiting myalgia shows a tiny interstitial perivascular infiltration between the muscle bundles, suggesting "myositis", although obvious muscular-degeneration was not found. The symptoms of the skin rash and myalgia of the extemities were improved temporary after treatment with oral PSL and NSAIDs. However, the patient died by lung cancer 2 years after his first visit to our clinic.

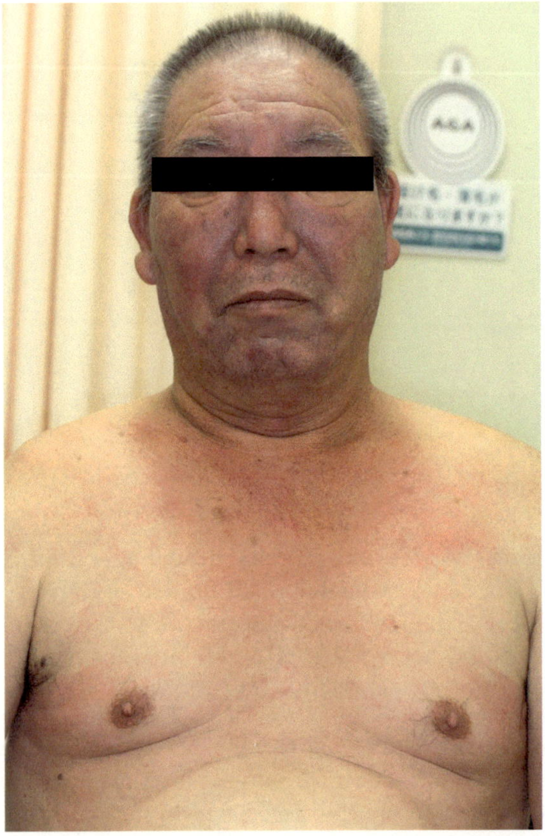

Fig. 5. A 66 years old patient with DM (Case 8) associated with lung cancer. Helio-trope-like erythema can be seen on the face and upper breast (so-called sun exposed areas).

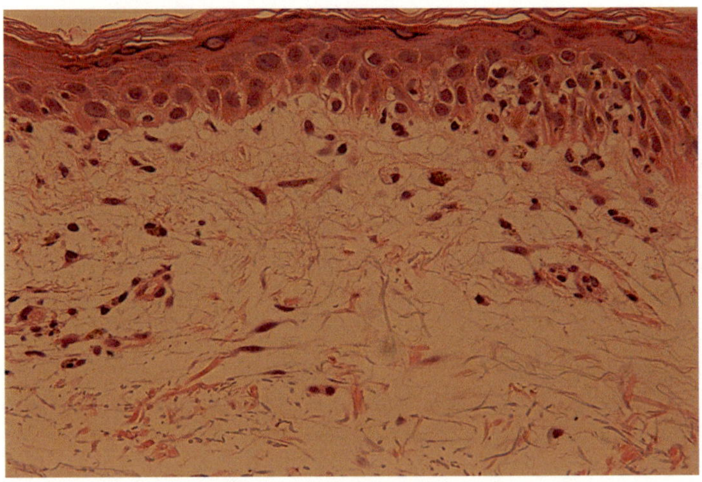

Fig. 6. A biopsy specimen of the helio-trope-like erythema from the upper chest. Liquefaction degeneration can be seen at the D-E junction and edema and a few lymphoid cell infiltration are present in the upper dermis (HE, 200x).

3. Discussion

It is rare to see the cases of pSjS with myalgia in Japan, but about 30 % of pSjS patients are reported to be associated with muscle involvement known as fibromyalgia in US and European countries (5, 6). The main cutaneous involvement is purpura, annular shaped erythema and/or macules, erythematous papules and ischemic ulcers due to microvasculitis in pSjS (7, 8). In this patient (Case 1 in Table 2), the cutaneous eruptions including the swollen and helio-trope-like colored erythema on the eye-lids, thin-reddish macules on the limbs, purpuric spots and Gottron's papule-like eruption on the dorsa of the fingers were recognized and quickly disappeared after administration with low dose of PSL. Although the clinical signs-like DM did not reappear by the treatment, the continuous treatment with PSL seems to be still needed. As reported that this disorder is a bothersome and slowly progressive disease (10-12), we should follow the clinical course whether the patient might develop lymphoproliferative disorders in a near future because the enlargement of the lymphnode and hepatosplenomegaly was noted initially. Regarding Case 2, the clinical symptoms and laboratory examination were suggestive of DM associated with SjS without the skin manifestations. We considered him as having pSjS associated with myopathy because dry-eye symptoms, positive anti-SSA Ab and no cutaneous symptom of DM were noted. Although these 2 cases of pSjS were associated with myalgia, the cause of their myopathy is not clear because no inflammation was found in the biopy specimens from their biceps muscle. However, it is reported that the myopathy might be due to small-vessel injury by auto-Abs or circulating immune complexes because electrondence deposits were noted (13). As to the infiltrated cells around the vessels in the cutaneous lesion, the $CD4^+$ T cells were dominant as similar to the findings in myositis of patients with DM.

DM is an idiopathic inflammatory disorder characterized by inflammatory myopathy, indicating myositis, and skin manifestations and it can be associated with the secondary SjS sometimes. The etiology is still unknown and the prevalence is estimated as 1-10 cases per million population, but in children 3.2 cases per million which are distributed in the whole world (3). The clinical types of DM are classified in Table 3 and the internal malignancies are frequently associated in the adult type of DM. The risk is reported to be a 6.5-fold higher than ordinary persons after 45 years of age (14). Regarding myopathy in DM patients it might be characterized by inflammatory myopathy progressing to myositis and degeneration of muscle fibers, and the helio-trope-like eruptions on the sun-exposed areas showed SLE-like changes histologically. On the other hand, there are the cases associated without myogenic symptoms in DM, which is called as "amyopathic DM" (DM sine myositis). However, these cases should be considered as "pre-myopathic DM" because they might Be rather early diagnosed (15). Though the direct cause of myopathy is still unknown, there are some pathogeneses reported, such as the presences of myositis- specific auto-Abs (15,16) and inflammatory cytokines from T cells including interleukin (IL)-17 and IL-23 in early stage of patients with DM (18). The study regarding Th1/Th2 balance showed that Th2 cell predominance was suggested in patients with active stage of DM (19). In plasma of patients with DM and/or polymyositis, microparticles derived from $CD14^+$ mononuclear cells, $CD3^+$ T cells and $CD19^+$ B cells were found to be elevated by electron microscopic examination, which suggests these diseases were immunological disorders (20). It is reported that $CD19^+CD23^+$ cells are increased and that $CD4^+CD45RO^+$ cells are decreased in the peripheral blood of patients with DM, suggesting reduction of regulatory T cells (21). It was also suggested that $CD4^+CD25^+$ cells, forkhead/winged helix transcription factor (Fox P3)$^+$, transforming growth factor$^+$ and IL-10$^+$ cells were reduced in peripheral blood of patients with DM (21). Actually, $CD4^+CD8^+$ cells were significantly distributed around vessels in the interstitial tissues of the muscle bundles in our patients with DM. These cells might be $CD4^+$CD 28^+ (null) cells and $CD8^+CD28^+$ (null) cell infiltration, as reported, and it is of interest that circulating $CD4^+CD28^+$ cells and $CD8^+CD28^+$ cells were significantly increased in seropositive individuals, responded to human cytomegalovirus antigen stimulation and correlated with disease duration (22).

As to treatment for myopathy of patients with pSjS and DM, adequate doses of NSAIDs and/or oral steroids were mainly used in corresponding to their clinical severities and these were considered to be effective. However, in addition to these drugs, the combination with immunosuppressive agents such as azathioprine, cyclosporine, mycophenolate or methotrexate should be used for the autoimmune diseases, if they were not clinically controlled. The biological agent, rituximab, and tacrolimus may offer additional benefit to some patients and emerging agents against T cells, B cells, transmigration or transduction molecules may be discussed as New treatments (23).

4. Conclusion

Myopathies are neuromuscular disorders exhibiting myalgia and muscular weakness due to dysfunction of muscle fibers which are frequently seen in autoimmune diseases. We here discussed about the non-inflammatory myopathy seen in patients with pSjS and the inflammatory myopathy, that is myositis, found in patients with DM is suggested to be Immunological dysfunction in pathogenesis. Although the mechanism of the myopathy is still unclear, it might be due to inflammatory cytokines released from $CD4^+$CD 28^+ (null) cells and $CD8^+CD28^+$ (null) cells infiltrated around vessels in the muscles of patients with MD.

5. Abbreviations

Ab, antibody; ALD, aldolase; ANA, anti-nuclear antibody; anti-SSA Ab, anti- Sjögren's syndrome A Ab; anti-SSB Ab, anti- Sjögren's syndrome B Ab; CK, creatine kinase; D-E junction, dermo-epidermal junction; DM, dermatomyositis; IL, interleukin; NSAID, non-steroidal anti-inflammatory drug; pSjS, primary Sjögren's syndrome; PSL, prednisolone; VAS, visual analog scale; WNL, within normal limit

6. References

[1] NINDS Myopathy Information Page: What is myopathy?, National Institute of Health, USA, December 10, 2010.

[2] Saito S, Togashi A, Kaneko F, Yamamoto T, Uchida T, Oyama N: Primary Sjögren's syndrome with myalgia mimicking dermatomyositis. J Dermatol 2010; 37: 837-839.

[3] Koler RA, Montemarano A: Dermatomyositis, Am Farm Physician 2001; 64: 1565-1573.

[4] Tishler M, Barak Y, Paran D, Yaron M. Sleep disturbances, fibromyalgia and primary Sjögren's syndrome. Clin Exp Rheumatol 1997; 15: 71-74.

[5] Pendarvis WT, Pillemer SR. Widespread pain and Sjögren's syndrome. J Rheumatol 2001; 28: 2657-2659.

[6] Lindvall B, Bengtsson A, Ernerudh J, Eriksson P. Subclinical myositis is common in primary Sjögren's syndrome and is related to muscle pain. J Rheumatol 2002; 29: 7-7-25.

[7] Eriksson P, Andersson C, Ekerfelt C, et al. Sjögren's syndrome with myalgia associated with subnormal secretion of cytokines by peripheral blood mononuclear cells. J Rheumatol 2004; 31: 729-735.

[8] Ramos-Casals M, Anaya J-M, Garcia-Carrasco M, et al. Cutaneous vasculitis in primary Sjögren syndrome-classification and clinical significance of 52 patients. Medicine 2004; 83: 96-106.

[9] Drake LA, Dinehart SM, Farma ER, Goltz RW, Graham GF, Hordinski MK, et al.: Guidlines of care of dermatomyositis, J Am Acad Dermatol 1996; 34: 824-829.

[10] Molina R, Provost TT, Alexander EL. Two histopathologic prototypes of inflammatory vascular disease in Sjögren's syndrome: Differential association with seroactivity to rheumatoid factor and antibodies to Ro (SS-A) and with hypocomplementemia. Arthritis Rheum 1985; 28: 1251-1258.

[11] Theander E, Anderson SI, Manthorpe R, Jacobson LT. Proposed core set of outcome measures in patients with primary Sjögren's syndrome:5 year follow up. J Rheumatol 2005; 32: 1495-1502.

[12] Champey J, Corruble E, Gottenberg JE, et al. Quality of life and psychological status in patients with primary Sjögren's syndrome and sicca symptoms without autoimmune features. Arthritis Rheum 2006; 55: 451-457.

[13] Ringle SP, Forestot JZ, Tan EM, Wehling C, Griggs RC, Butcher D. Sjögren's syndrome and polymyositis or dermatomyosistis. Arch Neurol 1982; 39: 157-163.

[14] Airio A, Pukkala E, Isomaki H. Elevated cancer incidence in patients with dermatomyositis: a population based study. J Rheumatol 1995; 22: 1300-1303.

[15] Gerami P, Schope JM, McDonald L, Walling HW, Sontheimer RD. A systemic review of adult-onset clinically amyopathic dermatomyositis (dermatomyosistitis sine myositis): a missing link within the spectrum of the idiopathic inflammatory myopathies. J Am Acad Dermatol 2006; 54: 597-613.

[16] Mammen AL. Dermatomyositis and polymyositis: clinical presentation, autoantibodies and pathogenesis. Ann N Y Acad Soc 2010; Jan: 1184; 134-153.

[17] Gherardi RK. Pathogenic aspects of dermatomyositis and overlap myositis. Press Med 2011; Apr: 40: e209-218.

[18] Shen H, Xia L, Lu J, Xiao W. Interleukin-17 and interleukin-23 in patients with polymyositis and dermatomyositis. Scand J Rheumatol 2011; 40: 217-220.

[19] Ishii W, Matsuda M, Shimojima Y, Iyoh S, Sumida T, Ikeda S. Flow cytometric analysis of lymphocyte subpopulations and Th1/Th2 balance in patients with polymyositis and dermatomyositis. Internal Medicine 2008; 47: 1593-1599.

[20] Baka Z, Senolt L, Vencovsky J, Mann IT, Simon PS, Kiltel A, Buzas E, Nagy G. Increase serum concentration of immune cell derived microparticles in polymyosisitis/ dematomyositis. Immunol Lett 2010; 128: 124-130.

[21] Antiga E, Kretz CC, Klembt R, Massi D, Ruland V. Characterization of regulatory T cells in patients with dermatomyositis. J Autoimmun 2010; 35: 342-350.

[22] Fasth AE, Dastmaich M, Rahbar A, Saiomonsson S, Pandya JM, Lindroos E, Nennesmo I, Malmberg KJ, Soderberg-Naucler C, Trollmo C, Lundberg IE, Malmstrom V. T cell infiltrates in the muscles of patients with dermatomyositis and polymyositis are dominated by CD28null T cells. J Immunol 2009; 183: 4792-4799.
[23] Dalakas MC. Immunotherapy of inflammatory myopathies: practical approach and future prospects. Curr Treat Options Neurol 2011; 13: 311-323.

7

Dermatomyositis

Fred van Gelderen
Radiology Department, Dunedin Hospital, Southern District Health Board & Clinical Senior Lecturer, University of Otago, Dunedin, New Zealand

1. Introduction

1.1 Dermatomyositis is an autoimmune inflammatory myopathy with diffuse nonsuppurative inflammation of the skin and striated muscles. {In polymyositis, skeletal muscles only are involved.]

1.2 The disease is uncommon, occurs twice as often in female patients, and most present between 40 and 60 years of age, with a smaller peak between the ages of 5 and 15. There is a two-to-seven fold increase in the frequency of malignancy, especially in older patients in the adult age group (about 21% for dermatomyositis and 15% for polymyositis) (Hansell, et al., 2005).

2. Clinical features

2.1 Nomenclature and classification

These different classifications are included:

2.1.1 Polymyositis and dermatomyositis (Hansell, et al., 2005)

- Primary idiopathic polymyositis
- Primary idiopathic dermatomyositis
- Amyopathic dermatomyositis
- Polymyositis/dermatomyositis associated with:
    i. malignant disease
    ii. other collagen vascular disease (overlap syndrome)
- Polymyositis/dermatomyositis of childhood

2.1.2 Inflammatory disease of muscle (Resnick & Kransdorf, 2005)

Idiopathic inflammatory myopathies:

- Polymyositis
- Dermatomyositis
- Juvenile (childhood) dermatomyositis

- Myositis associated with malignancy
- Inclusion body myositis

Other inflammatory myopathies:

- Myositis associated with eosinophilia
- Myositis ossificans
- Localized (focal) myositis
  Myopathies caused by infection
  Myopathies caused by drugs and toxins

2.1.3 Further classification (Resnick & Kransdorf, 2005)

Type I. Typical polymyositis (most common, 35% of patients)

Type II. Typical dermatomyositis (25% of patients)

Type III. Typical dermatomyositis with malignancy. (Malignancy occurs in 15-25%)

Type IV. Childhood dermatomyositis (20% of patients)

Type V. Acute myolysis (3% of patients)

Type VI. Polymyositis in Sjögren's syndrome and other connective tissue diseases (5%).

2.2.1 The most constant clinical finding is muscle weakness, the initial symptom in about 50% of patients. (Resnick & Kransdorf, 2005). Symmetric involvement of the proximal muscles is most characteristic. Clinical presentation may be with an acute, subacute or chronic illness, with progressive symmetric weakness of the girdle and neck muscles. In the acute form, muscle pain and tenderness are common features. Low grade fever and fatigue are further manifestations.

2.2.2 In children the acute form is more common with clinical features of fever, joint pain, lymphadenopathy, splenomegaly and subcutaneous oedema. The skin changes tend to be very severe, and prognosis is poor.

2.2.3 In adults the onset is often more insidious with periods of spontaneous remission. On relapse, skin changes are the first symptom in 25% of patients. These are more severe and more frequent in children. There are no skin changes in polymyositis, however, in dermatomyositis the changes are characteristic, with a heliotrope periorbital rash and violaceous/red papular rash over bony prominences.

2.2.4 In addition to the typical proximal muscle weakness and the skin rash, the raised muscle enzymes and characteristic electromyography and muscle biopsy, also contribute to characteristic clinical criteria.

2.2.5 Further clinical features include: Arthralgia and arthritis, with typical symmetrical involvement of the small joints of the fingers, the wrists and the knees. Permanent involvement is uncommon.

2.2.6.1 Visceral involvement due to dermatomyositis may include pharyngeal and oesophageal symptoms with dysphagia, pulmonary disease due to respiratory muscle weakness with aspiration pneumonia and/or interstitial lung disease. (Pulmonary involvement occurs in 50% of patients and contributes directly to death in about 10% of patients.)

2.2.6.2 Other systemic involvement includes myocardial disease, pericarditis, renal, neurological and ocular abnormalities.

2.2.7 In addition to typical muscular involvement with bilateral symmetric superficial oedema and palpable sheetlike confluent calcifications, especially in the thigh muscles, there may also be pointing and resorption of the terminal tufts of the fingers with distal soft tissue loss. The 'floppy-thumb' sign has been described as a common feature (Resnick & Kransdorf, 2005).

2.2.8 The aforementioned clinical features may be readily diagnosed on physical examination of the patient.

2.3 After effective treatment for dermatomyositis, the soft tissue oedema may decrease or disappear altogether, though fibrosis, muscle atrophy and contractures may become apparent in the later stages of the disease. With constant aggressive prednisone treatment, the development of progressive muscular weakness, contractures and disabling calcifications occur in less than 20% of patients with childhood dermatomyositis (Hesla, et al, 1990).

2.4 Polymyositis/dermatomyositis may precede, accompany or follow malignant disease, though usually found within one year of diagnosis. The course of the myopathy often follows the course of the malignancy, improving when the malignancy is treated, and increasing with relapse, suggesting that it is a true paraneoplastic symptom (Hansell, et al., 2005). There is an increased prevalence of malignant neoplasms of the breast, prostate, lung, ovary, gastrointestinal tract and kidney (Dähnert, 2007).

2.5.1 Furthermore for many patients, the manifestations of the disease process are incompatible with a single diagnosis. These patients appear to have more than one collagen vascular disease, and the diagnosis of an overlap syndrome (mixed connective tissue disease) is suggested to correlate the diverse clinical, imaging and laboratory findings. As many as 85% of patients with connective tissue disease may be included in this category. The existence of this entity is not universally accepted (Resnick & Kransdorf, 2005).

2.5.2 The overlap syndrome includes features similar to dermatomyositis, scleroderma, lupus erythematosus and rheumatoid arthritis, although Sjögren's syndrome and polyarteritis nodosa could also be included.

2.6 There is no cure for dermatomyositis, but the symptoms can be treated. Options include medication (e.g. corticosteroids or immunoglobulins), physical treatment (e.g. removal of calcium deposits that may cause nerve pain and recurrent infections), exercise, heat treatment, orthotics and assisting devices, and rest.

2.7 Other inflammatory diseases of muscles (Resnick & Kransdorf, 2005) include

2.7.1 Inclusion body myositis, occurs more often in men older than 55 years, the clinical findings resemble those of polymyositis, but there are distinctive microscopic findings with inclusion bodies noted.

2.7.2 Focal nodular myositis is a benign inflammatory muscle disorder, mostly affecting the thigh or lower extremity, and patients present with a painful, localised intramuscular mass. The histology of the small nodules or pseudotumours is similar to polymyositis, and the disease may progress to a more generalised distribution typical of polymyositis.

2.7.3 Eosinophilic myositis may present with an eosinophilic inflammatory infiltrate in skeletal muscle as a localised disorder, or as a generalised disease.

2.7.4 Drug-related myositis may vary from acute inflammatory changes to chronic fibrosis, the latter may appear as a consequence of direct intramuscular injection of drugs in the deltoid or quadriceps muscles. Alcohol, aspirin, penicillin and sulphonamides may also lead to myopathic changes.

3. Case reports

Three cases are included to highlight diverse and protean manifestations, also to demonstrate specific radiological investigations, with more advanced and specific tests for dermatomyositis now being available at many larger centres.

3.1 Case 1

A 17-year-old teenager was known to have dermatomyositis, having been diagnosed in 1978 at age 13. He had been treated since that time with prednisone (corticosteroid), alas, with little improvement. In 1981 he was referred for chest and pelvis X-rays, with increasing weakness, atrophy and contractures of the upper extremities. He furthermore experienced loss of strength in his legs and neck. The patient had extensive skin changes consistent with dermatomyositis and in addition was very emaciated. No clinical history of tuberculosis was elicited. The PA (posteroanterior) chest X-ray (Fig. 1a) demonstrated minimal left basal areas of opacification due to active lung disease; infective, inflammatory or due to aspiration. Hairline thickness fibrotic changes were identified in the left upper lobe due to longstanding disease, probably previous tuberculosis.

In the left supraclavicular region, the skin was noted to be retracted with soft tissue loss, and a subtle 2 cm long thin linear calcification was detected. (Fig.1b, magnified image). This finding is most suggestive of dermatomyositis, whereas the pulmonary changes are non-specific. [These images predate readily available high-resolution CT (computed tomography) of the chest.]

An AP (anteroposterior) view of the pelvis (Fig. 1c) demonstrated minimal and subtle calcification of the inner upper thighs, however, the diagnosis of dermatomyositis with multiple coarse linear calcifications overlying the outer aspect of the left iliac bone was clinched by observing this latter feature. There was an undisplaced fracture of the medial part of the left superior pubic ramus; this observation was unrelated to the known dermatomyositis.

3.2 Case 2

A 41-year-old woman with known dermatomyositis for many years (though not known whether she had had dermatomyositis as a child) was referred for radiographs of the chest, hands and thighs. She presented with cellulitis/myositis of the posterior aspect of the left thigh, with a possible abscess, despite 1 week of treatment with antibiotics. A shell of curvilinear calcification was noted around the chest on the PA chest radiograph (Fig. 2a). Predominant calcification was seen of the lateral chest wall, the axillary region and within the neck, superior and parallel to the first rib, with bilateral changes. Some tramline-like calcifications were detected overlying the peripheral midzones on both sides, thereby mimicking pleural or pulmonary parenchymal disease. However, these rather coarse calcifications were situated in the superficial soft tissue and superimposed on the lung fields. No bony abnormality was observed. No cardiac or pulmonary abnormalities were detected.

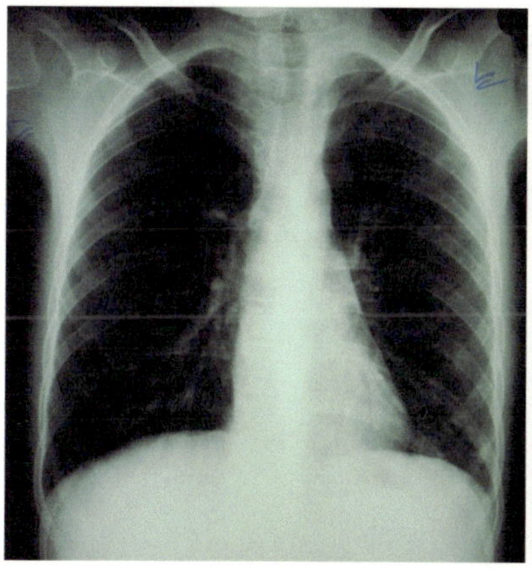

a.

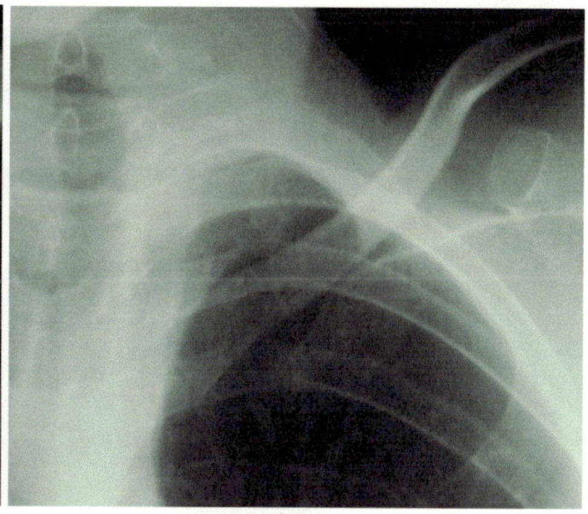

b.

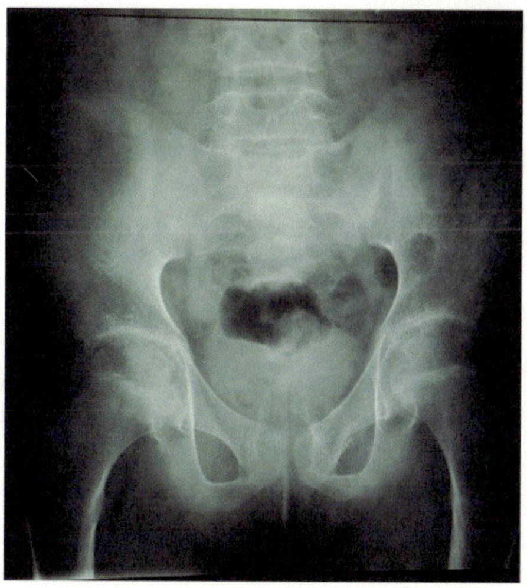

c.

Fig. 1. a.,b.,c. Case 1. A 17-year-old teenager with known dermatomyositis was referred for chest and pelvis radiographs. There is slight left based patchy opacification. Furthermore there is a minimal linear calcification of the left side of the neck (Fig. 1a,b). (Fig. 1b is a magnified image to demonstrate the calcification). The AP pelvis X-ray demonstrates extensive linear plaque-like calcification overlying the outer aspect of the left iliac bone (Fig. 1c). The radiological features correlate exactly with the clinical diagnosis of dermatomyositis.

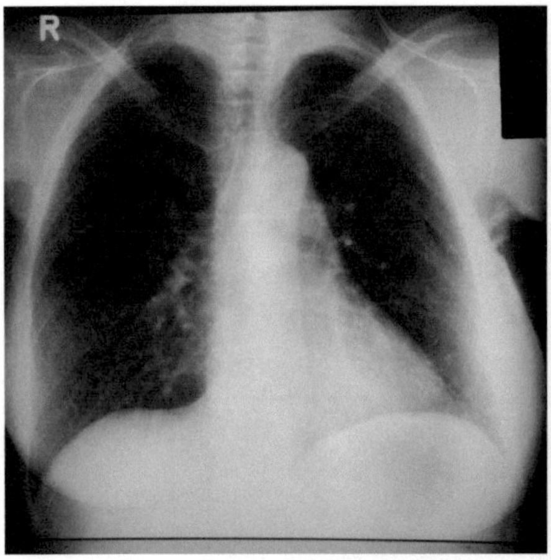

a.

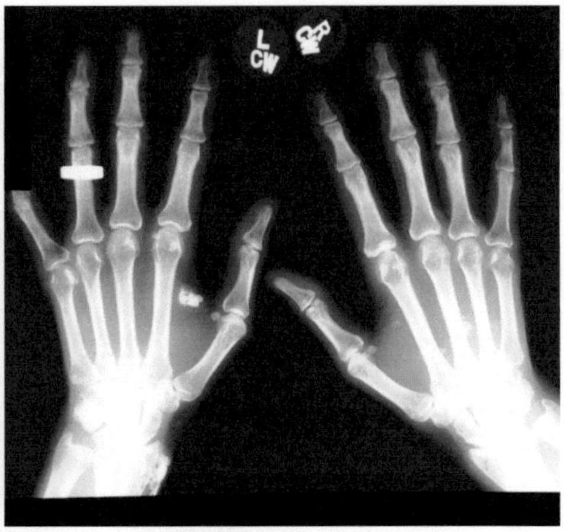

b.

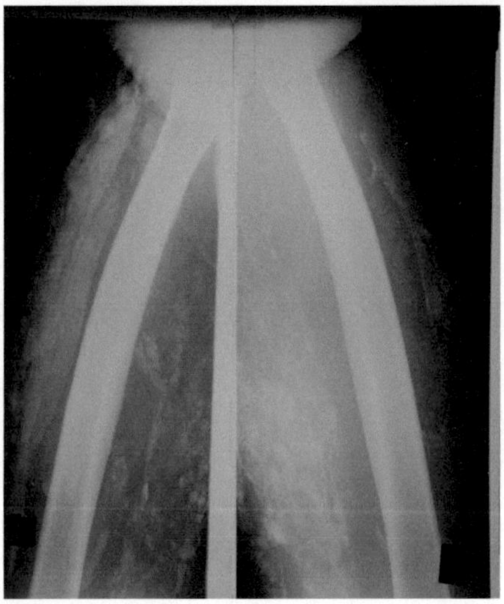

c.

Fig. 2. a.-c. Case 2. A 41-year-old woman with known clinical manifestations of dermatomyositis was referred for radiographs of the chest, hands, and thighs. Ultrasound of the thighs was also performed. The PA chest X-ray demonstrates a thick shell of plaque-like calcifications within the superficial soft tissue (Fig. 2a). The PA radiograph of the hands shows more discrete and dense calcific areas, and also soft tissue loss relating to the tips of some of the fingers (Fig. 2b). Radiography of the thighs reveals multiple dense calcified plaques involving the muscles of both thighs (Fig. 2c).

A PA radiograph of the hands (Fig. 2b) demonstrated a number of discrete, yet heavily calcified, foci in the soft tissue, involving both wrist areas (especially overlying the distal radius), intermetacarpal in position, and even more marked relating to the webspace between the left 1st and 2nd metacarpals. Juxtaarticular osteopaenia was noted, but no erosive articular changes were seen. Loss of soft tissue relating to the terminal tufts of the distal phalanges was detected, especially affecting the index fingers.

Layered dense plaques of calcification were observed relating to both thighs, both in the skin and in the deeper tissues, more extensive on the left posteriorly (Fig 2c). Ultrasound examination (US) of both thighs confirmed extensive subcutaneous and intermuscular plaque-like calcifications with marked shadowing from the superficial calcifications (Fig. 2d). Within the deeper tissues of the left thigh posteriorly, a flattered tubular, anechoic area was noted, with a long fluid level and high level echoes below the level (Fig. 2e). The hyperechoic material below the level was disturbed with transducer pressure. When the examination was subsequently continued in the erect position, a shorter fluid calcium level formed, along the short dimension of the collection.

The above features were reported as a fluid-calcium level because of the known dermatomyositis, but as the area was tender, a localized intermuscular abscess could not be excluded. Aspiration of the lesion yielded sterile, yellowish-white fluid with the consistency of toothpaste. After aspiration the signs and symptoms relating to the left thigh resolved and the patient made an uneventful recovery.

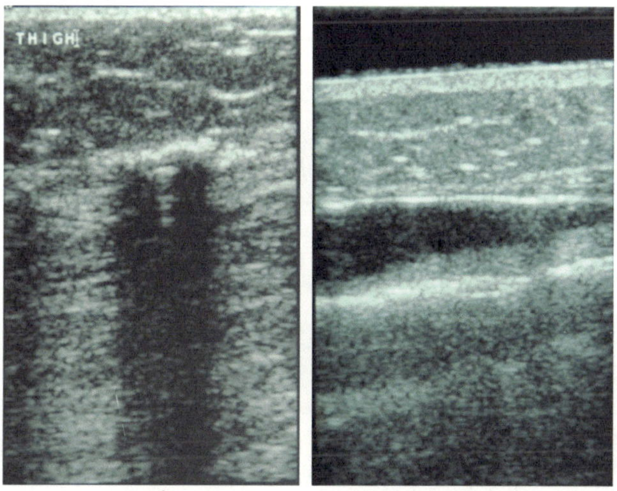

d. e.

Fig. 2. d.-e. Case 2. US of the thighs again demonstrates the superficial plaques with typical shadowing consistent with calcification. Fig. 2d shows the US appearance of the right thigh. Within the deep tissue on the left side, with the patient in the prone position, a flattened anechoic area was detected with a long fluid level and high level echoes below this level, due to a fluid-calcium level (Fig. 2e).

3.3 Case 3

A 46-year-old woman presented with severe proximal muscle weakness. An electromyogram demonstrated an active myopathy with neurophysiologic features of marked myopathic changes in the right deltoid muscle.

The diagnosis of dermatomyositis was made due to concomitant skin changes. The patient had also had difficulty swallowing. A limited speech language therapy barium swallow was performed. No abnormality was detected, except for uncoordination and slight aspiration into the trachea (Fig. 3a). Subsequent chest radiographs and high-resolution CT of the chest did not reveal an abnormality. MRI (magnetic resonance imaging) of the brain did not demonstrate any abnormal features of consequence.

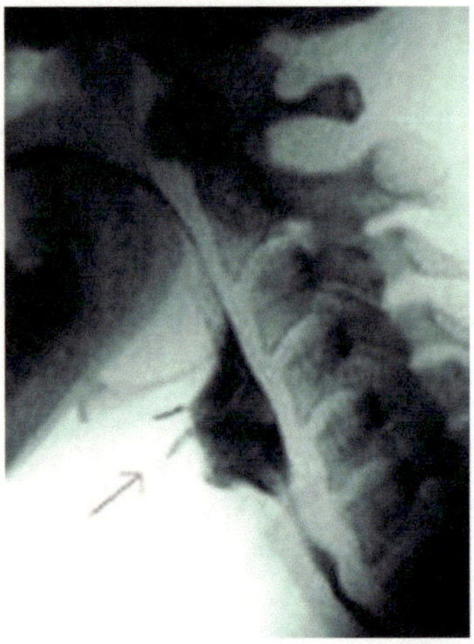

a.

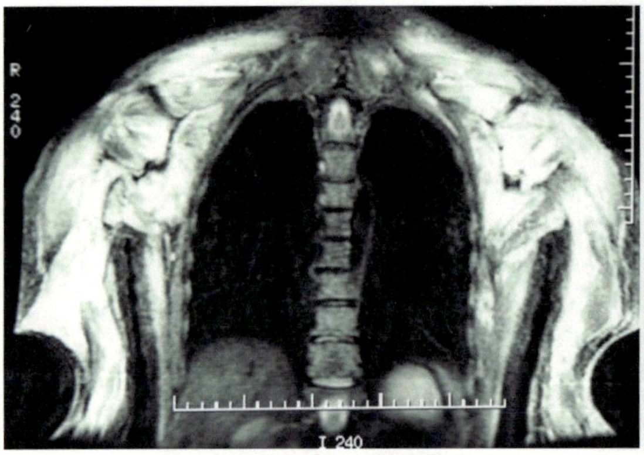

b.

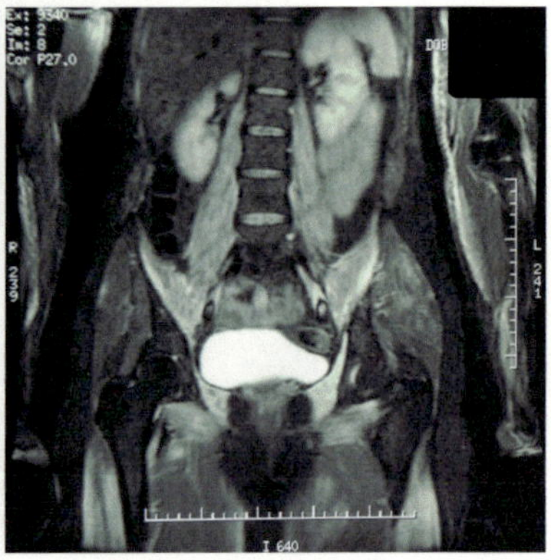

c.

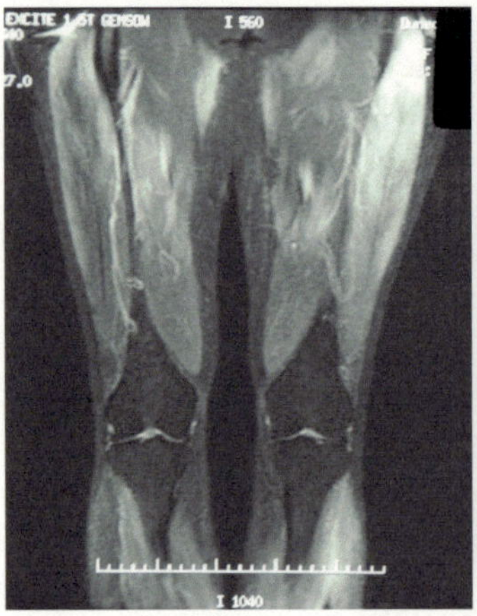

d.

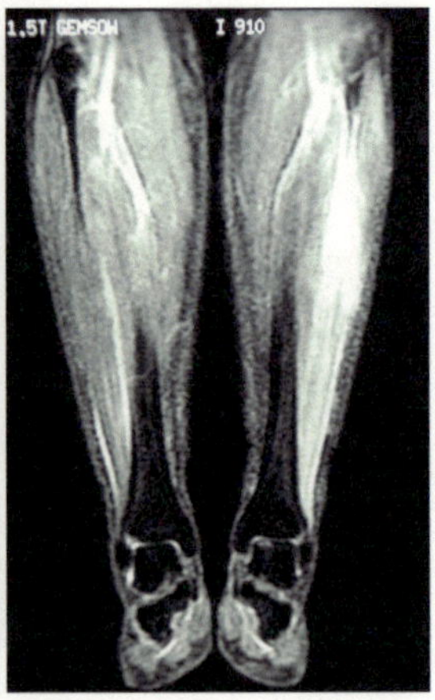

e.

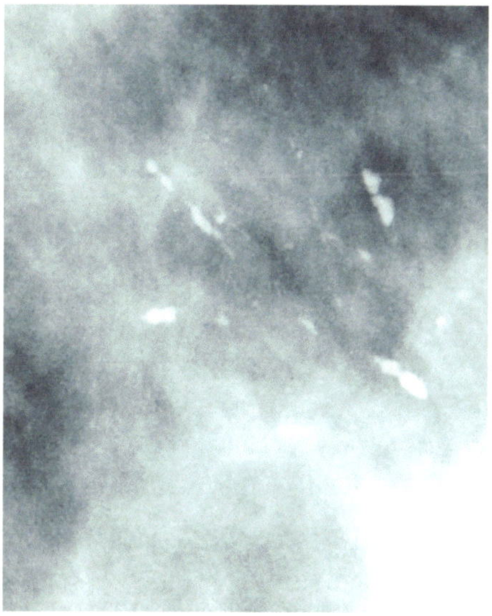

f.

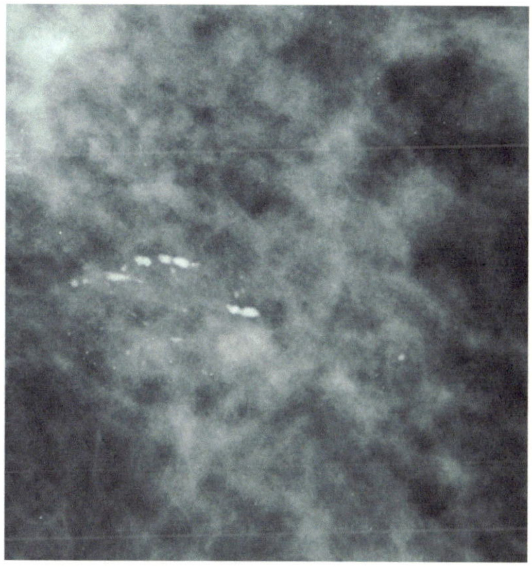

g.

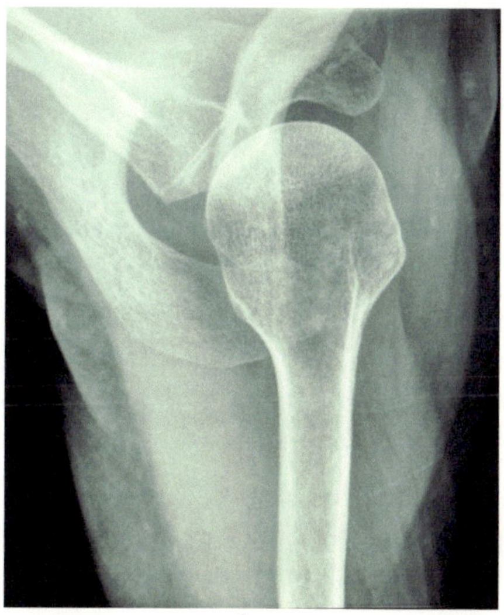

h.

Fig. 3. a.-h. Case 3. A 46-year-old woman was referred with typical skin lesions of dermatomyositis and dysphagia. A speech language therapy barium swallow reveals slight aspiration into the trachea (Fig. 3a). Four station STIR MRI (Fig. 3b-e) demonstrates features consistent with dermatomyositis, especially involving the shoulder girdles and trapezius muscles, the quadriceps musculature particularly the left vastus lateralis and the lateral head of the left gastrocnemius muscle. Subsequent X-ray mammography revealed a carcinoma in the superolateral quadrant of the left breast with typical minute malignant microcalcification (Fig. 3f,g). At the time of further follow-up, six years later, the patient experienced right shoulder girdle pain. No abnormality was demonstrated, except for a few small rounded superficial areas with faint rim calcification (Fig. 3h).

Four station whole body STIR (short tau inversion recovery) and T1-weighted MRI was performed on four occasions over a three year period. The later STIR MRI demonstrated more widespread low grade oedema within the muscles when compared to previous MRI. Initially the patient was treated with steroids, and later with methotrexate/plaquenil. The initial STIR MRI demonstrated marked increase in signal within the muscles of both shoulder girdles and trapezius muscles and to a lesser extent of the psoas muscles. Furthermore relatively symmetrical increased signal was noted in the quadriceps musculature, especially the left vastus lateralis. There was high signal intensity in the lateral head of the left gastrocnemius muscles. (Fig. 3b-e).

The patient had continued to be afflicted by severe dermatomyositis, with little response to treatment, and had had follow-up clinical management by the departments of rheumatology and neurology. There was concern that there might have been a concomitant underlying undetected malignancy; she had noted some tenderness of the left breast, though no lump had been palpable.

The patient was therefore referred for priority X-ray mammography and US of the breasts. Within the superolateral aspect of the left breast there was a group of dense linear casting type calcifications, but more concerning were some associated smaller, ill-defined, calcifications, the latter probably malignant. The magnification mediolateral oblique view (Fig. 3f) and craniocaudal view (Fig. 3g) demonstrated the microcalcifications to better advantage. No soft tissue mass, superficial skin thickening or retraction, or other features of malignancy were noted. US had not demonstrated a mass. Core biopsies were obtained of the calcifications under stereoradiographic guidance. The diagnosis of a carcinoma was confirmed and local excision of the tumour was performed (T_1 No, grade III). Following on surgery the patient developed infective changes of the superolateral quadrant of the left breast; these resolved with antibiotic treatment.

At a later stage the clinical diagnosis of a right ischial abscess had been considered, with the right buttock having become swollen, red and painful with point tenderness. However, US had demonstrated subcutaneous induration and oedema only (as compared to the opposite side) and no abscess or collection had been detected.

CT of the chest, abdomen and pelvis had not shown metastases from the breast carcinoma or other abnormality, except for postoperative appearances of the left breast. Specifically no soft tissue calcification had been seen relating to the subcutaneous tissues or muscles.

Six years after the initial diagnosis of dermatomyositis, the patient had experienced tightness and aching of the right shoulder girdle. Radiography of the shoulder had not revealed a bony abnormality or supraspinatus tendon calcification. However, multiple, small, rounded peripherally calcified lesions had been detected especially on the axial view of the shoulder (Fig. 3h). One of the larger calcifications anterior to the shoulder had measured 6 mm in long axis. These had been thought to be due to early changes of dermatomyositis, though rather atypical in shape and configuration.

At the same time as the shoulder pain, a palpable lump had been discovered clinically in the lateral part of the right breast. MRI, before and after the intravenous administration of 20 cc of gadolinium, had demonstrated the post surgical appearances of the left breast, and in addition a very small 4 mm simple cyst within the superolateral quadrant of the right breast.

Therefore, six years after the initial diagnosis of left breast cancer and dermatomyositis, no further malignant disease had been detected. The clinical and radiological features of dermatomyositis, however, had not improved, and appeared to be refractory to treatment, as had been shown at multiple follow-up STIR MRI.

4. Radiographic abnormalities

4.1 Musculoskeletal system

4.1.1 Soft tissue abnormalities

4.1.1.1 Soft tissue calcifications may be preceded by oedema of the subcutaneous tissue and muscle, causing increased muscular bulk and radiodensity, thickening of subcutaneous septa and poor definition of the subcutaneous tissue-muscle interface. These features may be detected on radiographs specifically exposed to show soft tissue to better advantage. Present day digital radiography generally shows the soft tissue far more optimally, as compared to film radiography, and even an incidental diagnosis of subtle changes of dermatomyositis may be established more readily with modern digital imaging (Fig. 3h). CT is more sensitive than MRI for demonstrating soft tissue calcifications, however, CT is rarely indicated.

4.1.1.2 The changes are more prominent in the proximal musculature, axilla, chest wall, forearms, thighs and calves (Fig. 3b-e).

4.1.1.3 Following on effective treatment, the soft tissue oedema may decrease or disappear entirely. However, fibrosis, muscle atrophy and contractures may develop later. There tends to be decreased soft tissue and muscular bulk, increased translucency of the soft tissue, osteopaenia, calcification and sometimes eventual contractures.

4.1.1.4 Soft tissue calcification occurs in 30—70% of children and 10% of adults, and may occur within the first year of the illness (Moses, 2008). The extent of calcification, especially within the muscles, appears to increase with the severity of the illness. Small or large calcareous intramuscular fascial plane calcification is distinctive of dermatomyositis and polymyositis, though subcutaneous calcification is more common. The large muscles of the proximal parts of the extremities are more frequently affected. Sheetlike confluent calcifications especially occur in the thigh (particularly the vastus lateralis) (Fig. 2c), the pelvic girdle, the upper extremity (deltoid muscles, especially), and the flexor muscles of the neck. Further areas include the elbows, knees, hands, chest and abdominal wall, axillary and inguinal regions.

4.1.1.5 There are four distinct patterns of soft tissue calcifications that occur in childhood dermatomyositis; deep calcareous masses, superficial calcareous masses, deep linear deposits and lacy, reticular, subcutaneous collections that encase the torso. The deep deposits are more commonly encountered (Resnick & Kransdorf, 2005).

4.1.1.6 The amorphous calcifications of dermatomyositis should be differentiated from the bone formation in myositis ossificans, where native bone with immature trabecular bone centrally surrounded by compact bone may be seen.

4.1.1.7.1 The term 'milk of calcium' has been used to describe calcium-laden fluid collections in the gall bladder and kidney and more recently by US, in the soft tissue of the subcutaneous and intermuscular regions of the thigh and calf in two patients with childhood dermatomyositis (Hesla, et al., 1990). Case 2 (Fig. 2e) presents similar features except that fluid-calcium layering (the sedimentation sign) was also demonstrated with an unusually long level indicating the flattened elongated shape of the collection. There was also localized tenderness and this prompted aspiration, even though from a US point of view the fluid-calcium level militated against a soft-tissue abscess.

4.1.1.7.2 Complications of diagnostic and therapeutic aspiration of such collections include introducing secondary infection and secondly the formation of a chronic sinus tract. The latter could result especially if a large bore needle was used to penetrate the frequently hard, brittle subcutaneous calcified tissues. If possible, formal surgical incision and drainage should therefore also be avoided.

4.1.1.7.3 Most conventional radiographic studies fail to show the layering as they are not taken with a horizontal ray beam.

4.1.1.7.4 The diagnosis of fluid-calcium layering can also be established by CT or MRI, when associated bony changes can also be assessed. However, in the absence of skeletal changes on conventional radiographs, US is thought to be more expeditious, less expensive, readily available and no ionizing radiation is involved, especially in childhood dermatomyositis. (Van Gelderen, 2007).

4.1.1.8 Abnormal accumulation of technetium polyphosphate in affected muscle (nuclear medicine study) was a useful technique, however this has now been superceded by MRI, with MRI more accurate and not employing ionizing radiation. Signal intensity would alternate according to the activity of the disease, and therefore changes in the signal pattern were useful to monitor response to treatment. MRI may allow the correct diagnosis of dermatomyositis (or polymyositis) to be made where muscle involvement is not detected clinically (Resnick & Kransdorf, 2005). T2-weighted imaging may be used, but fat-suppressed imaging and STIR-MRI are particularly optimal (Fig. 3b-e). The calcific mass might be of low signal but the affected muscle and perimuscular oedema would be hyperintense, and return to normal after treatment. Follow-up STIR MRI had shown no improvement in Case 3. Phosphorus-31 MR spectroscopy may be used for quantitative characterisation of inflammatory disease. (Park, et al., 1990). MRI may also aid in the clinical dilemma of differentiation between myositis from persistent steroid dermatomyositis.

4.1.2 Articular abnormalities

4.1.2.1 Transient radiographic features with soft tissue swelling and periarticular osteopaenia may be present, but bony erosive changes are uncommon and may involve the metacarpophalangeal and interphalangeal joints. Periosteal and soft tissue calcifications with flecks or small clumps of calcium may be detected on radiographs of the hands. (Fig. 2b). Rheumatoid-like changes are, however, uncommon. The 'floppy-thumb' sign may be detected with radial subluxation or dislocation of the interphalangeal joint of the thumb.

4.1.2.2 Acroosteolysis with pointing and resorption of the terminal tufts of the fingers may occur uncommonly, but reduced soft tissue relating to the tips of the fingers is less infrequent. (Fig. 2b). Flexion contractures and soft tissue ulceration may involve the fingers, though larger joints may be involved.

4.1.2.3 Arthralgias and arthritis are present in 20-50% of patients with the wrists, knees and small joints of the fingers affected symmetrically. Permanent joint changes are infrequently seen.

4.2 Pulmonary involvement

4.2.1 Lung changes will occur in up to 50% of patients, and aspiration pneumonia is probably the most common finding seen on chest X-rays (Fig. 1a). Aspiration is due to cough impairment, dysfunction of the pharynx and general weakness relating to body movement (Fig. 3a). Weakness of the respiratory muscles is associated with stiffness of the lungs, small lung volumes and diaphragmatic elevation with basal plate atelectasis. The myositis may, furthermore, affect the diaphragm directly.

4.2.2 Pulmonary arterial hypertension, with large main and proximal pulmonary arteries, may occur as a complication of interstitial lung disease, hypoventilation or vasculitis, however, may also be seen in isolation.

4.2.3 Interstitial fibrosis was first described in 1956, is now well recognised and occurs in 5-10% of patients (Hansell, et al., 2005). (It correlates strongly with the presence of anti-Jo-1, a myositis specific autoantibody.) The illness may be acute, rapidly fatal and resistant to therapy, or benign, indolent and asymptomatic, with favourable response to steroid treatment.

4.2.4 The more acute patients may demonstrate airspace opacity or even widespread groundglass shadowing, with alveolar opacities earlier in the course and more likely to be steroid responsive. These changes are likely to be predominantly due to organising pneumonia.

4.2.5 Radiographic changes often consist of symmetric reticulonodular changes, mostly in the base of the lungfields. In time the entire lungfields may be involved and a fine honeycomb pattern may form.

4.2.6 The chest X-ray may be normal, despite the presence of confirmed clinical disease. Multifocal dystrophic pulmonary ossifications, which have been demonstrated pathologically, are not detected radiographically.

4.2.7 High-resolution CT changes consist principally of groundglass opacification, diffuse but patchy, mostly peripheral, and also parenchymal bands and consolidation. Bronchiectasis occurs in 40% of patients, though honeycombing was uncommon. Pleural thickening and irregularity was frequently encountered.

4.3 Cardiac abnormalities

4.3.1 The myocardium may be affected in a similar way to the involvement of skeletal striated muscle. Cardiac complications include arrhythmias, congestive cardiac failure, and pericarditis (O'Brien & Kelleher, 2008).

4.4 Gastrointestinal abnormalities

4.4.1 Patients may complain of dysphagia and a barium swallow may reveal disordered peristalsis involving the upper oesophagus, that portion with striated muscle. [The lower oesophagus has smooth muscle, and is more likely to be affected by scleroderma.] Because of the progressive weakness of the proximal striated oesophageal muscle, there tends to be atony and dilatation. Aspiration into the tracheobronchial tree may occur during barium swallow examination (Fig. 3a). Atony of the small intestine and colon may furthermore be a feature. It should be emphasized that involvement of the gastrointestinal is not a common manifestation of dermatomyositis.

5. Conclusion

5.1 Some of the protean radiological manifestations of dermatomyositis in childhood and adults are illustrated, with the aid of various radiological examinations.

The superficial soft tissue changes may be very extensive and florid. In recent years MRI has become more important to demonstrate activity of disease.

The effect of treatment, for example, with corticosteroids, can be monitored by four-station STIR MRI. The very extensive disease with deformities and contractures, seen previously, are now less common as a consequence of more optimal management.

6. References

Dähnert, W. 2007. *Radiology Review Manual, 6th Ed.* pp. 64-65, Wolters Kluwer, ISBN 0 7817 6620 6, Philadelphia

Hansell, D., Armstrong, P., Lynch, D., & McAdams, H. 2005. In: *Imaging of Diseases of the Chest*, pp. 581-585, Elsevier Mosby, ISBN 0 3230 36600, Philadelphia

Hesla, R., Karlson, L, & McCauley, R. 1990. Milk of calcium collection in dermatomyositis : ultrasound findings. *Pediatr Radiol,* 20:, pp. 344-346

Moses, S. 2008. Dermatomyositis. *Family Practice Notebook.com. 2008*

O'Brien, J., & Kelleher, J. 2008. Calcinosis associated with dermatomyositis. *J. Belge de Radiol.,* 91. pp. 27

Park, J., Vansant, J, Kumar, N., Gibbs, S., Curvin, M., Price, D., Partain, C., & James, A. 1990. Dermatomyositis : correlatiive MR imaging and P-31 MR spectroscopy for quantitative characterisation of inflammatory disease. *Radiology,* 177(2), pp. 473-479

Resnick, D., & Kransdorf, M. 2005. *Bone and Joint Imaging, 3rd Ed.,* pp. 337-343; 349-352. Elsevier Saunders, ISBN 0 7216 0270 3, Philadelphia

van Gelderen, W., 2007. Fluid-calcium level in the thigh versus clinical diagnosis of a soft tissue abscess : ultrasound features of dermatomyositis. *Australasian Radiol,* 51, pp. B83-B85

8

Interstitial Pneumonia in Dermatomyositis

Tohru Takeuchi, Takuya Kotani and Shigeki Makino
Osaka Medical College
Japan

1. Introduction

Dermatomyositis (DM) and polymyositis (PM) are types of autoimmune inflammatory muscle disease that mainly damage proximal limb muscles, with DM involving characteristic skin findings such as Gottron's sign and heliotrope eruption (Bohan & Peter, 1975a, 1975b). Interstitial pneumonia (IP) is often associated with DM/PM and is one of the important prognostic factors. Above all, rapidly progressive IP (RPIP), which has the worst prognosis, is resistant to corticosteroid drugs and is strongly associated with clinical amyopathic DM (CADM), which is unlikely to show myositis (Kameda & Takeuchi, 2006). In response, combination therapies of corticosteroid drugs and immunosuppressive drugs have recently been administered early in the onset of IP, and outcomes have been improved. Here, we review the pathogenesis, the clinical and laboratory findings, and treatment of IP associated with DM/PM.

2. IP Associated with DM/PM

IP occurs in association with DM/PM in 40-50% of patients and is an important prognostic factor of DM/PM (Hidano, 1992, Marie, 2002, Fathi, 2004). In 2002, the American Thoracic Society and the European Respiratory Society jointly advocated classifying idiopathic IP into 7 types (American Thoracic Society & European Respiratory Society, 2002), which are applied to IP associated with connective tissue disease. Many cases of IP associated with DM/PM comprise one of 3 types: nonspecific interstitial pneumonia (NSIP), cryptogenic organizing pneumonia (COP), or diffuse alveolar damage (DAD) (Douglas, 2001, Fujisawa, 2005). Prognoses vary according to these types: cases of DAD are the most critical, but some cases of NSIP and COP also progress to unfortunate outcomes. IP is classified according to clinical course into 1 of 3 groups: acute/subacute IP (A/SIP) with rapidly progression over several weeks or months, chronic IP (CIP) with slowly progression over years, and asymptomatic type with only minor abnormalities on chest CT or in respiratory function tests (Frazier & Miller, 1974).

The histological features of muscle biopsies in DM and PM are different, as are the pathological features of the IP associated with each disease. PM mainly is associated with slowly progressive CIP, which histologically presents as fibrotic NSIP and which responds to corticosteroids. A/SIP also is associated with COP or cellular NSIP and shows good response to corticosteroids in many cases. In contrast, almost 50% of DM cases are associated with A/SIP, which histologically presents as fibrotic NSIP or DAD (Hirakata &

Nagai, 2000). It often evolves into corticosteroid-resistant RPIP, often progressing to acute or subacute disease in several weeks or months, and many patients die in spite of strong immunosuppressive therapies. There are many unclear points as to how certain cases evolve into RPIP. Some cases that were identified histologically as NSIP change to DAD. In addition, pathological findings can be mixed within the same patient, and the histological picture may vary according to the site of tissue sampling.

3. Laboratory findings

3.1 Pulmonary function tests

Pulmonary function tests (PFT) provide objective evaluation of respiratory symptoms and are important in determining the disease activity and therapeutic effects. However, in patients with severe respiratory failure such as that in RPIP, the tests cannot be performed or the results are not determined. Typically, a restrictive ventilatory impairment is present, and total lung capacity (TLC), vital capacity (VC), forced vital capacity (FVC), and the diffusing capacity for carbon monoxide (DLco) are decreased (Fathi, 2008). A decrease in DLco is one of the most sensitive indices showing a decrease in gas exchange. These abnormalities are improved by treatment. In cases without IP but with decreased FVC, it is necessary to also consider a decrease in ventilatory muscle strength.

3.2 Diagnostic Imaging

For imaging assessment of IP, the sensitivity of the chest X-ray is lower than that of high-resolution CT (HRCT) using less than 3-mm slices (Figure 1). When PM/DM or IP associated with PM/DM is suspected, the lung should be assessed by HRCT. However, because the chest X-ray is easy to use and radiation exposure is low, it is useful for following the course of the disease and for diagnosing complications such as infection.

HRCT findings observed in PM/DM are diverse. The most frequently observed findings are reticular opacity or ground-glass opacity with subpleural curvilinear shadow that is predominantly distributed just below the bilateral dorsal regions of the lungs, and the findings sometimes accompany consolidation (Mino, 1997, Douglas, 2001, Arakawa, 2003, Bonnefoy, 2004, Hayashi, 2008). Ground-glass opacity and consolidation are improved by treatment. The decreased lung volume and traction bronchiectasis (TBE) are sometimes observed, but patients with honeycomb lung are rare. It is difficult to predict the prognosis of IP associated with DM/PM and to select treatment based only on HRCT findings. However, HRCT are useful for the assessment of disease activity and therapeutic effect. IP that is distributed through a wide area of the lungs and accompanies TBE at the early onset or exacerbation has a poor prognosis.

3.3 Biomarkers of IP

Autoantibodies to various cell components are detected in 50 to 80% of PM/DM patients (Reichlin & Arnett, 1984, Love 1991). Myositis-specific autoantibodies such as anti-aminoacyl transfer RNA synthetase (ARS) antibody and anti-signal recognition particle (SRP) antibody are specifically detected in PM/DM, and myositis-related antigens, such as anti-Ku antibody and anti-U1-RNP antibody, are also detected in connective tissue diseases other

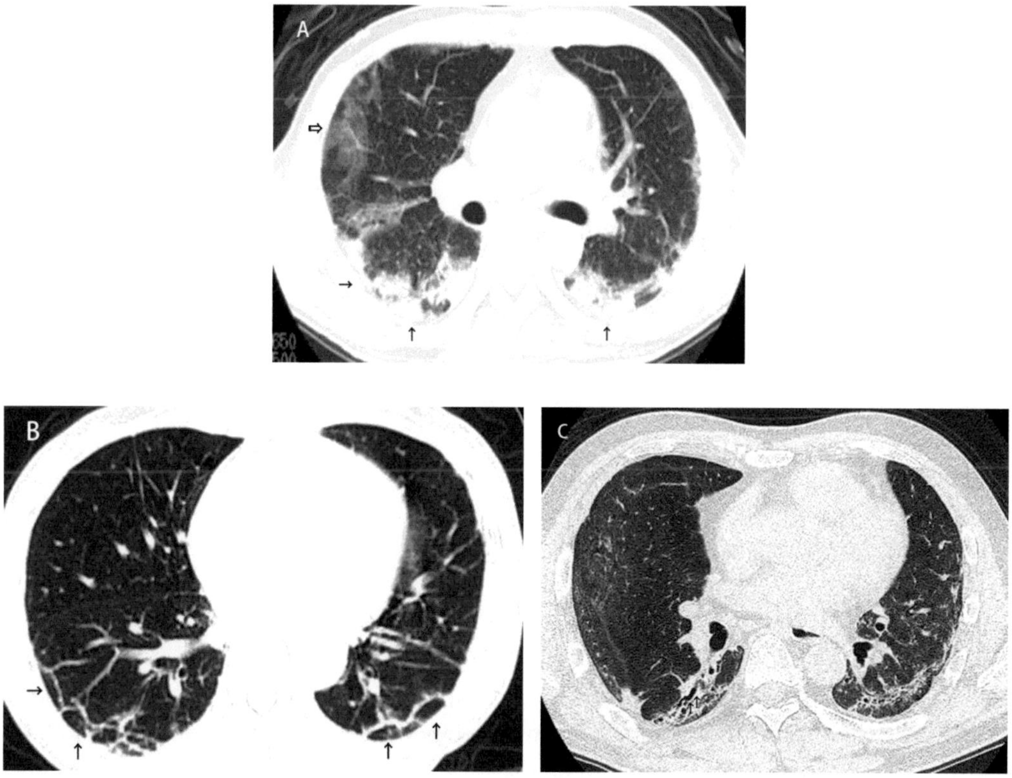

Fig. 1. Chest HRCT of IP associated with DM. (A) ground-glass opacity (open arrow) and consolidation (arrow); (B) subpleural curvilinear shadow (arrow); (C) Traction bronchiectasis.

than PM/DM. Patients from whom these autoantibodies are detected have respective clinical characteristics. Anti-ARS antibodies are detected in 25 to 30% of PM/DM patients, and of these anti-ARS antibodies, anti-Jo-1 antibody is most frequently detected and is closely related with myositis. Antibodies related to IP include anti-PL-12 antibody and anti-KS antibody (Friedman, 1996, Hirakata, 2007). Patients who test positive for anti-SRP antibody are considered to have fewer complications from IP (Targoff, 1990). Patients with CADM frequently complicate RPIP with poor prognosis and have been found to frequently test negative for antinuclear antibody. Recently, anti-CADM-140 (mda-5) antibody has been detected in the serum of patients with CADM (Sato, 2005). In the future, if a relation between this antibody and pathogenesis/clinical presentation is revealed, selection of treatment and prognosis are expected to improve.

Krebs von den Lungen-6 (KL-6) and surfactant D (SpD), which are produced and secreted on the epithelial surface by alveolar type II cells and bronchial epithelial cells, are useful markers for IP. These makers increase in the serum of patients with IP associated with PM/DM. The levels of these markers are inversely correlated with DLco and are useful in judging therapeutic effect (Kubo, 2000, Bandoh, 2000, Ihn, 2002). Not all patients with IP associated with PM/DM show increases in KL-6 and SpD, and there are patients without increased levels of KL-6 and SpD, especially in the acute phase.

Ferritin is the major molecule of iron storage, and it was reported that serum ferritin level increases in A/SIP associated with DM (Gono, 2010). Serum ferritin level is also useful as a predictive factor for onset of A/SIP and is related to its prognosis. Although it is not altogether clear why serum ferritin increases in A/SIP, it is considered to be related to activation of alveolar macrophages.

4. Treatment of IP

Therapy with massive doses of corticosteroids is used in the treatment of DM/PM-complicated IP. Although it is often effective in PM, IP associated with DM, especially in the initial treatment of RPIP, is often refractory to corticosteroid therapy . Nawata et al. reported on the prognosis of the treatment of IP in 31 cases of DM/PM using corticosteroid drugs along with pulse therapy (Nawata, 1999). The first-year survival rate after beginning the treatment was 50% in 20 patients with DM and 90% in 11 patients with PM. In addition, in all patients who died, death occurred within 12 weeks and was due to an exacerbation of IP or infection. Fujisawa et al. reported initial survival rates in 12 patients with DM and 16 patients with PM of 58% and 81%, respectively, when combining corticosteroids with an immunosuppressive agent such as cyclophosphamide (Fujisawa, 2005).

The combination of corticosteroids with immunosuppressive agents is currently the preferred method of treatment of DM/PM-complicated IP, especially in the early treatment of RPIP. Nagasawa et al. surveyed 32 facilities nationwide that specialize in the treatment of connective tissue diseases. The group analyzed clinical data from 38 patients with acute IP in DM/PM who were treated for 2 or more weeks with cyclosporine (Nagasawa, 2003). Among 25 patients who were initially treated for 2 weeks or longer using only corticosteroids following the addition of cyclosporine, the 2-year survival rate was 32%. Among the other13 patients who were treated with cyclosporine within 2 weeks of starting corticosteroid treatment, the average survival rate 2 years later was 69%. Takada et al. reported that when comparing the results from 20 active cases of DM/PM-complicated IP, in which only additional immunosuppressive agents were added if corticosteroid alone did not result in a favorable response, with 14 additional cases in which immunosuppressive agents were combined with corticosteroids, the combination therapy led to a higher survival rate (Takada, 2007). Other clinical trials reported similar results (Yamasaki, 2007, Kotani, 2008). These reports indicate that early combined therapy is more effective than combining additional agents at a later time; as a result, this maximizes the effectiveness of the immunosuppressant.

4.1 Immunosuppressants available for DM/PM-complicated IP

Currently, positive clinical trials are going forward for the following immunosuppressive drugs used in the treatment of DM/PM-complicated IP: cyclophosphamide, cyclosporine, and tacrolimus, amongst others. It is important to introduce treatment with the immunosuppressive agent at an early stage before remodeling the lung tissues, and the dosage and the mode of administration can also greatly influence the therapeutic effect. In addition, because of possible side effects, it is necessary to monitor renal function and carefully consider the dosages and effects of possible drug combinations. Specifically, infectious diseases are a critical side effect of each type of medicine. As reported by Kameda et al. and Kotani et al., through careful monitoring and early detection of infection, preventative treatments can be administered at an early stage leading to a decreased number of deaths due to infectious diseases (Kamdeda 2006, Kotani, 2008). In our facility, factors such as leukocyte count (lymphocyte count), CRP, IgG, β-D-glucan, CMV-C7-HRP, procalcitonin, are regularly measured, and Trimethoprim-sulfamethoxazole is administered to prevent *Pneumocystis jiroveci*.

4.2 Cyclosporine

Cyclosporine is a metabolic product of fungi and a hydrophobic cyclic polypeptide. When it is incorporated into T-lymphocytes, it binds to cyclophilin to form a complex, and when this complex inhibits the activity of calcineurin, expression of cytokine genes such as IL-2 and early activation genes is down-regulated. In DM/PM-complicated IP, because involvement of T-lymphocytes has been suggested from the lung biopsy and lymphocyte subset analysis of bronchoalveolar lavage fluid, concomitant therapy with steroids and cyclosporine has been conducted and has been shown to be efficacious (Nawata, 1999, Nagasawa, 2003, Kameda, 2005, Kotani, 2008). However, these various reports indicate variability in therapeutic effect as the reported survival rates range from 42 to 78%.

Cyclosporine is likely to be affected by food and the amount of bile acid secreted, and the absorbed amount of cyclosporine varies within and between individuals. Because the therapeutic efficacy of cyclosporine depends on the concentration of the drug in the body and not on the dose, therapeutic drug monitoring (TDM) to determine the method of administration based on the concentration of the drug in the blood of individual patients has been recommended. In the treatment of DM/PM-complicated IP, cyclosporine has been administered at doses between 100 and 300 g/day (3 to 5 mg/kg/day) and at a serum trough concentration (C0) between 150 and 250 ng/mL, but there are no specific guidelines.

Recently, Nagai et al. conducted and reported on TDM in 15 IP patients complicated with DM to determine the optimal method of cyclosporine administration (Nagai, 2010). It is known from organ transplantation that the immunosuppressive effect of cyclosporine correlates best with the area under the blood concentration curve (AUC), but this is not so suitable for use in daily management because frequent blood sampling is required. Therefore, the concentration of cyclosporine in the blood was determined before and after administration to determine which concentration correlates best with the AUC. As a result, the blood concentration at 2 hours after administration (C2) was the highest among all the patients, correlated best with AUC, and was considered to be an index of immunosuppressive effect (Figure 2). However, C0 did not correlate with the AUC. Moreover, when comparing between two postprandial doses and one preprandial dose, there was no difference in C2, but C0 was significantly lower when cyclosporine was administered once daily breakfast (Figure 3). Because the incidence of adverse events with cyclosporine increases when cyclosporine is used for a long time at a C0 of 200 ng/mL or higher (Min, 1998), the utility of the administration of one preprandial dose has been reported.

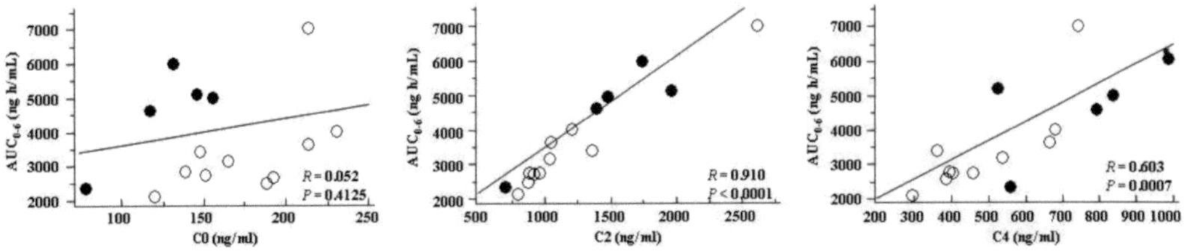

Fig. 2. Correlation of AUC0-6 with C0, C2 and C4 of cyclosporine. C0 presents the serum trough concentration. C2 and C4 present the blood concentration at 2 and 4 hours after administration, respectively. *Closed* and *Open circles* represent patients with preprandial and postprandial administration, respectively. Reproduced with permission from Nagai K, et al., Therapeutic drug monitoring of cyclosporine microemulsion in interstitial pneumonia with dermatomyositis. *Mod Rheumatol*, 2010 (21): 32-36.

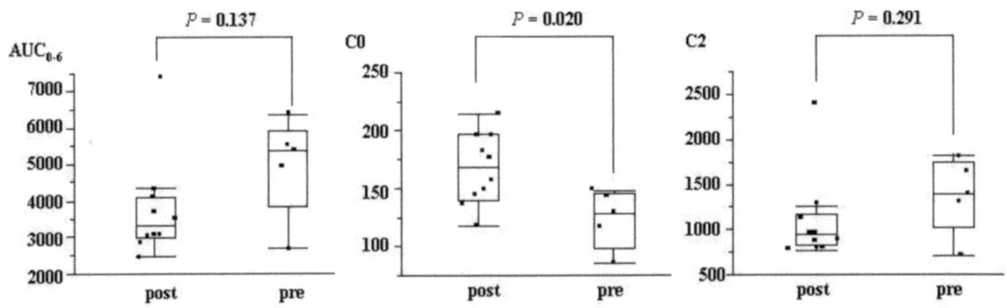

Fig. 3. Comparison of blood cyclosporine level between postprandial daily administration in two doses and preprandial, once daily administration; *Pre* preprandial, once daily before breakfast in a single dose; *Post* postprandial, twice daily in a divided dose. Reproduced with permission from Nagai K, et al., Therapeutic drug monitoring of cyclosporine microemulsion in interstitial pneumonia with dermatomyositis. *Mod Rheumatol*, 2010 (21): 32-36.

Adverse events to cyclosporine include infection as well as renal disorders, hypertension, diabetes mellitus, and hepatic disorders. Because the onset of adverse events is concentration-dependent, the dose is adjusted so that the C0 is 200 ng/mL or less, but it may be impossible to reduce the dose because of the high activity of IP. Nagai et al. reported that when the C2 was 1222.6±523.8 ng/mL, the C0 was 157.3±41.4 ng/mL (Nagai, 2010), so cyclosporine can be used relatively safely if the C2 is maintained at about 1200 ng/mL. If cyclosporine is used for a long time, however, the serum creatinine value gradually increases. Thus, monitoring of both C2 and C0 are required for the assessment of immunosuppressive effects and adverse events. Moreover, because cyclosporine is metabolized at cytochrome P450 (CYP) 3A4, concomitant use with tacrolimus, bosentan, pitavastatin, and rosuvastatin is contraindicated, and it is also necessary to pay attention to concomitant use with aminoglycoside antibiotics and amphotericin B, which have been known to induce renal disorders.

It has been reported that the immunosuppressive effect of cyclosporine reaches its maximum effects if the C2 exceeds 1000 ng/mL. The ideal dose of cyclosporine in the treatment of DM/PM-complicated IP has not been established yet. The dose is reported to be variable, which may affect its therapeutic effect. In the future, it will be necessary to evaluate not only dosage and C0 but also C2. Recently, Kotani et al. reported that the C2 of cyclosporine correlated with the HRCT findings and improvement of respiratory function instead of C0 (Kotani, 2011).

4.3 Tacrolimus

Tacrolimus is a metabolic product of an actinobacteria, *Streptomyces tsukubaensis*, and has a macrolide skeleton. When it is incorporated into T-lymphocytes, it forms a complex with the FK506-binding protein. As a cyclosporine, this complex shows immunosuppressive effects by inhibiting the activity of calcineurin. The activity of tacrolimus is 30- to 100-times higher than that of cyclosporine *in vitro,* and it inhibits mixed lymphocyte culture reaction, production of IL-2, expression of IL-2 receptor, and production of IFN-γ. Clinically, tacrolimus is used for inhibition of rejection after transplantation of kidneys, liver, heart, lung and pancreas and in rheumatic diseases such as systemic lupus erythematosus, rheumatoid arthritis, Behçet's disease, and myasthenia gravis.

Oddis et al. reported the utility of tacrolimus in 8 patients with refractory PM associated with IP (Oddis, 1999). When tacrolimus was orally administered to maintain the C0 at 5 to 20 ng/mL, recovery of muscle strength was observed in all 8 patients, and among 5 patients complicated with IP, 3 showed improvement, and 1 was stabilized. Thereafter, Wilkes et al. reported 13 patients with anti-tRNA synthase antibody-positive refractory DM/PM who were treated with tacrolimus (Wilkes, 2005). It was possible to rescue all the patients, to improve respiratory function, and to reduce the dose of corticosteroids administered. Takada et al. retrospectively examined the clinical effects of tacrolimus in 5 IP patients complicated with refractory DM/PM (Takada, 2005). As a result, they reported that all 5 patients could be rescued and that in 4 patients who could be evaluated by PFT before and after treatment, the PFT values were improved.

The treatment of DM/PM-complicated IP is conducted at a tacrolimus dose of 4 to 6 mg/day and a C0 of 5 to 10 ng/mL. Tacrolimus is also likely to be affected by food, and it is known that the AUC and the maximum blood concentration (Cmax) decrease with postprandial administration. For cyclosporine, C2 monitoring is required to evaluate immunosuppressive effects, but for tacrolimus, since both the blood concentrations before and at 0 to 7 hours after administration correlate well with the AUC, it is better to monitor C0 only. (Figure 4)

The adverse events of tacrolimus are infection as well as renal disorders, hypertension, diabetes mellitus, and hyperkalemia. The onset of adverse events depends on the concentration, and if the C0 is as high as 20 ng/mL for a long time, adverse reactions increase. Similar to cyclosporine, because tacrolimus is metabolized at CYP3A4, it is necessary to pay attention to concomitant drug use. Moreover, because hyperkalemia can be observed, attention must be paid to administration of potassium-conserving diuretics such as spironolactone and eplerenone.

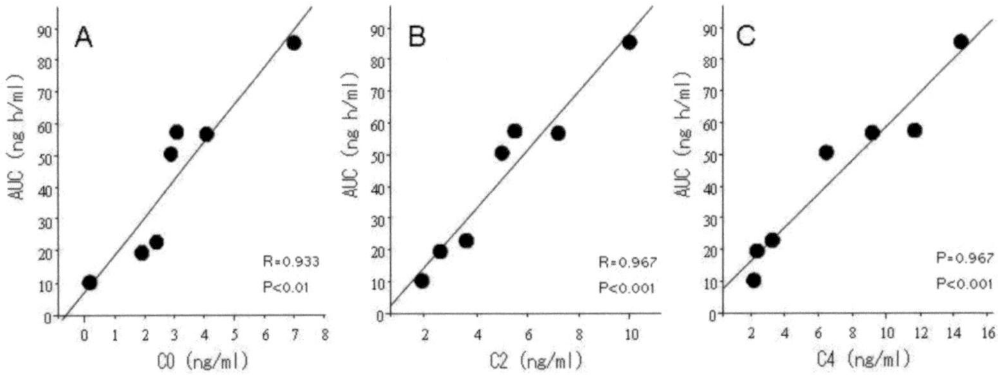

Fig. 4. Correlation of AUC0-6 with C0, C2 and C4 of Tacrolimus. C0 presents the serum trough concentration. C2 and C4 present the blood concentration at 2 and 4 hours after administration, respectively.

4.4 Cyclophosphamide

Cyclophosphamide is an alkylating agent that is used to inhibit rejection after renal transplantation and for the treatment of malignant tumors. Cyclophosphamide itself has no alkylating effect, but many of its metabolites have activities that alkylate guanine and inhibit replication of DNA chains and transcription to mRNA. To exert their immunosuppressive effects, these metabolites inhibit differentiation and proliferation of T-cells and B-cells and suppress antigen processes of antigen-presenting cells such as macrophages.

DM/PM-complicated IP is treated by pulse intravenous infusion of cyclophosphamide (IV-CY, 500 to 2,000 mg) in combination with corticosteroids. In the initial case reports, the effects of IV-CY were variable. Yamasaki et al. administered IV-CY at doses of 300 to 800 mg/m^2 6 times every 4 weeks in addition to steroids to 17 patients with DM/PM-complicated IP (Yamasaki, 2007). Dyspnea improved in 11 patients, %VC improved by 10% or more in 8 patients, and the chest CT score improved in 9 patients. Moreover, the number of days from the start of initial treatment and the rate of improvement in %VC showed a negative correlation, indicating the utility of early concomitant treatment.

Cyclophosphamide exerts strong immunosuppressive effects but is also accompanied by a number of adverse events including myelosuppression and following infections, hemorrhagic cystitis, ovarian insufficiency, azoospermia, and secondary carcinogenesis. It is therefore problematic whether cyclophosphamide may be used continuously for a long time in relapsed patients after remission induction or in patients with chronic advanced disease. It is considered useful to conduct initial treatment with concomitant use of corticosteroids and cyclophosphamide and then to switch to other immunosuppressive drugs, but this requires further evaluation. A prospective comparative study in which corticosteroids and IV-CY were administered 6 times every 4 weeks and then switched to azathioprine (2.5 mg/kg/day) was conducted in IP patients complicated with scleroderma[17)], which may be helpful for the treatment of DM/PM-complicated IP.

5. Conclusion

There are limitations in the treatment of DM/PM-complicated IP, and particularly RRIP, with corticosteroids alone; thus, immunosuppressive drugs should be introduced early and aggressively before remodeling of the lung tissues. Many challenges remain in determining what treatment should be started for which patient, how to perform maintenance therapy, and how to switch between immunosuppressive drugs. At this time, prospective clinical studies of various immunosuppressive drugs are ongoing, and the results are eagerly anticipated.

6. References

American Thoracic Society & European Respiratory Society. (2002) American Thoracic Society/ European Respiratory Society International Multidisciplinary Consensus Classification of the Idiopathic Interstitial Pneumonias. *Am J Respir Crit Care Med*, Vol. 165, No. 2, (Jan 2002), pp. 277-304, ISSN 1073-449X.

Arakawa H, Yamada H, Kurihara Y, Nakajima Y, Takeda A, Fukushima Y, Fujioka M. (2003). Nonspecific interstitial pneumonia associated with polymyositis and dermatomyositis. *Chest*, Vol. 123, No.4, (Apr 2003), pp.1096-1103, ISSN 0012-3692.

Bandoh S, Fujita J, Ohtsuki Y, Ueda Y, Hojo S, Tokuda M, Dobashi H, Kurata N, Yoshinouchi T, Kohno N, Takahara J. (2000). Sequential changes of KL-6 in sera of patients with interstitial pneumonia associated with polymyositis/ dermatomyositis. *Ann Rheum Dis*, Vol.59, No. 4, (Apr 2000), pp.257-262, ISSN 0003-4967.

Bohan A & Peter JB. (1975a). Polymyositis and dermatomyositis (first of two parts). *N Engl J Med*, Vol. 292, No. 7, (Feb 1975), pp. 344-347, ISSN 1533-4406.

Bohan A & Peter JB. (1975b). Polymyositis and dermatomyositis (second of two parts). *N Engl J Med*, Vol. 292, No. 8, (Feb 1975), pp. 403-407, ISSN 1533-4406.

Bonnefoy O, Ferreti G, Calaque O, Coulomb M Begueret H, Beylot-Barry M, Laurent F. (2004). Serial chest CT findings in interstitial lung disease associated with polymyositis-dermatomyositis. *Eur J Radiol*, Vol. 49, No. 3, (Mar 2004), pp. 235-244, ISSN 0720-048X.

Danko K, Ponyi A, Costantin T, Borgulya G, Szegedi G. (2004) Long-term survival of patients with idiopathic inflammatory myopathies according to clinical features: a longitudinal study of 162 cases. *Medicine (Baltimore)*, Vol. 83, No. 1, (Jan 2004), pp. 35-42, ISSN 0025-7974.

Douglas WW, Tazellar HD, Hartman TE, Hartman RE, Decker PA, Schroeder DR, Ryu JH. (2001). Polymyositis-dermatomyositis associated interstitial lung disease. *Am J Respir Crit Care Med*, Vol. 164, No. 7, (Oct 2001), pp.1182-1185, ISSN 1073-449X.

Fathi M, Dastmalchi M, Rasmussen E, Lundberg IE, Tornling. (2004). Interstitial lung disease, a common manifestation of newly diagnosed polymyositis and dermatomyositis. *Ann Rheum Dis*, Vol. 63, No. 3, (Mar 2004), pp. 297-301, ISSN 0003-4967

Fathi M, Vikgren J, Boijsen M, Tylen U, Jorfeldt L, Tornling G, Lundberg IE. (2008). Interstitial lung disease in polymyositis and dermatomyositis: longitudinal evaluation by pulmonary function and radiology. Arthritis Rheum, Vol. 59, No. 5, (Mar 2008), pp.677-685, ISSN 0004-3591.

Frazier AR & Miller RD. (1974). Interstitial pneumonitis in association with polymyositis and dermatomyositis. *Chest*, Vol. 65, No.4, (Apr 1974), pp. 403-407, ISSN 0012-3692.

Friedman AW, Targoff IN, Arnett FC. (1996). Interstitial lung disease with autoantibodies against aminoacyl-tRNA synthetase in the absence of clinically apparent myositis. Semin *Arthritis Rheum*, Vol. 26, No.1, (Aug 1996), pp. 459-467, ISSN 0004-3591.

Fujisawa T, Suda T, Nakamura Y, Enomoto N, Ide K, Toyoshima M, Uchiyama H, Tamura R, Ida M, Yagi T, Yasuda K, Genma H, Hayakawa H, Chida K, Nakamura H. (2005) Differences in clinical features and prognosis of interstitial lung disease between polymyositis and dermatomyositis. *J Rheumatol*, Vol. 32, No. 1, (Jan 2005), pp. 58-64, ISSN 0315-162X.

Gono T, Kawaguchi Y, Hara M, Masuda I, Katsumata Y, Shinozaki M, Ota Y, Ozeki E, Yamanaka H. (2010). Increased ferritin predicts development and severity of acute interstitial lung disease as a complication of dermatomyositis. Rheumatol (Oxford), Vol. 49, No. 7, (Apr 2010), pp. 1354-1360, ISSN 1462-0324.

Hayashi S, Tanaka M, Kobayashi H, Nakazono T, Satoh T, Fukuno Y, Aragane N, Tada Y, Koarada S, Ohta A, Nagasawa K.. (2008). High-resolution computed tomography characterization of interstitial lung diseases in polymyositis/ dermatomyositis. *J Rheumatol*, Vol. 35, No.2, (Dec 2007), pp.260-269, ISSN 0315-162X.

Hidano A, Torikai S, Uemura T, Shimizu S. (1992). Malignancy and interstitial pneumonia as fatal complications in dermatomyositis. *J Dermatol*, Vol. 19, No. 3, (Mar 1992), 153-160, ISSN 0385-2407.

Hirakata M & Nagai S. (2000) Interstitial lung disease in polymyositis and dermatomyositis. *Curr Opin Rheumatol*, Vol. 12, No. 6, (Nov 2000), pp. 501-508, ISSN 1040-8711.

Hirakata M, Suwa A, Takada T, Sato S, Nagai S, Genth E, Song YW, Mimori T, Targoff IN. (2007). Clinical and immunogenetic features of patients with autoantibodies to asparaginyl-transfer RNA synthetase. *Arthritis Rheum*, Vol.56, No. 4, (Apr 2007), pp. 1295-1303, ISSN 0004-3591.

Hoyles RK, Ellis RW, Wellsbury J, Lees B, Newlands P, Goh NS, Roberts C, Desai S, Herrick AL, McHugh NJ, Foley NM, Pearson SB, Emery P, Veale DJ, Denton CP, Wells AU, Black CM, du Bois RM. (2006). A multicenter, prospective, randomized, double-blind, placebo-controlled, trial of corticosteroids and intravenous cyclophosphamide followed by oral azathioprine for the treatment of pulmonary fibrosis in scleroderma. *Arthritis Rheum*, Vol. 54, No.12, (Dec 2006), pp. 3962-3970, ISSN 0004-3591.

Ihn H, Asano Y, Kubo M, Yamane K, Jinnin M, Yazawa N, Fujimoto M, Tamaki K.(2002). Clinical significance of serum surfactant protein D (Sp-D) in patients with polymyositis/dermatomyositis: correlation with interstitial lung disease. *Rheumatology (Oxford)*, Vol. 41, No. 11, (Nov 2002), pp.1268-1272, ISSN 1462-0324.

Kameda H, Nagasawa H, Ogawa H, Sekiguchi N, Takei H, Tokuhira M, Amano K, Takeuchi T. (2005). Combination therapy with corticosteroids, cyclosporine A, and intravenous cyclophosphamide for acute/ subacute interstitial pneumonia in patients with dermatomyositis. *J Rheumatol*, Vol. 32, No. 9, (Sep 2005), pp. 1719-1726,ISSN 0315-162X.

Kameda H & Takeuchi T. (2006) Recent advances in the treatment of interstitial lung disease in patients with polymyositis/dermatomyositis. *Endocr Metab Immune Disord Drug Targets*, Vol. 6, No. 4, (Dec 2006), pp. 409-415, ISSN 1871-5303.

Kotani T, Makino S, Takeuchi T, Kagitani M, Shoda T, Hata A, Tabushi Y, Hanafusa T. (2008). Early intervention with corticosteoids and cyclosporine A and 2-hour postdose blood concentration monitoring improves the prognosis of acute/ subacute interstitial pneumonia in dermatomyositis. *J Rheumatol*, Vol. 35, No. 2, (Dec 2007), pp.254-259, ISSN 0315-162X.

Kotani T, Takeuchi T, Makino S, Hata K, Yoshida S, Nagai K, Wakura D, Shoda T, Hanafusa T. (2011). Combination with corticosteroids and cyclosporine-A improves pulmonary function test results and chest HRCT findings in dermatomyositis patients with acute/subacute interstitial pneumonia. Clin Rheumatol, Vol. 30, No. 8, (Aug 2011), pp.1021-1028, ISSN 0770-3198.

Kubo M, Ihn H, Yamane K, Kikuchi K, Yazawa N, Soma Y, Tamaki K. (2000). Serum KL-6 in adult patients with polymyositis and dermatomyositis. *Rheumatology (Oxford)*, Vol. 39, No. 6, (Jan 2000), pp.632-636, ISSN 1462-0324.

Love LA, Leff RL, Fraser DD, Targoff IN, Dalakas M, Plotz PH, Miller FW. (1991). A new approach to the classification of idiopathic inflammatory myopathy: Myositis-specific autoantibodies define useful homogeneous patient groups. *Medicine (Baltimore)*, Vol. 70, No. 6, (Nov 1991), 360-374, ISSN 0025-7974.

Marie I, Hachulla E, Cherin P, Dominique S, Hatron PY, Hellot MF, Devulder B, Herson S, Levesque H, Courtois H. (2002). Interstitial lung disease in polymyositis and dermatomyositis. *Arthritis Rheum*, Vol. 47, No. 6, (Dec 2002), pp.614-622, ISSN 0004-3591.

Min DI, Perry PJ, Chen HY, Hunsicker LG. (1998). Cyclosporine trough concentrations in predicting allograft rejection and renal toxicity up to 12 months after renal transplantation. *Pharmacotherapy*, Vol. 18, No. 2, (Mar 1998), pp. 282-287, ISSN 0277-0008.

Mino M, Noma S, TaguchiY, Tomii K, Kohri Y, Oida K. (1997). Pulmonary involvement in polymyositis and dermatomyositis: sequential evaluation with CT. *Am J Rhoentgenol*, Vol.169, No. 1, (Jul 1997), pp. 83-87, ISSN 0361-803X.

Nagai K, Takeuchi T, Kotani T, Hata K, Yoshida S, Isoda K, Fujiki Y, Shiba H, Makino S, Hanafusa T. (2011). Therapeutic drug monitoring of cyclosporine microemulsion in interstitial pneumonia with dermatomyositis. *Mod Rheumatol*, Vol. 21, No. 1, (Jan 2011), pp. 32-36, ISSN 1439-7595.

Nagasawa K, Harigai M, Tateishi M, Hara M, Yoshizawa Y, Koike T, Miyasaka N. (2003). Efficacy of combination treatment with cyclosporin A and corticosteroids for acute interstitial pneumonitis associated with dermatomyositis. *Mod Rheumatol*, Vol. 13, No. 3, (Sep 2003), pp. 231-238, ISSN 1439-7595.

Nawata Y, Kurasawa K, Takabayashi, Miike S, Watanabe N, Hiraguri M, Kita Y, Kawai M Saito Y, Iwamoto I. (1999) Corticosteroid resistant interstitial pneumonitis in dermatomyositis/ polymyositis: prediction and treatment with cyclosporine. *J Rheumatol*, Vol. 26, No. 7, (Jul 1999), pp. 1527-1533, ISSN 0315-162X.

Oddis CV, Sciurba FC, Elmagd KA, Starzl TE. (1999). Tacrolimus in refractory polymyositis with interstitial lung disease. *Lancet*, Vol. 353, No. 9166, (May 1999), pp. 1762-1763, ISSN 0140-6736.

Reichlin M & Arnett FC. (1984). Multiplicity of antibodies in myositis sera. *Arthritis Rheum*, Vol. 27, No. 10, (Oct 1984), pp. 1150-1156, ISSN 0004-3591.

Sato S, Hirakata M, Kuwana M, Suwa A, Inada S, Mimori T, Nishikawa T, Oddis CV, Ikeda Y. (2005). Autoantibodies to a 140-kd polypeptide, CADM-140, in Japanese patients with clinically amyopathic dermatomyositis. *Arthritis Rheum*, Vol.52, No. 5, (May 2005), pp.1571-1576, ISSN 0004-3591.

Tagoff IN, Johnson AE, Miller FW. (1990). Antibody to signal recognition particle in polymyositis. *Arthritis Rheum*, Vol. 33, No. 9, (Sep 1990), pp.1361-1370, ISSN 0004-3591.

Takada K, Nagasaka K, Miyasaka N. (2005). Polymyositis / dermatomyositis and interstitial lung disease: a new therapeutic approach with T-cell-specific immunosuppressants. *Autoimmunity*, Vol. 38, No. 5, (Aug 2005), pp. 383-392, ISSN 0891-6934.

Takada K, Kishi J, Miyasaka N. (2007). Step-up versus primary intensive approach to the treatment of interstitial pneumonia associated with dermatomyositis/ polymyositis: a retrospective study. *Mod Rheumatol*, Vol. 17, No. 2, (Apr 2007), pp. 123-130, ISSN 1439-7595.

Wilkes MR, Sereika SM, Fertig N, Lucas MR, Oddis CV. (2005). Treatment of antisynthetase-associated interstitial lung disease with tacrolimus. *Arthritis Rheum*, Vol. 52, No. 8, (Aug 2005), pp. 2439-2446, ISSN 0004-3591.

Yamasaki Y, Yamada H, Yamasaki M, Ohkubo M, Azuma K, Matsuoka S, Kurihara Y, Osada H, Satoh M, Ozaki S. (2007) Intravenous cyclophosphamide therapy for progressive interstitial pneumonia in patients with polymyositis/dermatomyositis. *Rheumatol (Oxford)*, Vol. 46, No. 1, (Jun 2006), pp. 124-130, ISSN 1462-0324.

9

IBMPFD and p97, the Structural and Molecular Basis for Functional Disruption

Wai-Kwan Tang and Di Xia
Laboratory of Cell Biology, Center for Cancer Research, National Cancer Institute, National Institutes of Health, Bethesda, Maryland, USA

1. Introduction

Inclusion body myopathy associated with Paget's disease of the bone and frontotemporal dementia (IBMPFD, OMIM 167320) is an inherited, autosomal dominant, adult onset multi-disorder, which affects the muscle, bone and the brain (Watts et al., 2004). It is a rare condition with unknown worldwide prevalence. Affected individuals may display one or a combination of the following three symptoms which, however, are generally not recognized until patients are in their 40s or 50s (Weihl, 2011). (1) IBM (Inclusion body myopathy): About 90% of all patients develop proximal and distal muscle weakness initially with atrophy of the pelvic and shoulder girdle muscles (Kimonis et al., 2000; Kimonis et al., 2008b; Kovach et al., 2001; Watts et al., 2003). Cellular inclusion bodies and rimmed vacuoles are commonly found in these muscle tissues (Kimonis et al., 2008a; Kimonis et al., 2000; Watts et al., 2004). Characteristically, two proteins are most frequently found co-localized with the inclusion, ubiquitin and TDP-43 (TAR DNA binding protein-43) (Ritson et al., 2010; Weihl et al., 2008). Ubiquitin is a signaling molecule that directs protein substrates into a variety of cellular pathways, including protein degradation. Misfolded or unwanted proteins are labeled with ubiquitin, mostly in the form of polyubiquitin, and targeted for degradation (Clague and Urbe, 2010). TDP-43, on the other hand, is believed to be a substrate itself for either proteasome or autophagal degradation (Caccamo et al., 2009; Wang et al., 2010). Detection of these proteins in the inclusions suggests impairments in the protein degradation pathways. (2) PDB (Paget's disease of the bone): About half of IBMPFD patients develop PDB, which is caused by an imbalance in the activities between osteoblasts and osteoclasts. (3) FTD (Frontotemporal dementia): Only ~30% of patients develop FTD, which is characterized by language and/or behavioral dysfunction. Interestingly, clinical manifestation of these symptoms is rather random, and has no clear-cut correlation with family history or mutations. Even within isolated families bearing the same genetic mutation, individuals can exhibit different symptoms. These heterogeneities in clinical presentations cause frequent misdiagnoses of IBMPFD patients (van der Zee et al., 2009). Accurate diagnosis of IBMPFD often requires molecular genetic testing, in addition to a combined clinical diagnosis of myopathy, PDB and FTD.

2. What is p97?

In the year 2000, IBMPFD was recognized as a genetically distinct clinical syndrome (Kimonis et al., 2000) and was subsequently linked to heterozygous missense mutations in a highly abundant cellular protein called p97 (also called valosin-containing protein, VCP) (Watts et al., 2004). P97 belongs to the family of AAA^+ proteins (ATPases Associated with various cellular Activities), which use the energy from hydrolyzing ATP to drive mechanical work necessary for a host of functions including homotypic membrane fusion, cell cycle regulation and protein degradation (Wang et al., 2004; Woodman, 2003; Ye, 2006). The multi-functionality of p97 is consistent with its embryonic lethality when the p97 gene or its homologs are disrupted or knocked-out in the mouse, in yeast, in trypanosomes, and in Drosophila (Frohlich et al., 1991; Lamb et al., 2001; Leon and McKearin, 1999; Muller et al., 2007). Moreover, the functional versatility of p97 appears to lie in its ability to interact with a large variety of adaptor proteins. For instance, binding to the protein p47 incorporates p97 in the membrane fusion pathway (Kondo et al., 1997), whereas the p97-Ufd1-Npl4 complex participates in ER associated degradation (ERAD) (Richly et al., 2005). So far, more than twenty adaptor proteins have been identified that interact with p97 (Madsen et al., 2009), but detailed molecular mechanisms of these interactions remain elusive.

3. Structure of p97

Structurally, p97 is a homo-hexamer, each subunit (806 residues) consisting of three domains: a unique N-terminal domain (N-domain) followed by two conserved AAA^+ ATPase domains (D1- and D2-domain) in tandem (DeLaBarre and Brunger, 2003; Huyton et al., 2003) (Fig. 1A). The N-domain (residues 1-184) contains two sub-domains, an N-terminal double Ψ-barrel and a C-terminal four-stranded β-barrel, and is responsible for interacting with most adaptor proteins as well as with protein substrates. Both the D1- (residues 211-463) and D2-domains (residues 483-762) are typical AAA^+ ATPase domains comprised of two sub-domains: a large N-terminal RecA-like domain with an α/β fold and a smaller C-terminal α-helical bundle domain. The D1-domain is essential for hexamerization of p97 subunits (Wang et al., 2003) and the hexameric ring formation is predominantly mediated through interactions between the RecA-like sub-domains (Fig. 1B). However, unlike many members of the AAA^+ family proteins such as the *E. coli* ClpA unfoldase, the hexamerization of p97 subunits does not require the binding of nucleotide (ADP or ATP) at D1-domains, though it has been shown that nucleotide binding does accelerate p97 hexamer formation (Singh and Maurizi, 1994; Wang et al., 2003). Most of the ATPase activities of p97 involve the D2-domain, presumably required for the processing of substrates (Song & Li, 2003).

Connecting the domains are loops that have been shown to play important functions. The N-D1 loop is 27 residues long and is embedded at the interface between the N-domain and the D1-domain. The short peptide stretch (residues 763-806) immediately following the D2-domain is another region for adaptor protein binding. Although not as common as the N-domain, this C-terminal tail has been shown to interact with a number of proteins, such as Ubxd1 (Allen et al., 2006; Madsen et al., 2008). Similar to other Type-II AAA^+ assemblies, the p97 assembly was revealed by electron microscopy (EM) and crystallography to be a two-tiered concentric ring encircling a central pore or axial channel (Fig. 1B). The N-domains are attached to the periphery of the D1 ring, making one ring appear larger than the other. The central pore does not run unrestricted through the hexamer, but has a narrowing or a constriction point that is formed by a bound zinc ion (DeLaBarre and Brunger, 2003).

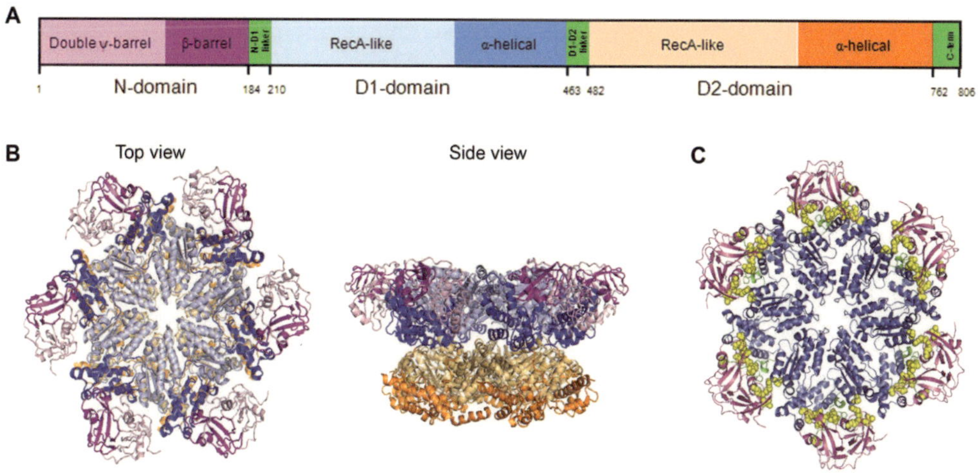

Fig. 1. **Structure of p97** (A) Domain organization of the full-length p97. (B) Ribbon representation of the crystal structure of p97 based on PDB: 1OZ4. Domains are color-coded using the scheme in (A) and two views are presented. (C) Locations of IBMPFD mutations are shown in the context of the p97 N-D1 structure (PDB: 1E32), which has the D1-domain bound with ADP. The IBMPFD mutations are represented by yellow balls. Thirteen positions representing twenty mutations are presented.

4. Mutations in p97 associated with IBMPFD

So far, only single amino acid substitutions in p97 have been identified from all the clinical IBMPFD specimens examined. Altogether, twenty missense mutations found in 13 different amino acid positions in p97 have been reported to be associated with the disease and the majority of them involve substitutions of arginine residues (Table 1) (http://www.molgen.ua.ac.be/FTDMutations). While more than half of these mutations are located in the N-domain (Ile^{27}, Arg^{93}, Arg^{95}, Pro^{137}, Arg^{155}, Gly^{157} and Arg^{159}), a few are found in the N-D1 linker region between the N- and D1-domains (Arg^{191} and Leu^{198}) and in the D1-domain (Ala^{232}, Thr^{262}, Asn^{387} and Ala^{439}). None has been found in the D2-domain. Among these, mutations at Arg^{155} are the most frequently observed in patients (Table 1). Interestingly, mapping these mutations onto the three-dimensional p97 structure in the ADP-bound form revealed that they all clustered at the interface between the N- and D1-domains (N-D1-interface, Fig. 1C).

5. Wild type vs. IBMPFD mutant p97: Structural characteristics

Changes in structure as a result of amino acid mutations can lead to a global disruption of the protein folding, resulting rapid clearance by cellular stress response mechanisms, or to localized structural changes that cause complete loss of the protein function, or to subtle conformational changes that alter the function of the protein. Structural changes in mutant proteins can be directly visualized by X-ray crystallography, NMR (nuclear magnetic resonance), and EM (electron microscopy) or inferred indirectly by biophysical and biochemical methods such as SAXS (small angle X-ray scattering). To understand how IBMPFD mutations lead to functional change in p97, it is absolutely necessary to know what structural changes these mutations entail. However, knowing what has changed in mutants depends heavily on our baseline knowledge of the wild type proteins.

	Change in amino acid	Change in gene	Location	References
1	I27V	79 A → G	N-domain	(Rohrer et al., 2011)
2	R93C	277 C → T		(Guyant-Marechal et al., 2006; Watts et al., 2004)
3	R95C	283 C → T		(Kimonis et al., 2008a)
	R95G	283 C → G		(Watts et al., 2004)
4	P137L	410 C → T		(Palmio et al., 2011; Stojkovic et al., 2009)
5	R155C	463 C → T		(Gidaro et al., 2008; Guyant-Marechal et al., 2006; Schroder et al., 2005; Watts et al., 2004)
	R155H	463 C → A		(Viassolo et al., 2008; Watts et al., 2004)
	R155P	463 C → C		(Watts et al., 2004)
	R155S	463 C → A		(Stojkovic et al., 2009)
	R155L	464 G → T		(Kumar et al., 2010)
6	G157R	469 G → C		(Djamshidian et al., 2009)
		469 G → A		(Stojkovic et al., 2009)
7	R159C	475 C → T		(Bersano et al., 2009)
	R159H	476 G → A		(Haubenberger et al., 2005; van der Zee et al., 2009)
8	R191Q	572 G → C	N-D1 linker	(Watts et al., 2004)
9	L198W	593 T → G		(Kumar et al., 2010; Watts et al., 2007)
10	A232E	695 C → A	D1-domain	(Watts et al., 2004)
11	T262A	784 A → G		(Spina et al., 2008)
12	N387H	1159 A → C		(Watts et al., 2007)
13	A439S	1315 G → T		(Stojkovic et al., 2009)

Table 1. IBMPFD mutations in p97.

5.1 Conformational changes in AAA$^+$ proteins

Studies of AAA$^+$ proteins have revealed conformational changes in various domains in response to changes in the environment, to substrate binding, and to various bound nucleotides. At least some of the observed conformational changes are believed to be necessary for function (Vale and Milligan, 2000). N-domains of ClpB were found in different positions in crystal structure even though all the subunits were bound with the ATP analog AMP-PNP (Lee et al., 2003); this conformational plasticity in N-domains is likely the result of different environments each subunit experienced in the crystal and may not be directly related to function. By far most of the observed conformational changes, though relatively subtle, are induced by binding of various nucleotides in the AAA$^+$ domains. Such nucleotide-driven conformational changes have been observed for both Type I (proteins with one AAA$^+$ domain) and Type II (proteins with two AAA$^+$ domains) AAA$^+$ proteins in crystal structures such as LTag (SV40 large tumor antigen) (Gai et al., 2004), FstH (Bieniossek et al., 2009) and HslU (Wang et al., 2001).

Conformational changes in AAA+ proteins have been probed by methods other than crystallography, which do not depend on obtaining 3-D crystals albeit at relatively lower resolutions. Such methods include cryo EM and SAXS. Cryo EM has revealed flexibility in the N-domains of *E. coli* AAA+ protein ClpA (Ishikawa et al., 2004) and SAXS experiments have shown large conformational changes in NtrC1 (Chen et al., 2010). Although in some cases conformational changes observed with different methods do not completely agree, it is widely accepted that AAA+ proteins undergo dynamic movements during their catalytic cycle. One general observation relating to structural movements among AAA+ proteins is the change in size of the axial pore where substrates enter. The "open-and-close" of the axial pore in AAA+ proteins is thought to provide the mechanical force needed to pull the substrates through the pore (Kravats et al., 2011; Zolkiewski, 2006).

5.2 Structural studies of wild type p97

Crystal structures of wild type p97 have been solved for both the full-length protein and a truncated N-D1 fragment (absent of the D2-domain) (DeLaBarre and Brunger, 2003; Huyton et al., 2003; Zhang et al., 2000). Although both D1- and D2-domains are capable of hydrolyzing ATP (Song et al., 2003), in all the wild type p97 crystal structures determined to date, ADP was invariably found in the D1-domains, while either ADP or ADP-AlFx (transitional analog) was observed in the D2-domain (DeLaBarre and Brunger, 2003; Huyton et al., 2003). These structures share an identical N-domain conformation with the N-domains attached to the periphery of the D1 ring, and in plane with it (Fig. 1B). Unsuccessful attempts have been made to crystallize wild type p97 with other forms of nucleotides trapped in the D1-domain (DeLaBarre and Brunger, 2003).

On a different front, studies using EM and SAXS to gain structural insights into the conformational changes of p97 have revealed rather dramatic changes in the positions of N-domains (Davies et al., 2005; Rouiller et al., 2002). In contrast to X-ray crystallography, these approaches are limited to providing molecular shapes without a clear delineation of bound nucleotides. Nevertheless, large conformational changes in the N-domains of p97 can be detected by modeling individual domains from crystal structures into these molecular envelopes to re-construct structures of p97 under various conditions, although lacking absolute certainty. In the presence of different nucleotides (ATP or ADP) and their non-hydrolysable or transitional analogs (ADP-AlFx, AMP-PNP or ATPγS), the N-domains of p97 were shown to undergo some of the most dramatic movements during the ATP cycle. Although some changes observed by different methods or in different laboratories were not always compatible with each other, it is generally agreed that N-domains of p97 are conformationally flexible. EM studies of p97 complexed with the adaptor protein p47 also showed the N-domains undergoing a large conformational change in the presence of different nucleotides (Beuron et al., 2006). However, conflicting results were reported in these low-resolution studies on the direction of the N-domain movement in response to binding of different nucleotides. An intrinsic difficulty with these studies is the uncertainty concerning the nucleotide states at the AAA+ ATPase domains due to the resolution limits of these methods. Compounding these problems, it has been known that at least half of the nucleotide-binding sites in the D1-domains of p97 are pre-occupied by ADP molecules, which are very difficult to remove (Briggs et al., 2008; Davies et al., 2005). Clearly, high-resolution structures of p97 in different nucleotide states are needed to unambiguously define the relationship of N-domain conformation with nucleotide-binding states.

5.3 Crystallographic studies of IBMPFD mutant p97

Recently, a new conformation of N-domains was observed by X-ray crystallography at 2 Å resolution with ATPγS (a non-hydrolysable ATP analog) bound at the D1-domains of two IBMPFD-associated p97 N-D1 mutants, R155H and R95G; both are N-domain mutations (Tang et al., 2010). With ATPγS bound at the D1-domain, the N-domain undergoes a rotational and translational movement to adopt a new position, which is in sharp contrast to the "in-plane" position with the D1-ring or Down-conformation, as observed previously in the ADP-bound form. In this new conformation, the N-domains uniformly occupy a position above the plane of the D1-ring or in the Up-conformation (Fig. 2), despite the fact that no detectable changes are seen in the N-domain itself due to either the R155H or R95G mutation (Data not shown) (Tang et al., 2010). Accompanying the transition of N-domain from the Down- to Up-conformation are two prominent structural rearrangements. One is the transition in secondary structure of the linker between N- and D1-domain (N-D1 linker), going from the random coil in the Down-conformation to the three-turn α-helix in the Up-conformation reminiscent of a contracted spring pulling the N-domains out of the planar conformation upon the binding of ATPγS (Fig. 3A). This novel conformation of p97 demonstrated for the first time the dynamic movement of the N-domain at near atomic resolution, although observed in p97 mutants. A second change is the re-ordering of the N-terminal fragment that encompasses residues 12 to 20, which was disordered in the ADP-bound structures (Fig. 3B). This re-ordering of the N-terminal peptide apparently protects the Lys18 from limited proteolysis by trypsin seen in the ADP form of p97 (Fernandez-Saiz and Buchberger, 2010).

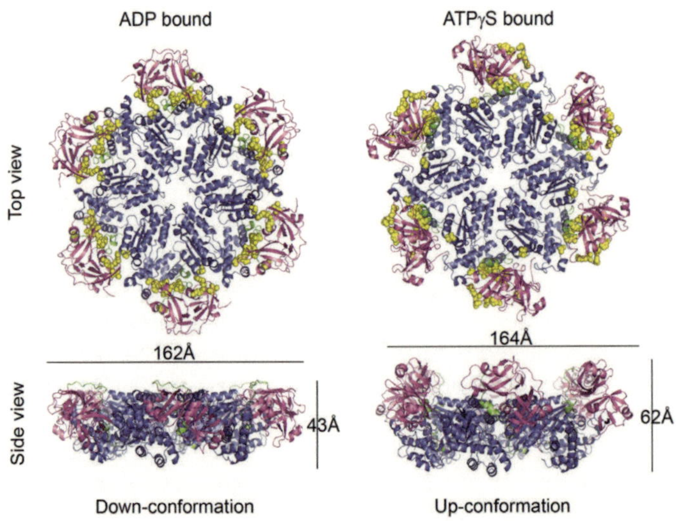

Fig. 2. **Changes in N-domain conformation in response to binding of different nucleotides to the D1 domain** Ribbon diagrams showing the two N-domain conformations of p97 N-D1 obtained from crystal structures. The N-domains, D1-domains and the IBMPFD mutations are colored in magenta and blue ribbons and in yellow balls, respectively.

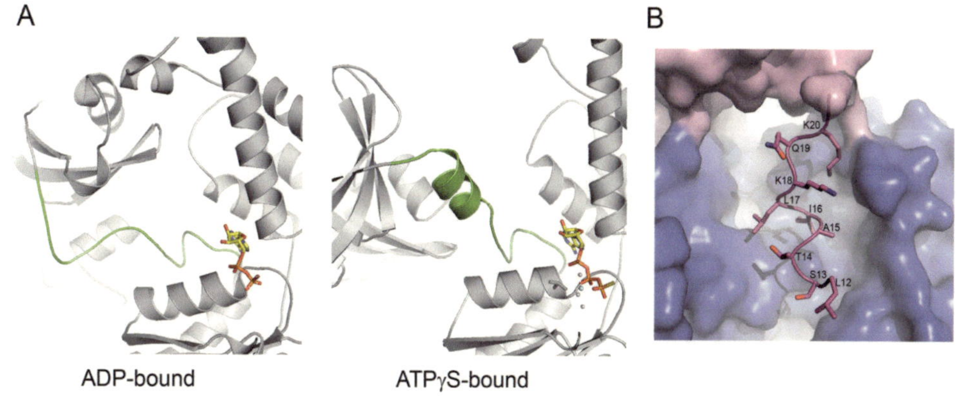

Fig. 3. **Observed structural re-arrangements in the N-D1 linker and N-terminal peptide in response to binding of different nucleotides in the D1-domain** (A) The secondary structure of the N-D1 linker undergoes a transition from a random coil to a three-turn helix as the N-domains move from the Down- to Up-conformation. A close-up view shows the two conformations of the N-D1 linker (in green) in the ADP-bound form (Down-conformation) and in the ATPγS-bound form (Up-conformation) of p97 N-D1. The nucleotides are represented by sticks with carbon atoms in yellow, oxygen in red, nitrogen in blue, phosphorous in orange, and sulfur in gold. (B) The reordering of N-terminal peptide Leu^{12} to Lys^{20} in the ATPγS-bound form (Up-conformation) is represented by stick model. The rest of the N-domain and D1-domain are shown as magenta and blue surfaces, respectively.

The above observation appears to favor the hypothesis that the Up and Down movement of N-domains is nucleotide dependent because the binding of ADP at the D1-domain of p97 results in a Down-conformation while binding of ATPγS leads to an Up-conformation. However, this nucleotide-driven movement may be arguable, as these two conformations were observed in two different systems - the wild type in ADP form and the IBMPFD mutants in ATPγS form. A subsequent structure determination using the same IBMPFD mutant and ADP showed that N-domains adopt the Down-conformation, just as the wild-type p97 in the presence of ADP (Tang et al., 2010), thus unequivocally confirming the dependency of N-domain conformation on the nucleotide binding states at the D1-domain.

5.4 Small angle X-ray scattering (SAXS) studies of wild type and IBMPFD mutant p97 in solution

Why crystallographic studies on wild type p97 can only reveal the Down-conformation, whereas IBMPFD p97 mutants can be crystallized in both Up- and Down-conformations was a paradox. One possible interpretation was that wild type and mutant p97 differ in nucleotide binding properties. Alternatively, this could be a crystallization effect. To investigate this, we performed SAXS experiments to identify conformational changes in IBMPFD mutants in solution. The results clearly demonstrated that in solution IBMPFD mutants undergo a nucleotide-dependent N-domain conformational change that is consistent with the Up- and Down-conformations observed in the crystals (Fig. 4). By serendipity, another major finding from this experiment was that wild type p97 also undergoes a similar nucleotide-driven conformational change as observed in IBMPFD mutants (Fig. 4) (Tang et al., 2010). Therefore, the lack of success in crystallizing the Up-conformation of wild type p97 suggests the presence of an intrinsic conformational heterogeneity or asymmetry in the N-domains of the homo-hexamer.

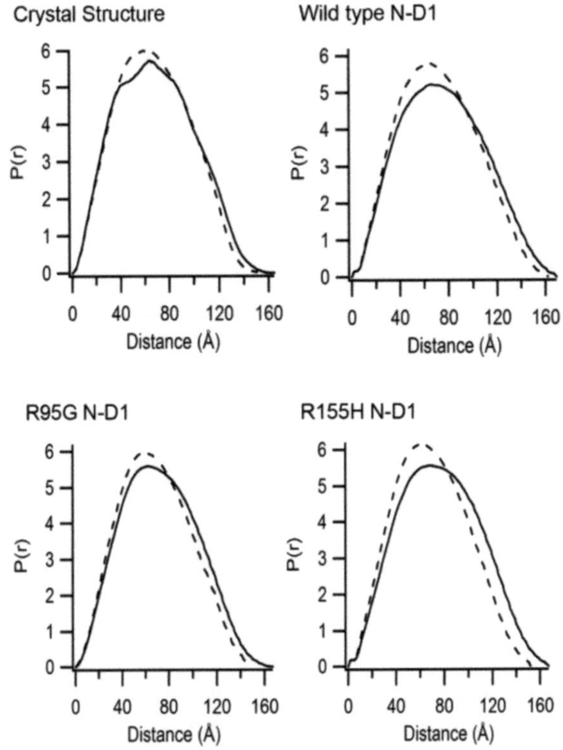

Fig. 4. **Nucleotide-driven conformational changes in solution observed by SAXS** Distance distribution functions, p(r), of p97 N-D1 normalized to a common total probability for wild type and mutant N-D1 fragments in the presence of ADP (solid line) ADP and ATPγS (dashed line). The calculated distribution (Glatter, 1980) is shown of the left based on the crystal structure in the absence of bound solvent molecules.

5.5 ADP and ATPγS binding at the D1-doamin

Although the binding of ATPγS to the D1-domain triggers a dramatic movement of the N-domain, the immediate vicinity of the D1 nucleotide-binding site shows only limited perturbations (Tang et al., 2010). When Cα atoms of the wild type and mutant N-D1 are superimposed, the adenosine moieties of the bound nucleotides align very well and the immediate environment around the adenosine moiety shows little change. By contrast, the phosphate groups in the alignment between ADP and ATPγS forms differ, even though the same set of residues are involved in contacting the α- and β-phosphate in both the wild type and mutant structures. The γ-phosphate in the ATPγS structure is stabilized by the ionic interaction with a magnesium ion (Mg^{2+}, see below), by hydrogen bonds with Gln^{348} and Lys^{251}, by Arg^{359}, an Arg finger residue from a neighboring subunit, and by two water molecules associated with the Mg^{2+} ion (Fig. 5). Perhaps due to better diffraction resolution, in the mutant structures of p97, a Mg^{2+} ion is present in the nucleotide-binding site of every subunit. The Mg^{2+} ion is at the center of an octahedral *mer*-triaquo complex with the additional three oxo ligands coming from the side chain of the highly conserved Thr[252] and from the β- and γ-phosphates. The acidic residues of the DEXX sequence (Asp[304] and Glu[305]) in the Walker B motif make hydrogen bonds with two of the water molecules in the Mg^{2+} coordination sphere and, additionally, Asp[304] stabilizes Thr[252]. As expected, most of the changes in the nucleotide-binding environment are a consequence of the introduction of the γ-phosphate.

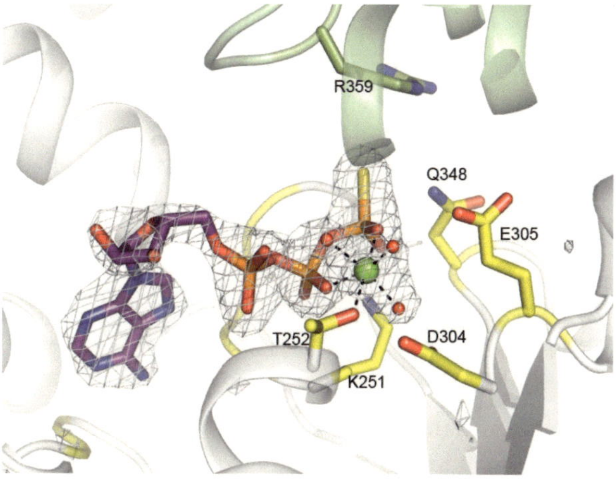

Fig. 5. **ATPγS binding vicinity of the D1-domain** The nucleotide-binding pocket is located at the subunit interface. The two subunits are in different colors, green and gray. The ATPγS molecule is shown as a stick model with carbon atoms in purple, oxygen in red, nitrogen in blue, phosphorous in magenta, and sulfur in yellow. The ATPγS molecule is enclosed in a difference electron density cage contoured at the 2.5 σ level. The Mg^{2+} ion is shown as a green ball with three coordinating water molecules in red.

6. Wild type vs. IBMPFD mutant p97: Biophysical and biochemical characteristics

Structurally observed differences in the N-domain conformation of p97 strongly suggest a change in nucleotide binding affinities between wild type and IBMPFD mutants, even though the binding environment for nucleotide seems unperturbed in mutant p97. The fact that mutant p97 can be crystallized in the presence of ATPγS suggests a few competing hypotheses: one of which is the possibility of IBMPFD mutants acquiring a higher affinity for ATPγS, leading to an alteration in ATPase activity. Alternatively, IBMPFD mutations could lead to a reduced ADP binding affinity. From structural studies, we can readily infer that the D1 nucleotide-binding site is seriously affected by IBMPFD mutations. However, how mutations at the N-D1 interface influence the D1 or D2 ATPase sites is not clear. Measuring the binding affinities of various nucleotides toward either D1 or D2 ATPase sites and the ATPase activities of the protein will provide biochemical indications as to how IBMPFD mutations might affect the biochemical properties of p97.

6.1 Nucleotide-binding affinity and ATPase activity

As mentioned earlier, p97 has two ATPase domains, D1 and D2; both are capable of hydrolyzing ATP. ATPase activity requires the presence of Mg^{2+} and is stimulated by high temperature (Song et al., 2003). While the D2-domain mediates most ATPase activity, the D1-domain contributes to heat-induced activity (Song et al., 2003). By using isothermal calorimetry (ITC) and Walker A mutants of either the D1- or D2-domains, it was shown that the binding of both domains to ATPγS is similar with dissociation constants in the range of 1 μM, but binding of ADP to the D1-domain is nearly 30-fold higher than that of the D2-domain, which is consistent with the higher ATPase activity of the D2-domain (Briggs et al., 2008).

Because the onset of IBMPFD is relatively late in life, the mutations in p97 are not expected to have dramatic defects in function. Indeed, IBMPFD equivalent mutations introduced into cdc48, a yeast homolog of p97, did not appear to interfere with normal cell growth (Esaki and Ogura, 2010). Although IBMPFD mutation sites are not in the immediate vicinity of the ATP-binding sites, as shown by crystal structures of p97, especially in the ATPγS bound form, reports on how mutations affect ATPase activity of p97 vary. Two reports showed that mutants exhibit higher ATPase activity than the wild type to various degrees (Manno et al., 2010; Weihl et al., 2006). One paper, by contrast, reported no significant alterations in ATPase activity of four IBMPFD mutants (Fernandez-Saiz and Buchberger, 2010). Mutant p97 also displayed an even higher level of heat-stimulated ATPase activity (Halawani et al., 2009).

ITC measurements in N-D1 fragments of p97 showed that instead of predicted higher affinity for ATPγS in the D1-domain, all mutants showed lowered affinity, up to five-fold weaker, towards ADP when compared to the wild type (Table 2) (Tang et al., 2010). More interestingly, all mutants displayed biphasic titration profiles toward ATPγS, suggesting two distinct binding sites, one high and one low affinity site.

N-D1 p97	ATPγS		ADP	
	K_d (μM)	N	K_d (μM)	N
Wild type	0.89 ± 0.28	0.12 ± 0.01	0.88 ± 0.18	0.35 ± 0.06
R95G	0.13 ± 0.02	0.56 ± 0.01	2.27 ± 0.11	0.62 ± 0.08
R155H	0.13 ± 0.01	0.61 ± 0.01	4.25 ± 0.54	0.72 ± 0.18

ITC with ATPγS for IBMPFD mutants showed biphasic titration curves and data were fitted with a 2-site model. The K_d values for mutants are derived from fitting to the first phase.

Table 2. Dissociation constants (K_d) and binding stoichiometry (N) of wild type and mutant p97 N-D1 fragments for ATPγS and ADP determined by ITC.

6.2 Pre-bound ADP in D1 nucleotide-binding sites

A unique characteristic of p97 was demonstrated by a urea denaturation experiment; the D1 sites are occupied by a significant portion of pre-bound ADP, which is difficult to release without denaturing the protein (Davies et al., 2005). ITC experiments with wild type p97 confirmed that a fraction of D1 sites are not accessible to nucleotide titration (Briggs et al., 2008). Consistent with the lowered K_d values for ADP binding in IBMPFD mutants, D1 sites were shown to be significantly more accessible to ADP titration by ITC and displayed a biphasic titration curve for ATPγS, reflecting the first phase binding of the empty sites and the second phase of the pre-bound sites (Table 2) (Tang et al., 2010). Extraction by heat denaturation experiments of pre-bound ADP from the D1 sites of p97 supported the observation by ITC that the number of titratable sites is inversely related to the amount of pre-bound ADP present at the D1-domain (Tang et al., unpublished data). These findings suggest that while in wild type p97 a significant number of sites with pre-bound ADP in D1-domains of p97 are not exchangeable by a different form of nucleotides present in solution, IBMPFD mutations have altered the environment and lowered binding affinity for ADP to allow exchange, even though the change in the ADP binding site is too subtle to be detected by crystal structures.

A consequence of lowered binding affinity for ADP in the D1-domain of IBMPFD mutants is the uniformly increased accessibility of D1 sites to various nucleotides present in solution such as ATPγS. Indeed, successful crystallization of mutant p97 in the presence of ATPγS is a result of this effect. On the contrary, the pre-bound ADP molecules in the D1-domains of some subunits of wild type p97 do not substitute for ATPγS, in spite of having a higher affinity towards ATPγS than ADP (Tang et al., 2010). Consequently, in the presence of excess ATPγS in solution, there will be an admixture of ADP- and ATPγS-bound D1 sites within a hexamer. Thus, the failure to crystallize wild type p97 in the presence of ATPγS is a manifestation of non-uniformity in binding to nucleotides by different subunits in the D1-domains of hexameric p97.

6.3 Changes in interaction with adaptor proteins

By interacting with various adaptor proteins, p97 is able to play a role in a number of important cellular pathways. Therefore, alterations in adaptor protein binding by IBMPFD mutants have been investigated in both *in vivo* and *in vitro* experiments. Again, results from different groups are not completely consistent (Fernandez-Saiz and Buchberger, 2010; Manno et al., 2010). Isolated mutant p97 exhibited the same binding as wild type p97 towards adaptor proteins p47, Ufd1-Npl4, E4B and the human UFD-2 homolog. However, mutants showed impaired binding to ubiquitin ligase E4B in the presence of Ufd1-Npl4. *In vivo* pull-down experiments using HEK293 cells showed reduced binding towards the E4B and enhanced binding towards ataxin 3, thus resembling the accumulation of mutant ataxin 3 on p97 in spinocerebellar ataxia type 3 (Fernandez-Saiz and Buchberger, 2010). However, similar *in vivo* studies were done showing enhanced binding of the Ufd1-Npl4 pair by IBMPFD mutants but not for p47 (Manno et al., 2010).

7. Implications concerning p97 function and disease

One major contribution of p97 to cellular processes is its apparent participation in protein quality control and homeostasis, involving the ubiquitin-proteasome degradation pathway, ER associated degradation, and formation of autophagosomes. The multifaceted clinical presentation of patients with IBMPFD is consistent with the broad spectrum of p97 functions. Indeed, pathology and the cellular hallmarks such as the accumulation of inclusion bodies and rimmed vacuoles of IBMPFD can be reproduced both in cell culture and in animal models (Custer et al., 2010; Ju and Weihl, 2010; Weihl et al., 2006; Weihl et al., 2007). However, the structural and molecular basis of how p97 is involved in these different pathways and the mechanism of how p97 mutations lead to dysfunction remain elusive.

7.1 IBMPFD mutations produce subtle structural and functional alteration in p97

Using structural, biophysical and biochemical approaches and through detailed comparative study of wild type and IBMPFD mutant p97, details of the molecular mechanisms of p97 at the most fundamental level are beginning to emerge. As a late onset disease, the IBMPFD mutations in p97 are not expected to dramatically disrupt cellular functions. Indeed, as shown from the cell biological, structural and biochemical data, all IBMPFD mutants (1) appear to have a normal phenotype at least in the early stage of life in cultured cells, in yeast, and in fruit flies, (2) do not have observable structural alterations in their constituent domains, as compared to the wild type, (3) can form proper hexameric ring structures, (4) have nucleotide-binding pockets indistinguishable from those of the wild type, and (5) are able to undergo nucleotide-driven conformational change in solution.

In spite of these similarities, subtle yet significant differences have also been detected in IBMPFD mutants, including (1) overall up-regulated ATPase activities, (2) ability to undergo uniform nucleotide-dependent N-domain conformational change that leads to its crystallization in the presence of ATPγS, (3) lowered binding affinity toward ADP in the D1-domain, (4) less non-exchangeable pre-bound ADP in the D1-domain, and (5) subtle differences in binding of adaptor proteins.

7.2 Asymmetry in p97 function

Enigmatic observations concerning the failure of wild type p97 to crystallize in the presence of ATPγS, yet being able to undergo nucleotide-dependent N-domain conformational change in solution suggest the functional importance of the non-uniform binding of nucleotides by p97 to the D1-domains and of the asymmetry in N-domain conformations among its six subunits. This asymmetry is a built-in property of wild type p97, as demonstrated by ITC and heat or urea denaturation experiments with characteristically pre-bound ADP at the D1-domain. Although a p97 hexamer is formed by six identical monomers, a fraction of the D1 sites is always pre-occupied by ADP, which is very difficult to release or exchange with other nucleotides. As a result, ATP in solution is only able to access the empty D1 sites, which drive the N-domain to the Up-conformation, whereas the N-domains remain in the Down-conformation for those subunits with pre-bound ADP. Although it is not yet clear how p97 maintains this asymmetry during its catalytic cycle, some level of communication must exist among subunits.

A model for the ATP cycle in the D1-domain and the corresponding N-domain conformation has been proposed by integrating the structural and biochemical data of wild type and mutant p97 (Fig. 6). The model proposes four nucleotide-binding states for the D1-domain. (1) There is the "ATP" state with ATP bound and the N-domain in the Up-conformation. Crystallographic and X-ray scattering experiments support the existence of this state in subunits of both mutant and wild type p97. It should be noted that due to non-exchangeable, pre-bound ADP in a wild type p97 hexamer, not all subunits can bring their N-domains to the Up-conformation, even with an excess of ATP in solution. (2) There is an "ADP-locked" state with non-exchangeable, pre-bound ADP at the D1 site and the N-domain in the Down-conformation. This state appears to be important for wild type p97 function and the pre-bound ADP is particularly difficult to release. The structure of the N-D1 fragment of wild type p97 may represent this conformation. (3) The "ADP-open" state is defined by the binding of exchangeable ADP. This state was observed for mutant p97 by its biphasic ITC titration profile and is presumably in equilibration with the ADP-locked state. The structure of R155H with bound ADP may represent this conformation. (4) Finally, there is the "Empty" state with nucleotide-binding sites unoccupied and the N-domain in an unknown position. For wild type p97, the transition between the "ADP-locked" and "ADP-open" states is thought to be tightly controlled, resulting in rare ADP-open states, leading to asymmetry in the nucleotide binding and N-domain conformation in a hexameric p97.

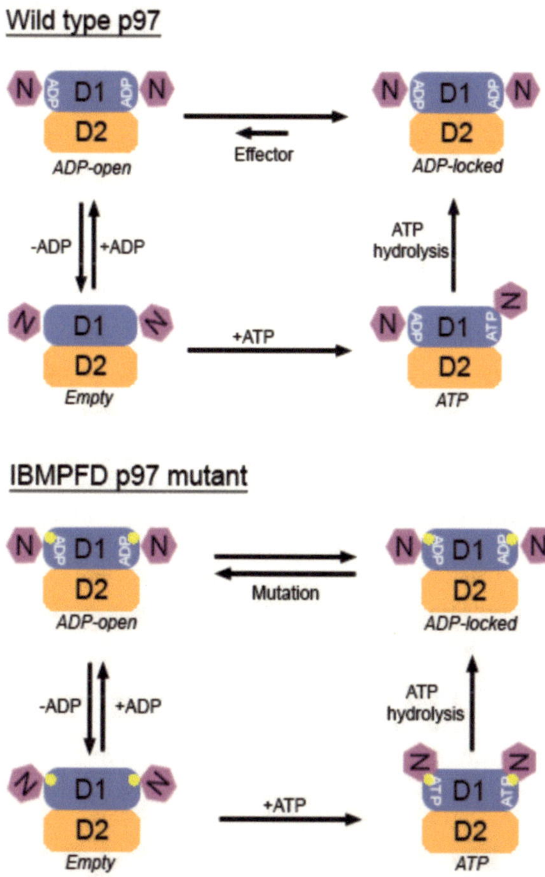

Fig. 6. **Models for the N-domain movement in p97 during ATP cycle** Schematic diagram for the control of the N-domain conformation in the wild type and IBMPFD associated N-D1 fragment of p97. Different domains are colored and labeled. The IBMPFD mutations are represented by yellow circles. Four states are defined for each nucleotide-binding site in D1: *Empty, ATP, ADP-locked* and *ADP-open* states, as labeled. The type of nucleotide bound at the D1-domain is labeled. Each subunit of the hexameric p97 is assumed to operate independently in this model.

From structural and molecular characterizations, we can infer that the non-uniform movement of p97 is essential to its function. In order to generate the up-and-down movement of the N-domain in a non-uniform fashion, the "ADP-locked" sites needed to be activated to the "ADP-open" state. It is thought that in wild type p97 control of the transition between the ADP-locked and ADP-open state in D1 could be achieved in two ways: (1) the binding of adaptor proteins to the N-domain, or (2) the hydrolysis of ATP in the D2-domain. The N-domain was shown to have an influence on the ATPase activity of both N-D1 and the full-length p97 ortholog, VAT, as the N-domain-deleted p97 mutants have higher ATPase activity (Gerega et al., 2005). The binding of adaptor protein p47 to the N-domain was shown to inhibit the ATPase activity of p97 (Meyer et al., 1998). Communication between D1 and D2 is also known to exist for p97 and other type II AAA^+ proteins. For example, it was shown that the absence of D2-domain inhibits the nucleotide exchange activity in D1 (Davies et al., 2005). The yeast Hsp104, another type II AAA^+ protein, displays cooperative kinetics and inter-domain communication for its two ATPase domains (Hattendorf and Lindquist, 2002). However, the exact details of these possible control mechanisms for the switching of D1 nucleotide states remain elusive. Like many AAA^+ proteins involved in protein quality control such as *E. coli* ClpA and yeast Hsp104, p97 functions in handling protein substrates to various pathways, which requires the presence of the N-domain. Although how p97 handles these substrates has yet to be defined, one advantage of asymmetric interaction over symmetric seems that the former ensures continuous contacts with the substrates.

7.3 Loss of asymmetry in IBMPFD mutant p97

Mapping the IBMPFD mutations to the Down-conformation of p97 reveals the clustering of these mutations at the interface between the N- and D1-domains. Site-directed mutagenesis of R86A, a residue present at the N-D1 interface but not identified as an IBMPFD mutation, showed to possess all the structural and biochemical characteristics of an IBMPFD mutant p97 (Tang et al., 2010). This suggests that the N-D1 interface residues are critical for the proper function of p97 by providing tight regulation of the movement of the N-domain and the nucleotide state of the D1-domain.

Instead of prominent structural changes, IBMPFD mutations introduce subtle modifications to p97, apparently disrupting communication among the monomers. Unlike the wild type p97, IBMPFD mutants allow easy displacement of pre-bound ADP at the D1-domain by ATPγS, resulting in a unified nucleotide state, and hence, a symmetric hexamer in the Up-conformation. Using the same ATP catalytic cycle model for the D1-domain shown above, it was postulated that the difference between the wild type and mutants lies in the transition between the "ADP-locked" state and the "ADP-open" state. While this transition is tightly regulated in wild type p97, this control mechanism is altered in IBMPFD mutants, leading to a high concentration of subunits in the "ADP-open" state (Fig. 6). Consequently, p97 mutants undergo a uniform N-domain conformational change in response to high concentrations of ATPγS, leading to a defective enzyme.

8. References

Allen, M.D.; Buchberger, A. & Bycroft, M. (2006). The PUB domain functions as a p97 binding module in human peptide N-glycanase. *J Biol Chem,* Vol.281, No.35, (Sep 1), pp. 25502-25508

Bersano, A.; Del Bo, R.; Lamperti, C.; Ghezzi, S.; Fagiolari, G.; Fortunato, F.; Ballabio, E.; Moggio, M.; Candelise, L.; Galimberti, D., *et al.* (2009). Inclusion body myopathy and frontotemporal dementia caused by a novel VCP mutation. *Neurobiol Aging,* Vol.30, No.5, (May), pp. 752-758

Beuron, F.; Dreveny, I.; Yuan, X.; Pye, V.E.; McKeown, C.; Briggs, L.C.; Cliff, M.J.; Kaneko, Y.; Wallis, R.; Isaacson, R.L., *et al.* (2006). Conformational changes in the AAA ATPase p97-p47 adaptor complex. *EMBO J,* Vol.25, No.9, (May 3), pp. 1967-1976

Bieniossek, C.; Niederhauser, B. & Baumann, U.M. (2009). The crystal structure of apo-FtsH reveals domain movements necessary for substrate unfolding and translocation. *Proc Natl Acad Sci U S A,* Vol.106, No.51, (Dec 22), pp. 21579-21584

Briggs, L.C.; Baldwin, G.S.; Miyata, N.; Kondo, H.; Zhang, X. & Freemont, P.S. (2008). Analysis of nucleotide binding to P97 reveals the properties of a tandem AAA hexameric ATPase. *J Biol Chem,* Vol.283, No.20, (May 16), pp. 13745-13752

Caccamo, A.; Majumder, S.; Deng, J.J.; Bai, Y.; Thornton, F.B. & Oddo, S. (2009). Rapamycin rescues TDP-43 mislocalization and the associated low molecular mass neurofilament instability. *J Biol Chem,* Vol.284, No.40, (Oct 2), pp. 27416-27424

Chen, B.; Sysoeva, T.A.; Chowdhury, S.; Guo, L.; De Carlo, S.; Hanson, J.A.; Yang, H. & Nixon, B.T. (2010). Engagement of arginine finger to ATP triggers large conformational changes in NtrC1 AAA+ ATPase for remodeling bacterial RNA polymerase. *Structure,* Vol.18, No.11, (Nov 10), pp. 1420-1430

Clague, M.J. & Urbe, S. (2010). Ubiquitin: same molecule, different degradation pathways. *Cell,* Vol.143, No.5, (Nov 24), pp. 682-685

Custer, S.K.; Neumann, M.; Lu, H.; Wright, A.C. & Taylor, J.P. (2010). Transgenic mice expressing mutant forms VCP/p97 recapitulate the full spectrum of IBMPFD including degeneration in muscle, brain and bone. *Hum Mol Genet,* Vol.19, No.9, (May 1), pp. 1741-1755

Davies, J.M.; Tsuruta, H.; May, A.P. & Weis, W.I. (2005). Conformational changes of p97 during nucleotide hydrolysis determined by small-angle X-Ray scattering. *Structure,* Vol.13, No.2, (Feb), pp. 183-195

DeLaBarre, B. & Brunger, A.T. (2003). Complete structure of p97/valosin-containing protein reveals communication between nucleotide domains. *Nat Struct Biol,* Vol.10, No.10, (Oct), pp. 856-863

Djamshidian, A.; Schaefer, J.; Haubenberger, D.; Stogmann, E.; Zimprich, F.; Auff, E. & Zimprich, A. (2009). A novel mutation in the VCP gene (G157R) in a German family with inclusion-body myopathy with Paget disease of bone and frontotemporal dementia. *Muscle Nerve,* Vol.39, No.3, (Mar), pp. 389-391

Esaki, M. & Ogura, T. (2010). ATP-bound form of the D1 AAA domain inhibits an essential function of Cdc48p/p97. *Biochem Cell Biol,* Vol.88, No.1, (Feb), pp. 109-117

Fernandez-Saiz, V. & Buchberger, A. (2010). Imbalances in p97 co-factor interactions in human proteinopathy. *EMBO Rep,* Vol.11, No.6, (Jun), pp. 479-485

Frohlich, K.U.; Fries, H.W.; Rudiger, M.; Erdmann, R.; Botstein, D. & Mecke, D. (1991). Yeast cell cycle protein CDC48p shows full-length homology to the mammalian protein VCP and is a member of a protein family involved in secretion, peroxisome formation, and gene expression. *J Cell Biol,* Vol.114, No.3, (Aug), pp. 443-453

Gai, D.; Zhao, R.; Li, D.; Finkielstein, C.V. & Chen, X.S. (2004). Mechanisms of conformational change for a replicative hexameric helicase of SV40 large tumor antigen. *Cell,* Vol.119, No.1, (Oct 1), pp. 47-60

Gerega, A.; Rockel, B.; Peters, J.; Tamura, T.; Baumeister, W. & Zwickl, P. (2005). VAT, the thermoplasma homolog of mammalian p97/VCP, is an N domain-regulated protein unfoldase. *J Biol Chem,* Vol.280, No.52, (Dec 30), pp. 42856-42862

Gidaro, T.; Modoni, A.; Sabatelli, M.; Tasca, G.; Broccolini, A. & Mirabella, M. (2008). An Italian family with inclusion-body myopathy and frontotemporal dementia due to mutation in the VCP gene. *Muscle Nerve,* Vol.37, No.1, (Jan), pp. 111-114

Glatter, O. (1980). Computation of distance distribution function and scattering function of models for small angle scattering experiments. *Acta Phys Austriaca,* Vol.52, pp. 243-256

Guyant-Marechal, L.; Laquerriere, A.; Duyckaerts, C.; Dumanchin, C.; Bou, J.; Dugny, F.; Le Ber, I.; Frebourg, T.; Hannequin, D. & Campion, D. (2006). Valosin-containing protein gene mutations: clinical and neuropathologic features. *Neurology,* Vol.67, No.4, (Aug 22), pp. 644-651

Halawani, D.; LeBlanc, A.C.; Rouiller, I.; Michnick, S.W.; Servant, M.J. & Latterich, M. (2009). Hereditary inclusion body myopathy-linked p97/VCP mutations in the NH2 domain and the D1 ring modulate p97/VCP ATPase activity and D2 ring conformation. *Molecular and cellular biology,* Vol.29, No.16, (Aug), pp. 4484-4494

Hattendorf, D.A. & Lindquist, S.L. (2002). Cooperative kinetics of both Hsp104 ATPase domains and interdomain communication revealed by AAA sensor-1 mutants. *EMBO J,* Vol.21, pp. 12-21

Haubenberger, D.; Bittner, R.E.; Rauch-Shorny, S.; Zimprich, F.; Mannhalter, C.; Wagner, L.; Mineva, I.; Vass, K.; Auff, E. & Zimprich, A. (2005). Inclusion body myopathy and Paget disease is linked to a novel mutation in the VCP gene. *Neurology,* Vol.65, No.8, (Oct 25), pp. 1304-1305

Huyton, T.; Pye, V.E.; Briggs, L.C.; Flynn, T.C.; Beuron, F.; Kondo, H.; Ma, J.; Zhang, X. & Freemont, P.S. (2003). The crystal structure of murine p97/VCP at 3.6A. *J Struct Biol,* Vol.144, No.3, (Dec), pp. 337-348

Ishikawa, T.; Maurizi, M.R. & Steven, A.C. (2004). The N-terminal substrate-binding domain of ClpA unfoldase is highly mobile and extends axially from the distal surface of ClpAP protease. *J Struct Biol,* Vol.146, No.1-2, (Apr-May), pp. 180-188

Ju, J.S. & Weihl, C.C. (2010). Inclusion body myopathy, Paget's disease of the bone and fronto-temporal dementia: a disorder of autophagy. *Hum Mol Genet,* Vol.19, No.R1, (Apr 15), pp. R38-45

Kimonis, V.E.; Fulchiero, E.; Vesa, J. & Watts, G. (2008a). VCP disease associated with myopathy, Paget disease of bone and frontotemporal dementia: review of a unique disorder. *Biochim Biophys Acta,* Vol.1782, No.12, (Dec), pp. 744-748

Kimonis, V.E.; Kovach, M.J.; Waggoner, B.; Leal, S.; Salam, A.; Rimer, L.; Davis, K.; Khardori, R. & Gelber, D. (2000). Clinical and molecular studies in a unique family with autosomal dominant limb-girdle muscular dystrophy and Paget disease of bone. *Genet Med,* Vol.2, No.4, (Jul-Aug), pp. 232-241

Kimonis, V.E.; Mehta, S.G.; Fulchiero, E.C.; Thomasova, D.; Pasquali, M.; Boycott, K.; Neilan, E.G.; Kartashov, A.; Forman, M.S.; Tucker, S., *et al.* (2008b). Clinical studies in familial VCP myopathy associated with Paget disease of bone and frontotemporal dementia. *Am J Med Genet A,* Vol.146A, No.6, (Mar 15), pp. 745-757

Kondo, H.; Rabouille, C.; Newman, R.; Levine, T.P.; Pappin, D.; Freemont, P. & Warren, G. (1997). p47 is a cofactor for p97-mediated membrane fusion. *Nature,* Vol.388, No.6637, (Jul 3), pp. 75-78

Kovach, M.J.; Waggoner, B.; Leal, S.M.; Gelber, D.; Khardori, R.; Levenstien, M.A.; Shanks, C.A.; Gregg, G.; Al-Lozi, M.T.; Miller, T., *et al.* (2001). Clinical delineation and localization to chromosome 9p13.3-p12 of a unique dominant disorder in four families: hereditary inclusion body myopathy, Paget disease of bone, and frontotemporal dementia. *Mol Genet Metab,* Vol.74, No.4, (Dec), pp. 458-475

Kravats, A.; Jayasinghe, M. & Stan, G. (2011). Unfolding and translocation pathway of substrate protein controlled by structure in repetitive allosteric cycles of the ClpY ATPase. *Proc Natl Acad Sci U S A,* Vol.108, No.6, (Feb 8), pp. 2234-2239

Kumar, K.R.; Needham, M.; Mina, K.; Davis, M.; Brewer, J.; Staples, C.; Ng, K.; Sue, C.M. & Mastaglia, F.L. (2010). Two Australian families with inclusion-body myopathy, Paget's disease of bone and frontotemporal dementia: novel clinical and genetic findings. *Neuromuscul Disord,* Vol.20, No.5, (May), pp. 330-334

Lamb, J.R.; Fu, V.; Wirtz, E. & Bangs, J.D. (2001). Functional analysis of the trypanosomal AAA protein TbVCP with trans-dominant ATP hydrolysis mutants. *J Biol Chem,* Vol.276, No.24, (Jun 15), pp. 21512-21520

Lee, S.; Sowa, M.E.; Watanabe, Y.; Sigler, P.B.; Chiu, W.; Yoshida, M. & Tsai, T.F. (2003). The structure of ClpB: a molecular chaperone that rescues proteins from an aggregated state. *Cell,* Vol.115, pp. 229-240

Leon, A. & McKearin, D. (1999). Identification of TER94, an AAA ATPase protein, as a Bam-dependent component of the Drosophila fusome. *Mol Biol Cell,* Vol.10, No.11, (Nov), pp. 3825-3834

Madsen, L.; Andersen, K.M.; Prag, S.; Moos, T.; Semple, C.A.; Seeger, M. & Hartmann-Petersen, R. (2008). Ubxd1 is a novel co-factor of the human p97 ATPase. *Int J Biochem Cell Biol,* Vol.40, No.12, pp. 2927-2942

Madsen, L.; Seeger, M.; Semple, C.A. & Hartmann-Petersen, R. (2009). New ATPase regulators--p97 goes to the PUB. *Int J Biochem Cell Biol,* Vol.41, No.12, (Dec), pp. 2380-2388

Manno, A.; Noguchi, M.; Fukushi, J.; Motohashi, Y. & Kakizuka, A. (2010). Enhanced ATPase activities as a primary defect of mutant valosin-containing proteins that cause inclusion body myopathy associated with Paget disease of bone and frontotemporal dementia. *Genes Cells,* Vol.15, No.8, (Aug), pp. 911-922

Meyer, H.H.; Kondo, H. & Warren, G. (1998). The p47 co-factor regulates the ATPase activity of the membrane fusion protein, p97. *FEBS Lett,* Vol.437, No.3, (Oct 23), pp. 255-257

Muller, J.M.; Deinhardt, K.; Rosewell, I.; Warren, G. & Shima, D.T. (2007). Targeted deletion of p97 (VCP/CDC48) in mouse results in early embryonic lethality. *Biochem Biophys Res Commun,* Vol.354, No.2, (Mar 9), pp. 459-465

Palmio, J.; Sandell, S.; Suominen, T.; Penttila, S.; Raheem, O.; Hackman, P.; Huovinen, S.; Haapasalo, H. & Udd, B. (2011). Distinct distal myopathy phenotype caused by VCP gene mutation in a Finnish family. *Neuromuscul Disord,* (Jun 17), pp.

Richly, H.; Rape, M.; Braun, S.; Rumpf, S.; Hoege, C. & Jentsch, S. (2005). A series of ubiquitin binding factors connects CDC48/p97 to substrate multiubiquitylation and proteasomal targeting. *Cell,* Vol.120, No.1, (Jan 14), pp. 73-84

Ritson, G.P.; Custer, S.K.; Freibaum, B.D.; Guinto, J.B.; Geffel, D.; Moore, J.; Tang, W.; Winton, M.J.; Neumann, M.; Trojanowski, J.Q., *et al.* (2010). TDP-43 mediates degeneration in a novel Drosophila model of disease caused by mutations in VCP/p97. *J Neurosci,* Vol.30, No.22, (Jun 2), pp. 7729-7739

Rohrer, J.D.; Warren, J.D.; Reiman, D.; Uphill, J.; Beck, J.; Collinge, J.; Rossor, M.N.; Isaacs, A.M. & Mead, S. (2011). A novel exon 2 I27V VCP variant is associated with dissimilar clinical syndromes. *J Neurol,* (Mar 9), pp.

Rouiller, I.; DeLaBarre, B.; May, A.P.; Weis, W.I.; Brunger, A.T.; Milligan, R.A. & Wilson-Kubalek, E.M. (2002). Conformational changes of the multifunction p97 AAA ATPase during its ATPase cycle. *Nat Struct Biol,* Vol.9, No.12, (Dec), pp. 950-957

Schroder, R.; Watts, G.D.; Mehta, S.G.; Evert, B.O.; Broich, P.; Fliessbach, K.; Pauls, K.; Hans, V.H.; Kimonis, V. & Thal, D.R. (2005). Mutant valosin-containing protein causes a novel type of frontotemporal dementia. *Ann Neurol,* Vol.57, No.3, (Mar), pp. 457-461

Singh, S.K. & Maurizi, M.R. (1994). Mutational analysis demonstrates different functional roles for the two ATP-binding sites in ClpAP protease from Escherichia coli. *J Biol Chem,* Vol.269, pp. 29537-29545

Song, C.; Wang, Q. & Li, C.C. (2003). ATPase activity of p97-valosin-containing protein (VCP). D2 mediates the major enzyme activity, and D1 contributes to the heat-induced activity. *J Biol Chem,* Vol.278, No.6, (Feb 7), pp. 3648-3655

Spina, S.; Van Laar, A.D.; Murrell, J.R.; De Courten-Myers, G.; Hamilton, R.L.; Farlow, M.R.; Quinlan, J.; DeKosky, S.T. & B., G. (2008). Frontotemporal dementia associated with a Valosin-Containing Protein mutation: report of three families. *FASEB Journal,* Vol.22, pp. 58.54

Stojkovic, T.; Hammouda el, H.; Richard, P.; Lopez de Munain, A.; Ruiz-Martinez, J.; Gonzalez, P.C.; Laforet, P.; Penisson-Besnier, I.; Ferrer, X.; Lacour, A., *et al.* (2009). Clinical outcome in 19 French and Spanish patients with valosin-containing protein myopathy associated with Paget's disease of bone and frontotemporal dementia. *Neuromuscul Disord,* Vol.19, No.5, (May), pp. 316-323

Tang, W.K.; Li, D.; Li, C.C.; Esser, L.; Dai, R.; Guo, L. & Xia, D. (2010). A novel ATP-dependent conformation in p97 N-D1 fragment revealed by crystal structures of disease-related mutants. *EMBO J,* Vol.29, No.13, (Jul 7), pp. 2217-2229

Vale, R.D. & Milligan, R.A. (2000). The way things move: looking under the hood of molecular motor proteins. *Science,* Vol.288, No.5463, (Apr 7), pp. 88-95

van der Zee, J.; Pirici, D.; Van Langenhove, T.; Engelborghs, S.; Vandenberghe, R.; Hoffmann, M.; Pusswald, G.; Van den Broeck, M.; Peeters, K.; Mattheijssens, M., *et al.* (2009). Clinical heterogeneity in 3 unrelated families linked to VCP p.Arg159His. *Neurology,* Vol.73, No.8, (Aug 25), pp. 626-632

Viassolo, V.; Previtali, S.C.; Schiatti, E.; Magnani, G.; Minetti, C.; Zara, F.; Grasso, M.; Dagna-Bricarelli, F. & Di Maria, E. (2008). Inclusion body myopathy, Paget's disease of the bone and frontotemporal dementia: recurrence of the VCP R155H mutation in an

Italian family and implications for genetic counselling. *Clin Genet,* Vol.74, No.1, (Jul), pp. 54-60

Wang, J.; Song, J.J.; Seong, I.S.; Franklin, M.C.; Kamtekar, S.; Eom, S.H. & Chung, C.H. (2001). Nucleotide-dependent conformational changes in a protease-associated ATPase HslU. *Structure,* Vol.9, No.11, (Nov), pp. 1107-1116

Wang, Q.; Song, C. & Li, C.C. (2003). Hexamerization of p97-VCP is promoted by ATP binding to the D1 domain and required for ATPase and biological activities. *Biochem Biophys Res Commun,* Vol.300, No.2, (Jan 10), pp. 253-260

Wang, Q.; Song, C. & Li, C.C. (2004). Molecular perspectives on p97-VCP: progress in understanding its structure and diverse biological functions. *J Struct Biol,* Vol.146, No.1-2, (Apr-May), pp. 44-57

Wang, X.; Fan, H.; Ying, Z.; Li, B.; Wang, H. & Wang, G. (2010). Degradation of TDP-43 and its pathogenic form by autophagy and the ubiquitin-proteasome system. *Neurosci Lett,* Vol.469, No.1, (Jan 18), pp. 112-116

Watts, G.D.; Thomasova, D.; Ramdeen, S.K.; Fulchiero, E.C.; Mehta, S.G.; Drachman, D.A.; Weihl, C.C.; Jamrozik, Z.; Kwiecinski, H.; Kaminska, A., *et al.* (2007). Novel VCP mutations in inclusion body myopathy associated with Paget disease of bone and frontotemporal dementia. *Clin Genet,* Vol.72, No.5, (Nov), pp. 420-426

Watts, G.D.; Thorne, M.; Kovach, M.J.; Pestronk, A. & Kimonis, V.E. (2003). Clinical and genetic heterogeneity in chromosome 9p associated hereditary inclusion body myopathy: exclusion of GNE and three other candidate genes. *Neuromuscul Disord,* Vol.13, No.7-8, (Sep), pp. 559-567

Watts, G.D.; Wymer, J.; Kovach, M.J.; Mehta, S.G.; Mumm, S.; Darvish, D.; Pestronk, A.; Whyte, M.P. & Kimonis, V.E. (2004). Inclusion body myopathy associated with Paget disease of bone and frontotemporal dementia is caused by mutant valosin-containing protein. *Nat Genet,* Vol.36, No.4, (Apr), pp. 377-381

Weihl, C.C. (2011). Valosin Containing Protein Associated Fronto-Temporal Lobar Degeneration: Clinical Presentation, Pathologic Features and Pathogenesis. *Curr Alzheimer Res,* (Jan 11), pp.

Weihl, C.C.; Dalal, S.; Pestronk, A. & Hanson, P.I. (2006). Inclusion body myopathy-associated mutations in p97/VCP impair endoplasmic reticulum-associated degradation. *Hum Mol Genet,* Vol.15, No.2, (Jan 15), pp. 189-199

Weihl, C.C.; Miller, S.E.; Hanson, P.I. & Pestronk, A. (2007). Transgenic expression of inclusion body myopathy associated mutant p97/VCP causes weakness and ubiquitinated protein inclusions in mice. *Hum Mol Genet,* Vol.16, No.8, (Apr 15), pp. 919-928

Weihl, C.C.; Temiz, P.; Miller, S.E.; Watts, G.; Smith, C.; Forman, M.; Hanson, P.I.; Kimonis, V. & Pestronk, A. (2008). TDP-43 accumulation in inclusion body myopathy muscle suggests a common pathogenic mechanism with frontotemporal dementia. *J Neurol Neurosurg Psychiatry,* Vol.79, No.10, (Oct), pp. 1186-1189

Woodman, P.G. (2003). p97, a protein coping with multiple identities. *J Cell Sci,* Vol.116, No.Pt 21, (Nov 1), pp. 4283-4290

Ye, Y. (2006). Diverse functions with a common regulator: ubiquitin takes command of an AAA ATPase. *J Struct Biol,* Vol.156, No.1, (Oct), pp. 29-40

Zhang, X.; Shaw, A.; Bates, P.A.; Newman, R.H.; Gowen, B.; Orlova, E.; Gorman, M.A.; Kondo, H.; Dokurno, P.; Lally, J., *et al.* (2000). Structure of the AAA ATPase p97. *Mol Cell,* Vol.6, No.6, (Dec), pp. 1473-1484

Zolkiewski, M. (2006). A camel passes through the eye of a needle: protein unfolding activity of Clp ATPases. *Mol Microbiol,* Vol.61, No.5, (Sep), pp. 1094-1100

Congenital Myasthenic Syndromes – Molecular Bases of Congenital Defects of Proteins at the Neuromuscular Junction

Kinji Ohno[1], Mikako Ito[1] and Andrew G. Engel[2]
[1]Division of Neurogenetics, Center for Neurological Diseases and Cancer, Nagoya University Graduate School of Medicine, Nagoya,
[2]Department of Neurology, Mayo Clinic, Rochester, Minnesota,
[1]Japan
[2]USA

1. Introduction

Congenital myasthenic syndromes (CMS) are heterogeneous disorders caused by mutations in molecules expressed at the neuromuscular junction (NMJ) (Fig. 1). Each mutation affects the expression level or the functional properties or both of the mutant molecule. No fewer than 11 defective molecules at the NMJ have been identified to date. The mutant molecules include (i) acetylcholine receptor (AChR) subunits that forms nicotinic AChR and generate endplate potentials (Ohno *et al.*, 1995; Sine *et al.*, 1995), (ii) rapsyn that anchors and clusters AChRs at the endplate (Ohno *et al.*, 2002; Milone *et al.*, 2009), (iii) agrin that is released from nerve terminal and induces AChR clustering by stimulating the downstream LRP4/MuSK/Dok-7/rapsyn/AChR pathway (Huze *et al.*, 2009), (iv) muscle-specific receptor tyrosine kinase (MuSK) that transmits the AChR-clustering signal from agrin/LRP4 to Dok-7/rapsyn/AChR (Chevessier *et al.*, 2004; Chevessier *et al.*, 2008), (v) Dok-7 that interacts with MuSK and exerts the AChR-clustering activity (Beeson *et al.*, 2006; Hamuro *et al.*, 2008), (vi) plectin that is an intermediate filament-associate protein concentrated at sites of mechanical stress (Banwell *et al.*, 1999; Selcen *et al.*, 2011), (vii) glutamine-fructose-6-phosphate aminotransferase 1 encoded by *GFPT1*, the function of which at the NMJ has not been elucidated (Senderek *et al.*, 2011), (viii) skeletal muscle sodium channel type 1.4 ($Na_V1.4$) that spreads depolarization potential from endplate throughout muscle fibers (Tsujino *et al.*, 2003), (ix) collagen Q that anchors acetylcholinesterase (AChE) to the synaptic basal lamina (Ohno *et al.*, 1998; Ohno *et al.*, 1999; Kimbell *et al.*, 2004), (x) β2-laminin that forms a cruciform heterotrimeric lamins-221, -421, and -521 and links extracellular matrix molecules to the β-dystroglycan at the NMJ (Maselli *et al.*, 2009), (xi) choline acetyltransferase (ChAT) that resynthesizes acetylcholine from recycled choline at the nerve terminal (Ohno *et al.*, 2001). AChR (Lang & Vincent, 2009), MuSK (Hoch *et al.*, 2001; Cole *et al.*, 2008), and LRP4 (Higuchi *et al.*, 2011) are also targets of myasthenia gravis, in which autoantibody against each molecule impairs the neuromuscular transmission.

CMS are classified into three groups of postsynaptic, synaptic, and presynaptic depending on the localization of the defective molecules. Among the eleven molecules introduced above, AChR, rapsyn, MuSK, Dok-7, plectin, and $Na_V1.4$ are associated with the postsynaptic membrane. Agrin, ColQ, and β2-laminin reside in the synaptic basal lamina. The only presynaptic disease protein identified to date is choline acetyltransferase (ChAT). A target molecule and its synaptic localization of glutamine-fructose-6-phosphate aminotransferase 1 (GFPT1) are still unresolved but the phenotypic consequence is the postsynaptic AChR deficiency. This chapter focuses on molecular bases of these three groups of CMS.

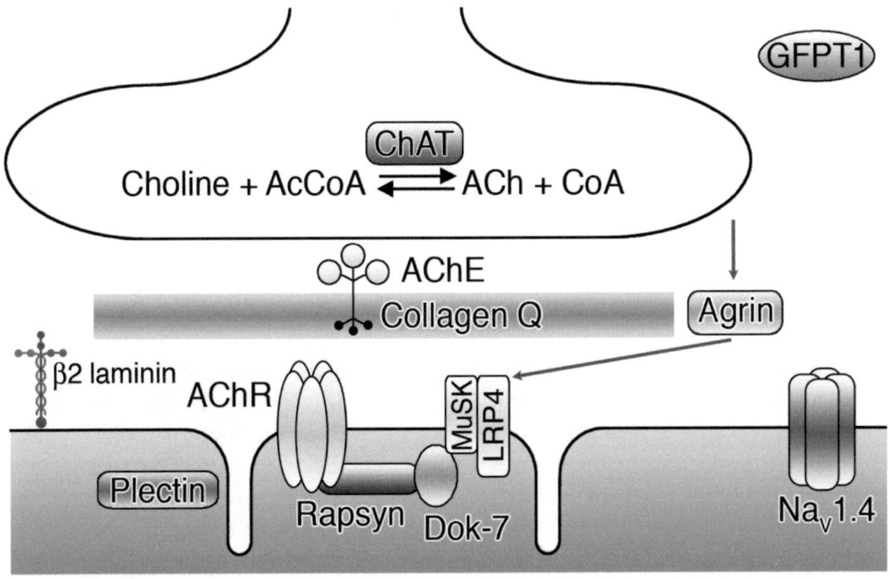

Fig. 1. Schematic of molecules expressed at the NMJ

2. Physiology of the NMJ

This section introduces molecular basis of development and maintenance of the NMJ, and physiological features of nicotinic muscle AChR.

2.1 NMJ synaptogenesis

At the NMJ, MuSK is an indirect receptor for agrin (Valenzuela *et al.*, 1995; Dechiara *et al.*, 1996). Agrin released from the nerve terminal binds to LRP4 on the postsynaptic membrane (Kim *et al.*, 2008; Zhang *et al.*, 2008). Binding of LRP4 to agrin phosphorylates MuSK. Phosphorylated MuSK recruits the noncatalytic adaptor protein Dok-7 (Okada *et al.*, 2006). Once recruited, Dok-7 further facilitates phosphorylation of MuSK, and induces clustering of rapsyn and AChR by phosphorylating the β subunit of AChR. Rapsyn self-associates and makes a homomeric cluster at the endplate, which serves as a scaffold for AChR. Rapsyn and AChR bind each other with a stoichiometry of 1:1. Rapsyn also binds to β-dystroglycan and links the rapsyn scaffold to the subsynaptic cytoskeleton (Froehner *et al.*, 1990; Cartaud *et al.*, 1998; Ramarao & Cohen, 1998; Ramarao *et al.*, 2001). Except for LRP4, each of the above molecules is a CMS target.

2.2 Physiology of the nicotinic muscle AChR

Nicotinic AChRs are pentameric ligand-gated ion channels. The family of pentameric ligand-gated ion channels includes cationic AChRs, cationic serotonergic receptors ($5HT_3$), anionic glycine receptors, and anionic $GABA_A$ and $GABA_C$ receptors (Keramidas *et al.*, 2004). Heteromeric neuronal nicotinic AChRs are comprised of various combinations of α (α2-α7) and β subunits (β2-β4), whereas homomeric AChRs are formed only by a single α subunit (e.g., α7-α9) (Mihailescu & Drucker-Colin, 2000). On the other hand, nicotinic muscle AChRs have only two forms: fetal AChR that carries the α, β, δ, and γ subunits encoded by *CHRNA1, CHRNB1, CHRND, CHRNG,* respectively, in the stoichiometry $\alpha_2\beta\delta\gamma$; and adult-type AChR that carries the ε subunit instead of the γ subunit in the stoichiometry $\alpha_2\beta\delta\varepsilon$ (Mishina *et al.*, 1986). The ε subunit is encoded by *CHRNE*. Nicotinic muscle AChR harbors two binding sites for ACh at the interfaces between the α–δ and α–γ/α–ε subunits (Lee *et al.*, 2009; Mukhtasimova *et al.*, 2009). Binding of a single ACh molecule opens the channel pore but for a short time. Binding of two ACh molecules stabilizes the open state of AChR, and AChR stays open for a longer time. Only cations pass through the channel pore of nicotinic AChRs. Unlike sodium, potassium, or calcium channels, AChRs, in general, have no selectivity for cations, but α7 AChRs have 10-20 times higher permeability for Ca^{2+} than for Na^+.

3. Postsynaptic CMS

Postsynaptic CMS is classified into four phenotypes: (i) endplate AChR deficiency due to defects in AChR, rapsyn, agrin, MuSK, Dok-7, plectin, glutamine-fructose-6-phosphate aminotransferase 1, (ii) slow-channel congenital myasthenic syndrome, (iii) fast-channel congenital myasthenic syndrome, and (iv) sodium channel myasthenia.

3.1 Endplate AChR deficiency

Endplate AChR deficiency is caused by defects in AChR, rapsyn, agrin, MuSK, Dok-7, plectin, and GFPT1.

3.1.1 Endplate AChR deficiency due to defects in AChR subunits

Endplate AChRs deficiency can arise from mutations in *CHRNA1, CHRNB1, CHRND,* and *CHRNE,* but not *CHRNG.*

Two different groups of mutations of the AChR subunit genes cause endplate AChR deficiency. The first group includes null mutations in *CHRNE* encoding the ε subunit. The null mutations are caused by frameshifting DNA rearrangements, *de novo* creation of a stop codon, and frameshifting splice-site mutations, or mutations involving residues essential for subunit assembly. Large-scale in-frame DNA rearrangements also abolish expression of the AChR ε subunit (Abicht *et al.*, 2002). Mutations in the promoter region (Ohno *et al.*, 1999) and most missense mutations (Ohno *et al.*, 1997) do not completely abolish expression of the ε subunit but the molecular consequences are indistinguishable from those of null mutations. Lack of the ε subunit can be compensated for by the presence of the fetal γ subunit that is normally expressed in embryos (Engel *et al.*, 1996). The patients can survive with γ-AChR even in the absence of ε-AChR. If a null mutation resides in the other AChR subunit genes, the affected individual will have no substituting subunit and cannot survive. Indeed, two homozygous missense low expressor or null mutations in *CHRNA1* and *CHRND* caused lethal fetal akinesia (Michalk *et al.*, 2008).

The second group of mutations affecting the AChR subunit genes includes missense mutations of *CHRNA1*, *CHRNB1*, and *CHRND*. These mutations compromise expression of the mutant subunit and/or the assembly of AChRs, but do not completely abolish AChRs expression. The main difference between mutations in *CHRNE* and those in *CHRNA1*, *CHRNB1*, and *CHRND* is tolerance to low or no expression of the ε subunit whereas similar mutations in other subunits generally have devastating consequences and cause high fatality. Some missense mutations in *CHRNA1*, *CHRNB1*, *CHRND*, and *CHRNE* also affect the AChR channel kinetics and vice versa. The kinetic effects will predominate if the second mutation is a low expressor, or if the kinetic mutation has slow-channel features with dominant gain-of function effects.

In endplate AChR deficiency, the postsynaptic membrane displays a reduced binding for peroxidase- or ^{125}I-labeled α-bungarotoxin and the synaptic response to ACh, reflected by the amplitude of the miniature endplate potential, endplate potential, and endplate current, is reduced. In some but not all cases the postsynaptic region is simplified. In most cases, the muscle fibers display an increased number of small synaptic contacts over an extended length of the muscle fiber. In some patients quantal release is higher than normal. In patients with null mutations in *CHRNE*, single channel recordings of AChRs at patient endplates reveal prolonged opening bursts that open to an amplitude of 60 pS, indicating expression of the fetal γ-AChR in contrast to the adult ε-AChR that has shorter opening bursts and opens to an amplitude of 80 pS. In contrast, in most patients with low-expressor mutations in the *CHRNA1*, *CHRNB1*, or *CHRND*, single channel recordings demonstrate no or minor kinetic abnormalities.

As in autoimmune myasthenia gravis, endplate AChR deficiency is generally well controlled by regular doses of anticholinesterases. Anticholinesterase medications inhibit the catalytic activity of AChE; this prolongs the dwell time of ACh in the synaptic space and allows each ACh molecule to bind repeatedly to AChR.

3.1.2 Endplate AChR deficiency due to defects in rapsyn

Congenital defects of rapsyn also cause endplate AChR deficiency. Rapsyn makes a homomeric cluster and binds to AChR as well as to β-dystroglycan, and forms AChR clusters at the endplate (Froehner *et al.*, 1990; Cartaud *et al.*, 1998; Ramarao & Cohen, 1998; Ramarao *et al.*, 2001). The structural domains of rapsyn include an N-terminal myristoylation signal required for membrane association (Ramarao & Cohen, 1998), seven tetratrico peptide repeats at codons 6 to 279 that subserve rapsyn self-association (Ramarao & Cohen, 1998; Ramarao *et al.*, 2001), a coiled-coil domain at codons 298 to 331 that binds to the long cytoplasmic loop of each AChR subunit (Bartoli *et al.*, 2001), a Cys-rich RING-H2 domain at codons 363-402 that binds to the cytoplasmic domain of β-dystroglycan (Bartoli *et al.*, 2001) and mediates the MuSK induced phosphorylation of AChR (Lee *et al.*, 2008), and a serine phosphorylation site at codon 406. Transcription of rapsyn in muscle is under the control of helix-loop-helix myogenic determination factors that bind to the *cis*-acting E-box sequence in the *RAPSN* promoter (Ohno *et al.*, 2003).

Loss-of-function mutations in *RAPSN* have been reported in the coding region (Ohno *et al.*, 2002; Burke *et al.*, 2003; Dunne & Maselli, 2003; Maselli *et al.*, 2003; Muller *et al.*, 2003; Banwell *et al.*, 2004; Yasaki *et al.*, 2004; Cossins *et al.*, 2006; Muller *et al.*, 2006) as we as in the promoter region (Ohno *et al.*, 2003). N88K in *RAPSN* is one of the most frequently observed mutations in CMS (Muller *et al.*, 2003; Richard et al., 2003). We reported lack of a founder haplotype for N88K (Ohno & Engel, 2004), but analysis of markers closer to *RAPSN* later revealed possible presence of a shared haplotype (Muller et al., 2004) suggesting that N88K is an ancient founder mutation but subsequent multiple recombination events and divergence of microsatellite markers have narrowed the shared haplotype region. Functional analysis L14P, N88K, and 553ins5 disclosed that these mutations have no effect on self-association of rapsyn but impair colocalization of rapsyn with AChR (Ohno *et al.*, 2002). Analysis of A25V, N88K, R91L, L361R, and K373del later revealed diverse molecular defects affecting colocalization of rapsyn with AChR, formation of agrin-induced AChR clusters, self-association of rapsyn, and expression of rapsyn (Cossins *et al.*, 2006). Although there are no genotype-phenotype correlations in mutations at the coding region, arthrogryposis at birth and other congenital malformations occurs in nearly a third of the patients. In addition, the -38A>G mutation affecting an E-box in the promoter region observed in Near-Eastern Jewish patients exhibits unique facial malformations associated with prognathism and malocclusion (Ohno *et al.*, 2003).

Most patients respond well to anticholinesterase medications. Some patients further improve with addition of 3,4-diaminopyridine, ephedrine, and albuterol (Banwell *et al.*, 2004). The drug 3,4-diaminopyridine blocks the presynaptic potassium channel, which slows the repolarization of the presynaptic membrane (Wirtz *et al.*, 2010) enhancing the influx of Ca^{2+} through the presynaptic voltage-gated P/Q-type and N-type channels. This, in turn, facilitates the exocytosis of synaptic vesicles and the quantal content of the endplate potential.

3.1.3 Endplate AChR deficiency due to a defect in agrin

Neural agrin released from the nerve terminal is a key mediator of synaptogenesis at the NMJ. A reported homozygous G1709R agrin mutation, however, did not cause AChR deficiency but mutations in agrin are potential causes of AChR deficiency by interfering with the activation of MuSK and by impeding synaptic maturation.

The patient harboring the G1709R mutation was a 42-year-old woman with right lid ptosis since birth, no oculoparesis, and mild weakness of facial, hip-girdle and anterior tibial muscles, and refractoriness to pyridostigmine or 3,4-diaminopyridine (Huze *et al.*, 2009). The mutation is in the laminin G-like 2 domain, upstream of the neuron-specific y and z exons that are required for MuSK activation and AChR clustering. AChR and agrin expression at the endplate were normal. Structural studies showed endplates with misshaped synaptic gutters partially filled by nerve endings and formation of new endplate regions. The postsynaptic regions were preserved. Expression studies in myotubes using a mini-agrin construct revealed the mutation did not affect MuSK activation or agrin binding to α-dystroglycan. Forced expression of the mutant mini-agrin gene in mouse soleus muscle induced changes similar to those at patient endplates. Thus, the observed mutation perturbs the maintenance of the endplate without altering the canonical function of agrin to induce development of the postsynaptic compartment.

3.1.4 Endplate AChR deficiency due to defects in MuSK

MuSK and LRP4 form a heteromeric receptor for agrin. Five *MUSK* mutations have been reported in three papers. The first report describes heteroallelic frameshift (220insC) and missense (V790M) mutations in a patient with respiratory distress in early life, mild ptosis, decreased upward gaze, and fatigable weakness of the cervical and proximal more than distal muscles. The symptoms were worsened by pregnancy. Treatment with pyridostigmine and 3,4-diaminopyridine was ineffective (Chevessier *et al.*, 2004). The frameshift mutation prevents MuSK expression and the missense mutation decreases MuSK expression and impairs its interaction with Dok-7. Forced expression of the mutant protein in mouse muscle decreased AChR expression at the endplate and caused aberrant axonal outgrowth (Chevessier *et al.*, 2004). Interestingly, mice homozygous for MuSK V789M (which corresponds to the human MuSK V790M) are normal but mice hemizygous for V789M are severely affected suggesting that MuSK V790M in humans is a haploinsufficient only when accompanied by a null mutation (Chevessier *et al.*, 2008).

A second report describes heteroallelic M605I and A727V mutations in MuSK in a patient with severe myasthenic symptoms since early life that improved after puberty but worsened after menstrual periods. The MEPP and MEPC amplitudes in anconeus muscle were reduced to about 30% of normal and the EPP quantal content was half-normal. Synaptic contacts were small and electron microscopy showed simplified postsynaptic regions with too few secondary synaptic clefts. The patient failed to respond to pyridostigmine, ephedrine or 3,4-diaminopyuridine but responded partially to albuterol (Maselli *et al.*, 2010).

A third report describes a homozygous P31L mutation in the extracellular domain of MuSK in 5 patients in a consanguineous Sudanese kinship. The findings included ptosis from an early age, partial ophthalmoparesis, and weakness of torso and limb girdle muscles. Pyridostigmine therapy gave only slight benefit (Mihaylova *et al.*, 2009).

3.1.5 Endplate AChR deficiency due to defects in Dok-7

Phosphorylated MuSK recruits a noncatalytic adaptor protein, Dok-7. Recruited Dok-7 further facilitates phosphorylation of MuSK (Okada *et al.*, 2006). Dok-7 is highly expressed at the postsynaptic region of skeletal muscle and in heart. It harbors an N terminal pleckstrin homology domain (PH) important for membrane association, a phosphotyrosine-binding (PTB) domain, and C-terminal sites for phosphorylation. The PH and PTB domains are required for association with and phosphorylation of MuSK. Phosphorylation of two C terminal residues is a requisite for Dok-7 activation by Crk and Crk-L (Hallock *et al.*, 2010).

Numerous mutations have been identified in *DOK7* (Beeson *et al.*, 2006; Muller *et al.*, 2007; Anderson *et al.*, 2008; Selcen *et al.*, 2008; Vogt *et al.*, 2009; Ben Ammar *et al.*, 2010). Nearly all patients carry a common 1124_1127dupTGCC mutation in exon 7. This and other mutations upstream of the C-terminal phosphorylation sites abrogate the ability of Dok-7 to associate with Crk1/Crk1L and hence its activation (Hallock *et al.*, 2010; Wu *et al.*, 2010). Mutations disrupting or eliminating the PH and PTB domains of Dok-7 prevent dimerization and association of Dok-7 with MuSK (Bergamin *et al.*, 2010).

3.1.6 Endplate AChR deficiency due to defects in plectin

Plectin, encoded by *PLEC*, is a highly conserved and ubiquitously expressed intermediate filament-linking protein concentrated at sites of mechanical stress, such as the postsynaptic membrane of the endplate, the sarcolemma, Z-disks in skeletal muscle, hemidesmosomes in skin, and intercalated disks in cardiac muscle. Pathogenic mutations in *PLEC* result in epidermolysis bullosa simplex, a progressive myopathy (Smith *et al.*, 1996), and, in some patients, myasthenic syndrome (Banwell *et al.*, 1999; Selcen *et al.*, 2011). We reported two cases of CMS associated with plectin deficiency (Banwell *et al.*, 1999; Selcen *et al.*, 2011). The dystrophic changes in muscle are attributed to dislocation of the fiber organelles no longer anchored by the cytoskeletal intermediate filaments and to sarcolemmal defects allowing Ca^{2+} ingress into the muscle fibers. The myasthenic syndrome is attributed to destruction of the junctional folds lacking adequate cytoskeletal support.

3.1.7 Endplate AChR deficiency due to defects in glutamine-fructose-6-phosphate aminotransferase 1 (GFPT1)

Glutamine-fructose-6-phosphate transaminase 1, encoded by *GFPT1*, catalyzes transfer of an amino group from glutamine onto fructose-6-phosphate, yielding glucosamine-6-phosphate and glutamate. GFPT1 is a rate-limiting enzyme that controls the flux of glucose into the hexosamine biosynthesis pathway. GFPT1 thus initiates formation of UDP-N-acetylglucosamine (UDP-GlcNAc), which is a source of multiple glycosylation processes including addition of N-acetylglucosamine to serine or threonine residues (O-linked GlcNAc) (Wells *et al.*, 2001). The disease gene was discovered by linkage analysis and homozygosity mapping of 13 kinships with a limb-girdle CMS often associated with tubular aggregates in skeletal muscle (Senderek *et al.*, 2011). Immunoblots of muscle of affected patients revealed decreased expression of O-linked GlcNAc, but the responsible molecule(s) causing CMS remain elusive.

3.2 Slow-channel congenital myasthenic syndrome (SCCMS)

The second class of postsynaptic CMS due to mutations in the AChR subunit genes is SCCMS. SCCMS is an autosomal dominant disorder, in which a gain-of-function mutation on a single allele compromises the neuromuscular signal transduction (Ohno *et al.*, 1995). The mutation causes prolonged AChR channel openings and increases the synaptic response to ACh (Fig. 2). There is a single reported case of autosomal recessive SCCMS, in which an εL78P mutation minimally prolongs channel opening events but the mutant channel arising from a single allele is not sufficient to cause disease (Croxen *et al.*, 2002). In general, dominantly inherited disorders, including SCCMS, tend to present after adolescence and have a relatively mild course. Some patients with SCCMS, however, present early in life and become severely disabled even in the first decade.

In SCCMS, neuromuscular transmission is compromised by three distinct mechanisms. First, staircase summation of endplate potentials causes depolarization block of the postsynaptic membrane by rendering the voltage-gated skeletal muscle sodium channel go into an inactivated state and thereby inhibit action potential generation (Maselli & Soliven, 1991). Second, some mutant AChRs are prone to become desensitized (Milone *et al.*, 1997), which reduces the number of AChRs that respond to the released ACh quanta. Third, prolonged opening of AChR causes excessive influx of extracellular calcium, which results in focal degeneration of the junctional folds as well as apoptosis of some of the junctional nuclei (Groshong *et al.*, 2007). In normal adult human ε-AChR, 7% of the synaptic current is carried by Ca^{2+}, which is higher than that carried by the human fetal γ-AChR or by muscle AChRs of other species (Fucile *et al.*, 2006). This predisposes endplate to Ca^{2+} overloading when the channel opening events are prolonged. In addition, at least two SCCMS mutations, εT264P (Ohno *et al.*, 1995) and αV259F (Fidzianska *et al.*, 2005), increase the Ca^{2+} permeability 1.5- and 2-fold, respectively (Di Castro *et al.*, 2007).

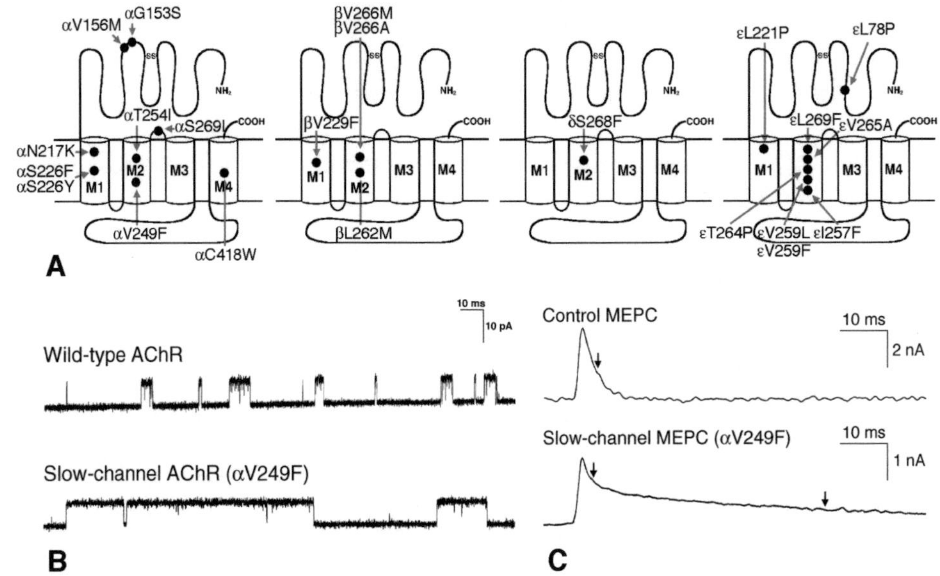

Fig. 2. Slow channel CMS. (A) Schematic diagram of AChR subunits with SCCMS mutations. (B) Single channel currents from wild-type and slow channel (αV249F) AChRs expressed on HEK293 cells. (C) Miniature endplate current (MEPC) recorded from endplates of a control and a patient harboring αV249F. The patient's MEPC decays biexponentially (arrows) due to expression of both wild-type and mutant AChRs.

Slow channel mutations can be divided into two groups. The first group includes mutations at the extracellular domain like αG153S (Sine *et al.*, 1995), as well as at the N-terminal part of the first transmembrane domain like αN217K (Wang *et al.*, 1997) and εL221F (Hatton *et al.*, 2003). These mutations increase the affinity for ACh binding, probably by retarding the dissociation of ACh from the binding site, which gives rise to repeated channel openings after a single event of ACh binding. The second group includes mutations at the second transmembrane domain (M2) that lines the ion channel pore. These mutations mostly introduce a bulky amino acid into the channel lining face, but εT264P (Ohno *et al.*, 1995) introduces a kink into the channel pore, whereas βV266A (Shen *et al.*, 2003) and εV265A (Ohno *et al.*, 1998) introduce a smaller amino acid into the pore. Mutations in M2 retard the channel closing rate α and variably enhance the channel opening rate β. Some mutations in M2 also increase affinity for ACh, which include αV249F (Milone *et al.*, 1997), εL269F (Engel *et al.*, 1996), and εT264P (Ohno *et al.*, 1995).

SCCMS can be treated with conventional doses of long-lived open channel blockers of AChR, such as the antiarrhythmic agent quinidine (Fukudome *et al.*, 1998; Harper & Engel, 1998) and the antidepressant fluoxetine (Harper *et al.*, 2003). Quinidine reduces the prolonged burst duration of SCCMS to the normal level at 5 μM (Fukudome *et al.*, 1998). As the concentration of quinidine in the treatment of cardiac arrhythmia is 6-15 μM, 5 μM is readily attainable in clinical practice and indeed demonstrates significant effects (Harper & Engel, 1998). Similarly, fluoxetine reduces the prolonged burst duration to the normal level at 10 μM, which is clinically attainable without adverse effects at 80 to 120 mg/day of fluoxetine (Harper *et al.*, 2003).

3.3 Fast-channel congenital myasthenic syndrome (FCCMS)

The third class of postsynaptic CMS due to mutations in AChR subunit genes is FCCMS. FCCMS is kinetically opposite to SCCMS (Fig. 3). In FCCMS, the closed state of AChR is stabilized compared to the open state which results in abnormally brief channel opening events which, in turn, reduces the amplitude of the endplate potential and impair the safety margin of neuromuscular transmission. The resulting pathophysiology is thus similar to endplate AChR deficiency, but abnormally small endplate potential is a qualitative instead of a quantitative defect in AChR.

FCCMS is an autosomal recessive disorder. One allele carries a missense mutation that confers a fast closure of AChRs, and the other allele usually harbors a low-expressor or null mutation, or the fast channel mutation occurs at homozygosity. As in heterozygous healthy parents of endplate AChR deficiency, we humans may completely lack 50% of each AChR subunit without any clinical symptoms. In FCCMS, a low-expressor or null mutation on one allele unmasks the deleterious effect of the fast-channel mutation on the second allele. Detailed kinetic analyses of FCCMS mutations have revealed special insights into the molecular architectures of the AChR subunits. Three such examples are presented here.

The ε1254ins18 mutation causes a duplication of STRDQE codons at positions 413 to 418 close to the C-terminal end of the long cytoplasmic loop (LCP) linking the third (M3) and fourth (M4) transmembrane domains of the receptor. ε1254ins18-AChR expressed on HEK293 cells opens in three different modes. The opening probabilities of normal AChRs are clustered into a single large peak, whereas the ε1254ins18-AChR shows three different peaks (Milone *et al.*, 1998). In all the three modes, the AChR is activated slowly and inactivated rapidly, which gives rise to an inefficient synaptic response to ACh. Another FCCMS mutation, εA411P in the LCP also destabilizes the channel opening kinetics. The channel opening probabilities of εA411P-AChRs are widely distributed and do not form any discernible peaks (Wang *et al.*, 2000). Our analysis first disclosed that the function of LCP is to stabilize the open conformation of the AChR.

εN436del is a deletion of Asn at the C-terminal end of the LCP. The deletion shortens the LCP and shifts a negatively charged Asp residue at codon 435 against M4. εN436del-AChR decreases the duration of channel opening bursts 2.7-fold compared to the wild type due to a 2.3-fold decrease in gating efficiency and a 2.5-fold decrease in agonist affinity of the diliganded closed state. A series of artificial mutations established that the effects of εN436del are not due to juxtaposition of a negative charge against M4 but to the shortening of the LCP. Deletion of the C-terminal residue of the LCP of the β and δ subunits also results in fast-channel kinetics, but that in the α subunit dictates slow-channel kinetics. Thus, the LCPs of four AChR subunits contribute in an asymmetric manner to optimize the activation of AChRs through allosteric links to the channel and to the agonist binding sites (Shen *et al.*, 2005).

The mutation αV285I introduces a bulky amino acid into the M3 transmembrane domain and causes FCCMS (Fig. 3). Kinetic studies demonstrate that the mutation slows the channel opening rate β and speeds the channel closing rate α, resulting in a 15.1-fold reduction in the channel gating equilibrium constant θ (= β/α). On the other hand, the mutation minimally affects affinity for ACh. The probability of channel openings decreased when we introduced Leu, a bulky amino acid, at position V285, but rather increased when we introduced smaller amino acids such as Thr and Ala. We observed similar effects when we introduced similar substitutions into the β, δ, and ε subunits. Thus, introduction of bulky amino acids narrows the channel pore, while introduction of smaller amino acids widens the channel pore. Our analysis thus revealed that the M3 domain backs up the channel-lining pore lined by the M2 transmembrane domains and has stereochemical effects on channel gating kinetics (Wang *et al.*, 1999).

FCCMS can be effectively treated with anticholinesterases and 3,4-diaminopyridine. The pharmacologic effects of these drugs were discussed in the section of endplate AChR deficiency (Section 3.1.2).

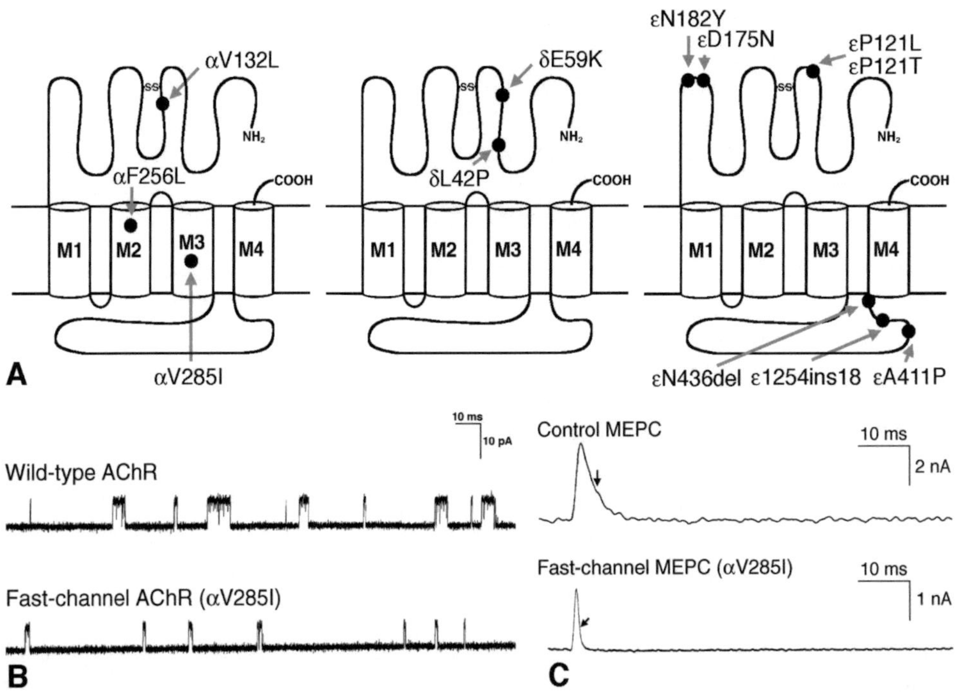

Fig. 3. Fast channel CMS. (A) Schematic diagram of AChR subunits with FCCMS mutations. (B) Single channel currents from wild-type and fast channel (αV285I) AChRs expressed on HEK293 cells. (C) Miniature endplate current (MEPC) recorded from endplates of a control and a patient harboring αV285I. The patient's MEPC decays faster than that of the normal control.

3.4 CMS due to defects in skeletal muscle sodium channel, $Na_V1.4$

Another class of postsynaptic CMS is due to mutations in skeletal muscle sodium channel, $Na_V1.4$, encoded by *SCN4A* (Tsujino *et al.*, 2003). Dominant gain-of-function mutations in this gene cause hyperkalemic periodic paralysis (Ptacek *et al.*, 1991), paramyotonia congenita (McClatchey *et al.*, 1992; Ptacek *et al.*, 1992), potassium-aggravated myotonia (Lerche *et al.*, 1993), and hypokalemic periodic paralysis type 2 (Bulman *et al.*, 1999). On the other hand, loss-of-function mutations cause a CMS.

Failure of normal-amplitude endplate potential depolarizing the resting potential to -40 mV in intercostal muscle of a CMS patient with episodes of apnea and myasthenic symptoms since birth prompted us to search for mutations in *SCN4A*. We identified two heteroallelic missense mutations, S246L and V1442E (Tsujino *et al.*, 2003). Activation kinetics of the mutant $Na_V1.4$ was normal for both S246L and V1442E, but the fast inactivation curves were shifted to hyperpolarization by 7.3 mV for S246L and 33.2 mV for V1442E, indicating that both mutations enhance fast inactivation of the $Na_V1.4$ immediately after it is activated. Moreover, a high proportion of the V1442 channel was in the inactivated state even at a normal resting membrane potential. Recovery from the fast-inactivated state was slowed for both mutations. This was in contrast to gain-of-function mutations in other diseases, which shift the fast inactivation curves to depolarization. Neither S246L nor V1442E affected slow inactivation. Analysis of use-dependent inactivation in HEK293 cells by stimulating at 50 Hz for 3 ms revealed that wild-type and S246L channels decreased the peak current only by 5% and V1442E channel decreased it by 30% during the first few pulses and suggested that the S246L mutation is relatively benign.

4. Synaptic CMS

Defects in three components of the synaptic basal lamina, AChE, β2 laminin and neural agrin, are associated with CMS. The CMS caused by mutations in agrin was discussed above under the postsynaptic CMS (Section 3.1.3) because the site of action of agrin is the LRP4/MuSK complex at the endplate.

4.1 Endplate AChE deficiency due to defects in collagen Q

Three tetramers of catalytic AChE subunits are linked by a triple helical collagen Q (ColQ) to constitute an asymmetric ColQ-tailed AChE (Krejci *et al.*, 1997). ColQ carries three domains (i) an N-terminal proline-rich attachment domain (PRAD) that organizes the catalytic AChE subunits into a tetramer, (ii) a collagenic domain that forms a triple helix, and (iii) a C-terminal domain enriched in charged residues and cysteines. ColQ-tailed AChE is organized in the secretory pathway, excreted, and anchored into the synaptic basal lamina using two domains of ColQ (Fig. 4). First, the collagen domain harbors two heparan sulfate proteoglycan (HSPG) binding domains (Deprez *et al.*, 2003) that bind to HSPG, such as perlecan (Peng *et al.*, 1999). Second, the C-terminal domain binds to MuSK (Cartaud *et al.*, 2004).

Endplate AChE deficiency is caused by congenital defects of ColQ (Donger *et al.*, 1998; Ohno *et al.*, 1998; Ohno *et al.*, 2000). Congenital defects of ColQ cause endplate AChE deficiency. No mutations have been detected in a gene encoding the catalytic subunit of AChE in CMS or in any other disease. There are three classes of ColQ mutations. First, mutations in the proline-rich attachment domain (PRAD) hinder binding of ColQ to AChE. Sedimentation analysis of AChE species of the patient muscle and transfected cells shows complete lack of ColQ-tailed AChE. Second, mutations in the collagen domain, most of which are truncation mutations, hinder formation of triple helix of ColQ. Sedimentation analysis of muscle and transfected cells demonstrate a truncated single-stranded ColQ associated with a homotetramer of AChE. Third, the mutations in the C-terminal domain have no deleterious effect on formation of the asymmetric ColQ-tailed AChE, but they compromise anchoring of ColQ-tailed AChE to the synaptic basal lamina as elegantly shown in vitro overlay binding of mutant and wild-type human recombinant ColQ-tailed AChE to the frog endplate (Kimbell *et al.*, 2004).

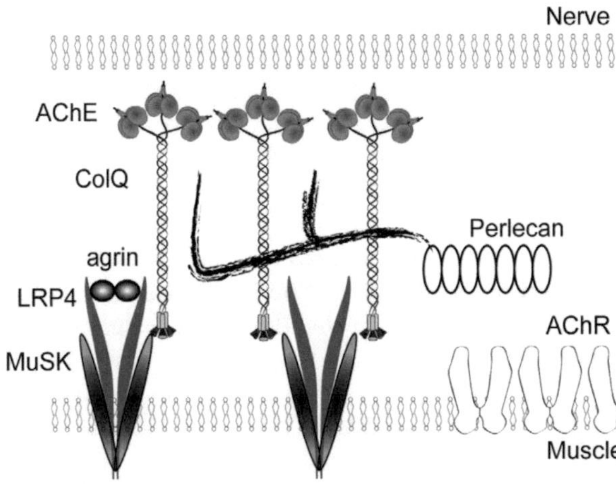

Fig. 4. ColQ anchors to the synaptic basal lamina by binding to perlecan and MuSK.

EMG studies show a decremental response as in other CMS. In addition, most patients have a repetitive CMAP response on a single nerve stimulus. The repetitive CMAP decrements faster than the primary CMAP. It can be overlooked unless a well rested muscle is tested by single nerve stimuli. The prolonged dwell time of unhydrolyzed ACh in the synaptic space prolongs the endplate potential; when this exceeds the absolute refractory period of the muscle fiber action potential, it elicits a repetitive CMAP. As mentioned above, a repetitive CMAP also occurs in slow channel syndrome.

Some aspects of the pathophysiology of endplate AChE deficiency resemble those of the SCCMS. As in the SCCMS, neuromuscular transmission is compromised by three distinct mechanisms. First, staircase summation of endplate potentials causes a depolarization block, which inactivates a proportion the voltage-gated skeletal sodium channel, $Na_V1.4$. (Maselli & Soliven, 1991). Second, prolonged exposure of AChR to ACh during physiologic activity desensitizes a fraction of the available AChRs (Milone *et al.*, 1997). Third, repeated openings of AChR cause calcium overloading to the endplate, which culminates in an endplate myopathy (Groshong *et al.*, 2007). Unlike in the SCCMS, the nerve terminals are abnormally small and often encased by Schwann cells. This decreases the quantal content and hence the amplitude of the endplate potential (Engel *et al.*, 1977).

Anticholinesterase medications have no effect on neuromuscular transmission and can cause excessive muscarinic side effects. Quinidine (Fukudome *et al.*, 1997; Harper & Engel, 1997) and fluoxetine (Harper *et al.*, 2003), which shorten the open duration of the AChR channel and benefit the slow-channel syndrome, can increase muscle weakness. A respirator dependent infant with severe endplate AChE deficiency was improved by intermittent blockade of AChR by atracurium, an agent that protects AChR from overexposure to ACh (Breningstall *et al.*, 1996). Ephedrine sulfate at a dose of 150 to 200 mg per day in adults is effective for myasthenic symptoms (Bestue-Cardiel *et al.*, 2005; Mihaylova *et al.*, 2008). Although high concentrations of ephedrine are able to block AChR openings (Milone & Engel, 1996), molecular bases of ephedrine effects in clinical practice remain elusive. As an alternative to ephedrine, albuterol sulfate 8 to 16 mg per day also shows benefit (Liewluck *et al.*, in press).

4.2 CMS due to a defect in β2 laminin

Laminins are cruciform heterotrimeric glycoproteins composed of α, β, and γ chains and are assembled from products of five α, four β, and three γ genes. The laminin molecules are named according to their chain composition. For example, laminin-321 contains α3, β2, and γ1 chains (Aumailley *et al.*, 2005). Three laminins are present at the synaptic basal lamina, laminin-221, laminin-421, and laminin-521. Each contains the β2 subunit. Laminin-421 is restricted to the primary synaptic cleft and promotes the precise alignment of pre- and postsynaptic specializations. Laminin-521 lines the primary and secondary clefts, promotes presynaptic differentiation, and prevents Schwann cells from entering the synaptic cleft. The synaptic laminins provide a stop signal for axons at developing endplates and organize presynaptic differentiation (Sanes, 1997). Mice deficient for *Lamb2* that encodes β2 laminin show reduced terminal branching of presynaptic motor axons, with a decreased number of active zones, no clustering of the synaptic vesicles above the active zones, and extension of Schwann cell processes into the primary synaptic cleft, and decreased spontaneous and evoked quantal release (Noakes *et al.*, 1995; Patton *et al.*, 1998). In addition to its presence at the endplate, β2-laminin is also highly expressed in renal glomeruli and the eye. *LAMB2* mutations in humans cause Pierson syndrome characterized by ocular malformation including small non-reactive pupils, loss of accommodation, and abnormalities of the lens, cornea and retina and by fatal nephrotic syndrome that requires renal transplantation (Zenker *et al.*, 2004).

Maselli and coworkers reported a 20-year-old woman with Pierson syndrome caused by two heteroallelic frameshifting mutations (1478delG and 4804delC) in *LAMB2* who also had a severe CMS (Maselli *et al.*, 2009). The nephrotic syndrome was corrected by a renal transplant at age 15 months. The patient had respiratory distress in infancy, delayed motor milestones, a decremental EMG response, limited ocular ductions, bilateral ptosis, severe proximal limb weakness, scoliosis, and required assisted ventilation at night and sometimes during the day. AChE activity was spared at the NMJ. Electron microscopy of the NMJ showed small axon terminal size and encasement of nerve endings by the Schwann cell, widening of the primary synaptic clefts with invasion of the synaptic space by processes of Schwann cells, moderate simplification of postsynaptic membranes, and decreased number of synaptic vesicles. Both morphological and microelectrode studies were similar to those observed in *Lamb2*-mice (Noakes *et al.*, 1995). Notably, symptoms were worsened by pyridostigmine but were improved by ephedrine.

5. Presynaptic CMS

Choline acetyltransferase (ChAT) is the only presynaptic molecule that is known to be defective in CMS.

5.1 CMS with episodic apnea due to defects in choline acetyltransferase (ChAT)

ACh released from the nerve terminal is hydrolyzed into choline and acetate by AChE at the synaptic basal lamina. Choline is taken up by the nerve terminal by a high-affinity choline transporter on the presynaptic membrane (Apparsundaram *et al.*, 2000; Okuda *et al.*, 2000). ChAT resynthesizes ACh from choline and acetyl-CoA (Oda *et al.*, 1992). After the synaptic vesicles are acidified by the vesicular proton pump (Reimer *et al.*, 1998), the resynthesized cationic ACh is packed into a synaptic vesicle by the vesicular ACh transporter (vAChT) in exchange for protons (Erickson *et al.*, 1994).

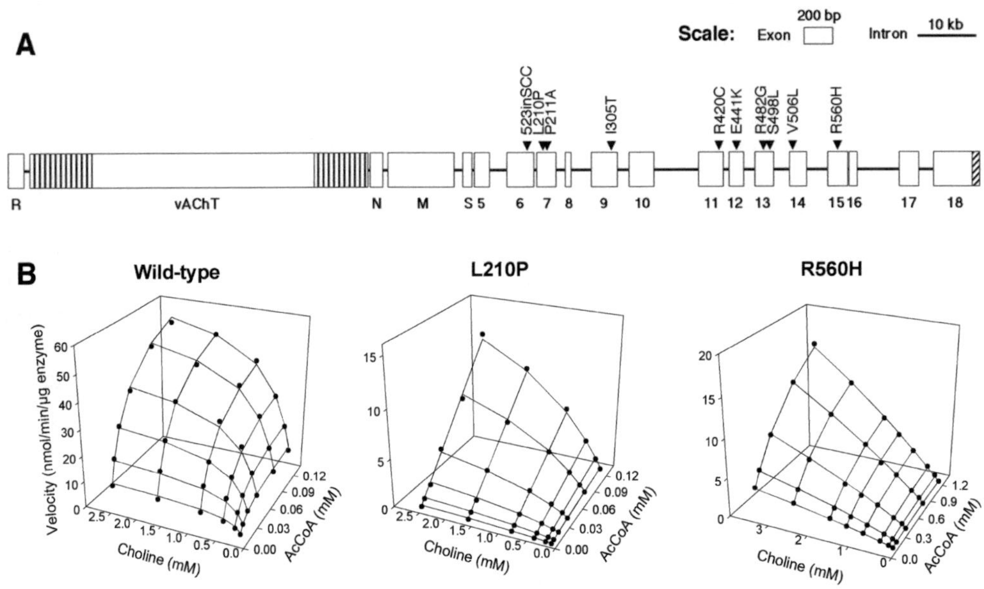

Fig. 5. Choline acetyltransferase (ChAT). (A) Genomic structure of *CHAT* and identified mutations. A gene for vesicular acetylcholine transporter (vAChT) is in the first intron of *CHAT*. (B) Kinetics of wild-type and mutant ChAT enzymes. ChAT synthesizes acetylcholine using choline and acetyl-CoA. L210P abrogates an affinity of ChAT for acetyl-CoA (AcCoA), and R560H abolishes an affinity of ChAT for choline.

We determined the complete genomic structure of *CHAT* encoding ChAT, and identified ten mutations in five CMS patients with the characteristic clinical features of sudden episodes of apnea associated with variable myasthenic symptoms (Ohno *et al.*, 2001). Additional *CHAT* mutations were later reported by other groups (Maselli *et al.*, 2003; Schmidt *et al.*, 2003; Barisic *et al.*, 2005; Mallory *et al.*, 2009; Yeung *et al.*, 2009; Schara *et al.*, 2010). All of our patients showed a marked decrease of the endplate potential after subtetanic stimulation that recovered slowly over 5 to 10 min, which pointed to a defect in the resynthesis or vesicular packaging of ACh at the nerve terminal. Kinetic studies of mutant ChAT enzymes disclosed variable decreases in affinity for choline and/or acetyl-CoA, as well as variable reduction the catalytic rate (Ohno *et al.*, 2001) (Fig. 5). Moreover, some recombinant mutants expressed at a reduced level in COS cells. Two patients carried a functionally null mutation on one allele, but ChAT encoded on the other allele was partially functional. Heterozygous parents that carried the null allele were asymptomatic indicating that humans can tolerate up to but not exceeding 50% reduction of presynaptic ChAT activity. None of our patients has autonomic symptoms or signs of central nervous system involvement other than that attributed to anoxic episodes. This suggests that the ChAT activity and/or substrate availability are rate limiting for ACh synthesis at the motor nerve but not at other cholinergic synapses. Indeed, stimulated quantal release at the endplate is higher than at other cholinergic synapses, which points to selective vulnerability of the NMJ to reduced ACh resynthesis. Crystal structure of ChAT resolved at 2.2 Å revealed that some of the reported *CHAT* mutations in CMS patients are not at the substrate-binding or the catalytic site of ChAT. Hence these mutation exert their effect by an allosteric mechanism or render the enzyme structurally unstable (Cai *et al.*, 2004).

In most patients, anticholinesterase medications are of benefit in ameliorating the myasthenic symptoms and preventing the apneic crises but few patients fail to respond to cholinergic therapy remaining permanently paralyzed and remain respirator dependent. Prophylactic anticholinesterase therapy is advocated even for patients asymptomatic between crises. Parents of affected children must be indoctrinated to anticipate sudden worsening of the weakness and possible apnea with febrile illnesses, excitement, or overexertion. Long-term nocturnal apnea monitoring is indicated in any patient in whom ChAT deficiency is proven or suspected (Byring *et al.*, 2002).

6. Conclusions

We reviewed the clinical and molecular consequences of defects in 11 genes associated with CMS. Molecular studies of CMS began with identification of a missense mutation in the AChR ε subunit in a SCCM patient (Ohno *et al.*, 1995). Since then, mutations in seven postsynaptic, three synaptic, and one presynaptic proteins have been discovered. In some CMS the disease gene has been elusive and await discovery. Resequencing analysis with the next generation sequencers may speed this effort.

7. Acknowledgments

Works in our laboratories were supported by Grants-in-Aid from the MEXT and the MHLW of Japan to K.O., and by NIH Grant NS6277 and a research Grant from Muscular Dystrophy Association to A.G.E.

8. References

Abicht, A., Stucka, R., Schmidt, C., Briguet, A., Höpfner, S., Song, I.-H., Pongratz, D., Müller-Felber, W., Ruegg, M. A. & Lochmüller, H. (2002). A newly identified chromosomal microdeletion and an N-box mutation of the AChR gene cause a congenital myasthenic syndrome. *Brain*, Vol. 125, No., pp. 1005-1013, ISSN 0006-8950

Anderson, J. A., Ng, J. J., Bowe, C., McDonald, C., Richman, D. P., Wollmann, R. L. & Maselli, R. A. (2008). Variable phenotypes associated with mutations in DOK7. *Muscle and Nerve*, Vol. 37, No. 4, pp. 448-456, ISSN 0148-639X

Apparsundaram, S., Ferguson, S. M., George, A. L., Jr. & Blakely, R. D. (2000). Molecular cloning of a human, hemicholinium-3-sensitive choline transporter. *Biochemical and Biophysical Research Communications*, Vol. 276, No. 3, pp. 862-867, ISSN 0006-291X

Aumailley, M., Bruckner-Tuderman, L., Carter, W. G., Deutzmann, R., Edgar, D., Ekblom, P., Engel, J., Engvall, E., Hohenester, E., Jones, J. C., Kleinman, H. K., Marinkovich, M. P., Martin, G. R., Mayer, U., Meneguzzi, G., Miner, J. H., Miyazaki, K., Patarroyo, M., Paulsson, M., Quaranta, V., Sanes, J. R., Sasaki, T., Sekiguchi, K., Sorokin, L. M., Talts, J. F., Tryggvason, K., Uitto, J., Virtanen, I., von der Mark, K., Wewer, U. M., Yamada, Y. & Yurchenco, P. D. (2005). A simplified laminin nomenclature. *Matrix Biology*, Vol. 24, No. 5, pp. 326-332, ISSN 0945-053X

Banwell, B. L., Russel, J., Fukudome, T., Shen, X. M., Stilling, G. & Engel, A. G. (1999). Myopathy, myasthenic syndrome, and epidermolysis bullosa simplex due to plectin deficiency. *Journal of Neuropathology and Experimental Neurology*, Vol. 58, No. 8, pp. 832-846, ISSN 0022-3069

Banwell, B. L., Ohno, K., Sieb, J. P. & Engel, A. G. (2004). Novel truncating RAPSN mutations causing congenital myasthenic syndrome responsive to 3,4-diaminopyridine. *Neuromuscular Disorders*, Vol. 14, No. 3, pp. 202-207, ISSN 0960-8966

Barisic, N., Muller, J. S., Paucic-Kirincic, E., Gazdik, M., Lah-Tomulic, K., Pertl, A., Sertic, J., Zurak, N., Lochmuller, H. & Abicht, A. (2005). Clinical variability of CMS-EA (congenital myasthenic syndrome with episodic apnea) due to identical CHAT mutations in two infants. *Eur J Paediatr Neurol*, Vol. 9, No. 1, pp. 7-12, ISSN 1570-9639

Bartoli, M., Ramarao, M. K. & Cohen, J. B. (2001). Interactions of the rapsyn RING-H2 domain with dystroglycan. *Journal of Biological Chemistry*, Vol. 276, No. 27, pp. 24911-24917, ISSN 0021-9258

Beeson, D., Higuchi, O., Palace, J., Cossins, J., Spearman, H., Maxwell, S., Newsom-Davis, J., Burke, G., Fawcett, P., Motomura, M., Muller, J. S., Lochmuller, H., Slater, C., Vincent, A. & Yamanashi, Y. (2006). Dok-7 mutations underlie a neuromuscular junction synaptopathy. *Science*, Vol. 313, No. 5795, pp. 1975-1978, ISSN 0036-8075

Ben Ammar, A., Petit, F., Alexandri, N., Gaudon, K., Bauche, S., Rouche, A., Gras, D., Fournier, E., Koenig, J., Stojkovic, T., Lacour, A., Petiot, P., Zagnoli, F., Viollet, L., Pellegrini, N., Orlikowski, D., Lazaro, L., Ferrer, X., Stoltenburg, G., Paturneau-Jouas, M., Hentati, F., Fardeau, M., Sternberg, D., Hantai, D., Richard, P. & Eymard, B. (2010). Phenotype genotype analysis in 15 patients presenting a congenital myasthenic syndrome due to mutations in DOK7. *J Neurol*, Vol. 257, No. 5, pp. 754-766, ISSN 0340-5354

Bergamin, E., Hallock, P. T., Burden, S. J. & Hubbard, S. R. (2010). The cytoplasmic adaptor protein Dok7 activates the receptor tyrosine kinase MuSK via dimerization. *Molecular Cell*, Vol. 39, No. 1, pp. 100-109, ISSN 1097-2765

Bestue-Cardiel, M., Saenz de Cabezon-Alvarez, A., Capablo-Liesa, J. L., Lopez-Pison, J., Pena-Segura, J. L., Martin-Martinez, J. & Engel, A. G. (2005). Congenital endplate acetylcholinesterase deficiency responsive to ephedrine. *Neurology*, Vol. 65, No. 1, pp. 144-146, ISSN 0028-3878

Breningstall, G. N., Kurachek, S. C., Fugate, J. H. & Engel, A. G. (1996). Treatment of congenital endplate acetylcholinesterase deficiency by neuromuscular blockade. *Journal of Child Neurology*, Vol. 11, No. 4, pp. 345-346, ISSN 0883-0738

Bulman, D. E., Scoggan, K. A., van Oene, M. D., Nicolle, M. W., Hahn, A. F., Tollar, L. L. & Ebers, G. C. (1999). A novel sodium channel mutation in a family with hypokalemic periodic paralysis. *Neurology*, Vol. 53, No. 9, pp. 1932-1936, ISSN 0028-3878

Burke, G., Cossins, J., Maxwell, S., Owens, G., Vincent, A., Robb, S., Nicolle, M., Hilton-Jones, D., Newsom-Davis, J., Palace, J. & Beeson, D. (2003). Rapsyn mutations in hereditary myasthenia: Distinct early- and late-onset phenotypes. *Neurology*, Vol. 61, No., pp. 826-828, ISSN 0028-3878

Byring, R. F., Pihko, H., Tsujino, A., Shen, X.-M., Gustafsson, B., Hackman, P., Ohno, K., Engel, A. G. & Udd, B. (2002). Congenital myasthenic syndrome associated with episodic apnea and sudden infant death. *Neuromuscular Disorders*, Vol. 12, No. 6, pp. 548-553, ISSN 0960-8966

Cai, Y., Cronin, C. N., Engel, A. G., Ohno, K., Hersh, L. B. & Rodgers, D. W. (2004). Choline acetyltransferase structure reveals distribution of mutations that cause motor disorders. *EMBO Journal*, Vol. 23, No. 10, pp. 2047-2058, ISSN 0261-4189

Cartaud, A., Coutant, S., Petrucci, T. C. & Cartaud, J. (1998). Evidence for in situ and in vitro association between beta-dystroglycan and the subsynaptic 43k rapsyn protein - consequence for acetylcholine receptor clustering at the synapse. *Journal of Biological Chemistry*, Vol. 273, No. 18, pp. 11321-11326, ISSN 0021-9258

Cartaud, A., Strochlic, L., Guerra, M., Blanchard, B., Lambergeon, M., Krejci, E., Cartaud, J. & Legay, C. (2004). MuSK is required for anchoring acetylcholinesterase at the neuromuscular junction. *Journal of Cell Biology*, Vol. 165, No. 4, pp. 505-515, ISSN 0021-9525

Chevessier, F., Faraut, B., Ravel-Chapuis, A., Richard, P., Gaudon, K., Bauche, S., Prioleau, C., Herbst, R., Goillot, E., Ioos, C., Azulay, J. P., Attarian, S., Leroy, J. P., Fournier, E., Legay, C., Schaeffer, L., Koenig, J., Fardeau, M., Eymard, B., Pouget, J. & Hantai, D. (2004). MUSK, a new target for mutations causing congenital myasthenic syndrome. *Human Molecular Genetics*, Vol. 13, No. 24, pp. 3229-3240, ISSN 0964-6906

Chevessier, F., Girard, E., Molgo, J., Bartling, S., Koenig, J., Hantai, D. & Witzemann, V. (2008). A mouse model for congenital myasthenic syndrome due to MuSK mutations reveals defects in structure and function of neuromuscular junctions. *Human Molecular Genetics*, Vol. 17, No. 22, pp. 3577-3595, ISSN 0964-6906

Cole, R. N., Reddel, S. W., Gervasio, O. L. & Phillips, W. D. (2008). Anti-MuSK patient antibodies disrupt the mouse neuromuscular junction. *Annals of Neurology*, Vol. 63, No. 6, pp. 782-789, ISSN 0364-5134

Cossins, J., Burke, G., Maxwell, S., Spearman, H., Man, S., Kuks, J., Vincent, A., Palace, J., Fuhrer, C. & Beeson, D. (2006). Diverse molecular mechanisms involved in AChR deficiency due to rapsyn mutations. *Brain*, Vol. 129, No. Pt 10, pp. 2773-2783, ISSN 0006-8950

Croxen, R., Hatton, C., Shelley, C., Brydson, M., Chauplannaz, G., Oosterhuis, H., Vincent, A., Newsom-Davis, J., Colquhoun, D. & Beeson, D. (2002). Recessive inheritance and variable penetrance of slow-channel congenital myasthenic syndromes. *Neurology*, Vol. 59, No. 2, pp. 162-168, ISSN 0028-3878

Dechiara, T. M., Bowen, D. C., Valenzuela, D. M., Simmons, M. V., Poueymirou, W. T., Thomas, S., Kinetz, E., Compton, D. L., Rojas, E., Park, J. S., Smith, C., Distefano, P. S., Glass, D. J., Burden, S. J. & Yancopoulos, G. D. (1996). The receptor tyrosine kinase MuSK is required for neuromuscular junction formation in vivo. *Cell*, Vol. 85, No. 4, pp. 501-512, ISSN 0092-8674

Deprez, P., Inestrosa, N. C. & Krejci, E. (2003). Two different heparin-binding domains in the triple-helical domain of ColQ, the collagen tail subunit of synaptic acetylcholinesterase. *Journal of Biological Chemistry*, Vol. 278, No. 26, pp. 23233-23242, ISSN 0021-9258

Di Castro, A., Martinello, K., Grassi, F., Eusebi, F. & Engel, A. G. (2007). Pathogenic point mutations in a transmembrane domain of the epsilon subunit increase the Ca2+ permeability of the human endplate ACh receptor. *J Physiol*, Vol. 579, No. Pt 3, pp. 671-677, ISSN 0022-3751

Donger, C., Krejci, E., Pou Serradell, A., Eymard, B., Bon, S., Nicole, S., Chateau, D., Gary, F., Fardeau, M., J., M. & Guicheney, P. (1998). Mutation in the human acetylcholinesterase-associated collagen gene, *COLQ*, is responsible for congenital myasthenic syndrome with end-plate acetylcholinesterase deficiency (Type Ic). *Am J Hum Genet*, Vol. 63, No., pp. 967-975, ISSN 0002-9297

Dunne, V. & Maselli, R. A. (2003). Identification of pathogenic mutations in the human rapsyn gene. *Journal of Human Genetics*, Vol. 48, No. 4, pp. 204-207, ISSN 1434-5161

Engel, A. G., Lambert, E. H. & Gomez, M. R. (1977). A new myasthenic syndrome with end-plate acetylcholinesterase deficiency, small nerve terminals, and reduced acetylcholine release. *Annals of Neurology*, Vol. 1, No. 4, pp. 315-330, ISSN 0364-5134

Engel, A. G., Ohno, K., Bouzat, C., Sine, S. M. & Griggs, R. C. (1996). End-plate acetylcholine receptor deficiency due to nonsense mutations in the epsilon subunit. *Annals of Neurology*, Vol. 40, No. 5, pp. 810-817, ISSN 0364-5134

Engel, A. G., Ohno, K., Milone, M., Wang, H. L., Nakano, S., Bouzat, C., Pruitt, J. N., 2nd, Hutchinson, D. O., Brengman, J. M., Bren, N., Sieb, J. P. & Sine, S. M. (1996). New mutations in acetylcholine receptor subunit genes reveal heterogeneity in the slow-channel congenital myasthenic syndrome. *Human Molecular Genetics*, Vol. 5, No. 9, pp. 1217-1227, ISSN 0964-6906

Erickson, J. D., Varoqui, H., Schafer, M. K., Modi, W., Diebler, M. F., Weihe, E., Rand, J., Eiden, L. E., Bonner, T. I. & Usdin, T. B. (1994). Functional identification of a vesicular acetylcholine transporter and its expression from a "cholinergic" gene locus. *Journal of Biological Chemistry*, Vol. 269, No. 35, pp. 21929-21932, ISSN 0021-9258

Fidzianska, A., Ryniewicz, B., Shen, X. M. & Engel, A. G. (2005). IBM-type inclusions in a patient with slow-channel syndrome caused by a mutation in the AChR epsilon subunit. *Neuromuscular Disorders*, Vol. 15, No. 11, pp. 753-759, ISSN 0960-8966

Froehner, S. C., Luetje, C. W., Scotland, P. B. & Patrick, J. (1990). The postsynaptic 43K protein clusters muscle nicotinic acetylcholine receptors in Xenopus oocytes. *Neuron*, Vol. 5, No. 4, pp. 403-410, ISSN 0896-6273

Fucile, S., Sucapane, A., Grassi, F., Eusebi, F. & Engel, A. G. (2006). The human adult subtype ACh receptor channel has high Ca2+ permeability and predisposes to endplate Ca2+ overloading. *J Physiol*, Vol. 573, No. Pt 1, pp. 35-43, ISSN 0022-3751

Fukudome, T., Ohno, K., Brengman, J. M. & Engel, A. G. (1997). Quinidine sulfate normalizes the open duration of slow channel congenital myasthenic syndrome acetylcholine receptor channels expressed in human embryonic kidney cells. *Neurology*, Vol. 48, No., pp. A72, ISSN 0028-3878

Fukudome, T., Ohno, K., Brengman, J. M. & Engel, A. G. (1998). Quinidine normalizes the open duration of slow-channel mutants of the acetylcholine receptor. *Neuroreport*, Vol. 9, No. 8, pp. 1907-1911, ISSN 0959-4965

Groshong, J. S., Spencer, M. J., Bhattacharyya, B. J., Kudryashova, E., Vohra, B. P., Zayas, R., Wollmann, R. L., Miller, R. J. & Gomez, C. M. (2007). Calpain activation impairs neuromuscular transmission in a mouse model of the slow-channel myasthenic syndrome. *Journal of Clinical Investigation*, Vol. 117, No. 10, pp. 2903-2912, ISSN 0021-9738

Hallock, P. T., Xu, C. F., Park, T. J., Neubert, T. A., Curran, T. & Burden, S. J. (2010). Dok-7 regulates neuromuscular synapse formation by recruiting Crk and Crk-L. *Genes & Development*, Vol. 24, No. 21, pp. 2451-2461, ISSN 0890-9369

Hamuro, J., Higuchi, O., Okada, K., Ueno, M., Iemura, S., Natsume, T., Spearman, H., Beeson, D. & Yamanashi, Y. (2008). Mutations causing DOK7 congenital myasthenia ablate functional motifs in Dok-7. *Journal of Biological Chemistry*, Vol. 283, No. 9, pp. 5518-5524, ISSN 0021-9258

Harper, C. M. & Engel, A. G. (1997). Quinidine sulfate in the treatment of the slow channel congenital myasthenic syndrome. *Neurology*, Vol. 48, No., pp. A72, ISSN 0028-3878

Harper, C. M. & Engel, A. G. (1998). Quinidine sulfate therapy for the slow-channel congenital myasthenic syndrome. *Annals of Neurology*, Vol. 43, No. 4, pp. 480-484, ISSN 0364-5134

Harper, C. M., Fukodome, T. & Engel, A. G. (2003). Treatment of slow-channel congenital myasthenic syndrome with fluoxetine. *Neurology*, Vol. 60, No. 10, pp. 1710-1713, ISSN 0028-3878

Hatton, C. J., Shelley, C., Brydson, M., Beeson, D. & Colquhoun, D. (2003). Properties of the human muscle nicotinic receptor, and of the slow-channel myasthenic syndrome mutant epsilonL221F, inferred from maximum likelihood fits. *J Physiol*, Vol. 547, No. Pt 3, pp. 729-760, ISSN 0022-3751

Higuchi, O., Hamuro, J., Motomura, M. & Yamanashi, Y. (2011). Autoantibodies to low-density lipoprotein receptor-related protein 4 in myasthenia gravis. *Annals of Neurology*, Vol. 69, No. 2, pp. 418-422, ISSN 0364-5134

Hoch, W., McConville, J., Helms, S., Newsom-Davis, J., Melms, A. & Vincent, A. (2001). Auto-antibodies to the receptor tyrosine kinase MuSK in patients with myasthenia gravis without acetylcholine receptor antibodies. *Nature Medicine*, Vol. 7, No. 3, pp. 365-368, ISSN 1078-8956

Huze, C., Bauche, S., Richard, P., Chevessier, F., Goillot, E., Gaudon, K., Ben Ammar, A., Chaboud, A., Grosjean, I., Lecuyer, H. A., Bernard, V., Rouche, A., Alexandri, N., Kuntzer, T., Fardeau, M., Fournier, E., Brancaccio, A., Ruegg, M. A., Koenig, J., Eymard, B., Schaeffer, L. & Hantai, D. (2009). Identification of an agrin mutation that causes congenital myasthenia and affects synapse function. *American Journal of Human Genetics*, Vol. 85, No. 2, pp. 155-167, ISSN 0002-9297

Keramidas, A., Moorhouse, A. J., Schofield, P. R. & Barry, P. H. (2004). Ligand-gated ion channels: mechanisms underlying ion selectivity. *Progress in Biophysics and Molecular Biology*, Vol. 86, No. 2, pp. 161-204, ISSN 0079-6107

Kim, N., Stiegler, A. L., Cameron, T. O., Hallock, P. T., Gomez, A. M., Huang, J. H., Hubbard, S. R., Dustin, M. L. & Burden, S. J. (2008). Lrp4 Is a Receptor for Agrin and Forms a Complex with MuSK. *Cell*, Vol. 135, No. 2, pp. 334-342, ISSN 0092-8674

Kimbell, L. M., Ohno, K., Engel, A. G. & Rotundo, R. L. (2004). C-terminal and heparin-binding domains of collagenic tail subunit are both essential for anchoring acetylcholinesterase at the synapse. *Journal of Biological Chemistry*, Vol. 279, No. 12, pp. 10997-11005, ISSN 0021-9258

Krejci, E., Thomine, S., Boschetti, N., Legay, C., Sketelj, J. & Massoulié, J. (1997). The mammalian gene of acetylcholinesterase-associated collagen. *Journal of Biological Chemistry*, Vol. 272, No. 36, pp. 22840-22847, ISSN 0021-9258

Lang, B. & Vincent, A. (2009). Autoimmune disorders of the neuromuscular junction. *Curr Opin Pharmacol*, Vol. 9, No. 3, pp. 336-340, ISSN 1471-4892

Lee, W. Y., Free, C. R. & Sine, S. M. (2009). Binding to gating transduction in nicotinic receptors: Cys-loop energetically couples to pre-M1 and M2-M3 regions. *Journal of Neuroscience*, Vol. 29, No. 10, pp. 3189-3199, ISSN 0270-6474

Lee, Y., Rudell, J., Yechikhov, S., Taylor, R., Swope, S. & Ferns, M. (2008). Rapsyn carboxyl terminal domains mediate muscle specific kinase-induced phosphorylation of the muscle acetylcholine receptor. *Neuroscience*, Vol. 153, No. 4, pp. 997-1007, ISSN 0306-4522

Lerche, H., Heine, R., Pika, U., George, A. L., Jr., Mitrovic, N., Browatzki, M., Weiss, T., Rivet-Bastide, M., Franke, C., Lomonaco, M. & et al. (1993). Human sodium channel myotonia: slowed channel inactivation due to substitutions for a glycine within the III-IV linker. *J Physiol*, Vol. 470, No., pp. 13-22, ISSN 0022-3751

Liewluck, T., Selcen, D. & Engel, A. G. (in press). Beneficial effects of albuterol in congenital endplate acetylcholinesterase deficiency and DOK-7 myasthenia. *Muscle and Nerve*, Vol., No., pp., ISSN 0148-639X

Mallory, L. A., Shaw, J. G., Burgess, S. L., Estrella, E., Nurko, S., Burpee, T. M., Agus, M. S., Darras, B. T., Kunkel, L. M. & Kang, P. B. (2009). Congenital myasthenic syndrome with episodic apnea. *Pediatric Neurology*, Vol. 41, No. 1, pp. 42-45, ISSN 0887-8994

Maselli, R. A. & Soliven, B. C. (1991). Analysis of the organophosphate-induced electromyographic response to repetitive nerve stimulation: paradoxical response to edrophonium and D-tubocurarine. *Muscle & Nerve*, Vol. 14, No. 12, pp. 1182-1188, ISSN 0148-639X

Maselli, R. A., Chen, D., Mo, D., Bowe, C., Fenton, G. & Wollmann, R. L. (2003). Choline acetyltransferase mutations in myasthenic syndrome due to deficient acetylcholine resynthesis. *Muscle and Nerve*, Vol. 27, No. 2, pp. 180-187, ISSN 0148-639X

Maselli, R. A., Dunne, V., Pascual-Pascual, S. I., Bowe, C., Agius, M., Frank, R. & Wollmann, R. L. (2003). Rapsyn mutations in myasthenic syndrome due to impaired receptor clustering. *Muscle and Nerve*, Vol. 28, No. 3, pp. 293-301, ISSN 0148-639X

Maselli, R. A., Ng, J. J., Anderson, J. A., Cagney, O., Arredondo, J., Williams, C., Wessel, H. B., Abdel-Hamid, H. & Wollmann, R. L. (2009). Mutations in *LAMB2* causing a severe form of synaptic congenital myasthenic syndrome. *Journal of Medical Genetics*, Vol. 46, No. 3, pp. 203-208, ISSN 0022-2593

Maselli, R. A., Arredondo, J., Cagney, O., Ng, J. J., Anderson, J. A., Williams, C., Gerke, B. J., Soliven, B. & Wollmann, R. L. (2010). Mutations in MUSK causing congenital myasthenic syndrome impair MuSK-Dok-7 interaction. *Human Molecular Genetics*, Vol., No., pp., ISSN 0964-6906

McClatchey, A. I., McKenna-Yasek, D., Cros, D., Worthen, H. G., Kuncl, R. W., DeSilva, S. M., Cornblath, D. R., Gusella, J. F. & Brown, R. H., Jr. (1992). Novel mutations in families with unusual and variable disorders of the skeletal muscle sodium channel. *Nature Genetics*, Vol. 2, No. 2, pp. 148-152, ISSN 1061-4036

Michalk, A., Stricker, S., Becker, J., Rupps, R., Pantzar, T., Miertus, J., Botta, G., Naretto, V. G., Janetzki, C., Yaqoob, N., Ott, C. E., Seelow, D., Wieczorek, D., Fiebig, B., Wirth, B., Hoopmann, M., Walther, M., Korber, F., Blankenburg, M., Mundlos, S., Heller, R. & Hoffmann, K. (2008). Acetylcholine receptor pathway mutations explain various fetal akinesia deformation sequence disorders. *American Journal of Human Genetics*, Vol. 82, No. 2, pp. 464-476, ISSN 0002-9297

Mihailescu, S. & Drucker-Colin, R. (2000). Nicotine, brain nicotinic receptors, and neuropsychiatric disorders. *Archives of Medical Research*, Vol. 31, No. 2, pp. 131-144, ISSN 0188-4409

Mihaylova, V., Muller, J. S., Vilchez, J. J., Salih, M. A., Kabiraj, M. M., D'Amico, A., Bertini, E., Wolfle, J., Schreiner, F., Kurlemann, G., Rasic, V. M., Siskova, D., Colomer, J., Herczegfalvi, A., Fabriciova, K., Weschke, B., Scola, R., Hoellen, F., Schara, U., Abicht, A. & Lochmuller, H. (2008). Clinical and molecular genetic findings in COLQ-mutant congenital myasthenic syndromes. *Brain*, Vol. 131, No. Pt 3, pp. 747-759, ISSN 0006-8950

Mihaylova, V., Salih, M. A., Mukhtar, M. M., Abuzeid, H. A., El-Sadig, S. M., von der Hagen, M., Huebner, A., Nurnberg, G., Abicht, A., Muller, J. S., Lochmuller, H. & Guergueltcheva, V. (2009). Refinement of the clinical phenotype in musk-related congenital myasthenic syndromes. *Neurology*, Vol. 73, No. 22, pp. 1926-1928, ISSN 0028-3878

Milone, M. & Engel, A. G. (1996). Block of the endplate acetylcholine receptor channel by the sympathomimetic agents ephedrine, pseudoephedrine, and albuterol. *Brain Research*, Vol. 740, No. 1-2, pp. 346-352, ISSN 0006-8993

Milone, M., Wang, H. L., Ohno, K., Fukudome, T., Pruitt, J. N., Bren, N., Sine, S. M. & Engel, A. G. (1997). Slow-channel myasthenic syndrome caused by enhanced activation, desensitization, and agonist binding affinity attributable to mutation in the M2 domain of the acetylcholine receptor alpha subunit. *Journal of Neuroscience*, Vol. 17, No. 15, pp. 5651-5665, ISSN 0270-6474

Milone, M., Wang, H.-L., Ohno, K., Prince, R., Fukudome, T., Shen, X.-M., Brengman, J. M., Griggs, R. C., Sine, S. M. & Engel, A. G. (1998). Mode switching kinetics produced by a naturally occurring mutation in the cytoplasmic loop of the human acetylcholine receptor epsilon subunit. *Neuron*, Vol. 20, No. 3, pp. 575-588, ISSN 0896-6273

Milone, M., Shen, X. M., Selcen, D., Ohno, K., Brengman, J., Iannaccone, S. T., Harper, C. M. & Engel, A. G. (2009). Myasthenic syndrome due to defects in rapsyn: Clinical and molecular findings in 39 patients. *Neurology*, Vol. 73, No. 3, pp. 228-235, ISSN 0028-3878

Mishina, M., Takai, T., Imoto, K., Noda, M., Takahashi, T., Numa, S., Methfessel, C. & Sakmann, B. (1986). Molecular distinction between fetal and adult forms of muscle acetylcholine receptor. *Nature*, Vol. 321, No. 6068, pp. 406-411, ISSN 0028-0836

Mukhtasimova, N., Lee, W. Y., Wang, H. L. & Sine, S. M. (2009). Detection and trapping of intermediate states priming nicotinic receptor channel opening. *Nature*, Vol. 459, No. 7245, pp. 451-454, ISSN 0028-0836

Muller, J. S., Mildner, G., Muller-Felber, W., Schara, U., Krampfl, K., Petersen, B., Petrova, S., Stucka, R., Mortier, W., Bufler, J., Kurlemann, G., Huebner, A., Merlini, L., Lochmuller, H. & Abicht, A. (2003). Rapsyn N88K is a frequent cause of congenital myasthenic syndromes in European patients. *Neurology*, Vol. 60, No. 11, pp. 1805-1810, ISSN 0028-3878

Muller JS, Abicht A, Burke G, Cossins J, Richard P, Baumeister SK, et al. The congenital myasthenic syndrome mutation RAPSN N88K derives from an ancient Indo-European founder. J Med Genet 2004; 41: e104.

Muller, J. S., Baumeister, S. K., Rasic, V. M., Krause, S., Todorovic, S., Kugler, K., Muller-Felber, W., Abicht, A. & Lochmuller, H. (2006). Impaired receptor clustering in congenital myasthenic syndrome with novel RAPSN mutations. *Neurology*, Vol. 67, No. 7, pp. 1159-1164, ISSN 0028-3878

Muller, J. S., Herczegfalvi, A., Vilchez, J. J., Colomer, J., Bachinski, L. L., Mihaylova, V., Santos, M., Schara, U., Deschauer, M., Shevell, M., Poulin, C., Dias, A., Soudo, A., Hietala, M., Aarimaa, T., Krahe, R., Karcagi, V., Huebner, A., Beeson, D., Abicht, A. & Lochmuller, H. (2007). Phenotypical spectrum of DOK7 mutations in congenital myasthenic syndromes. *Brain*, Vol. 130, No. Pt 6, pp. 1497-1506, ISSN 0006-8950

Noakes, P. G., Gautam, M., Mudd, J., Sanes, J. R. & Merlie, J. P. (1995). Aberrant differentiation of neuromuscular junctions in mice lacking s-laminin laminin beta 2. *Nature*, Vol. 374, No., pp. 258-262, ISSN 0028-0836

Oda, Y., Nakanishi, I. & Deguchi, T. (1992). A complementary DNA for human choline acetyltransferase induces two forms of enzyme with different molecular weights in cultured cells. *Brain Research Molecular Brain Research*, Vol. 16, No. 3-4, pp. 287-294, ISSN 0006-8993

Ohno, K., Hutchinson, D. O., Milone, M., Brengman, J. M., Bouzat, C., Sine, S. M. & Engel, A. G. (1995). Congenital myasthenic syndrome caused by prolonged acetylcholine receptor channel openings due to a mutation in the M2 domain of the epsilon subunit. *Proceedings of the National Academy of Sciences of the United States of America*, Vol. 92, No. 3, pp. 758-762, ISSN 0027-8424

Ohno, K., Quiram, P. A., Milone, M., Wang, H.-L., Harper, M. C., Pruitt, J. N., 2nd, Brengman, J. M., Pao, L., Fischbeck, K. H., Crawford, T. O., Sine, S. M. & Engel, A. G. (1997). Congenital myasthenic syndromes due to heteroallelic nonsense/missense mutations in the acetylcholine receptor epsilon subunit gene: identification and functional characterization of six new mutations. *Human Molecular Genetics*, Vol. 6, No. 5, pp. 753-766, ISSN 0964-6906

Ohno, K., Brengman, J., Tsujino, A. & Engel, A. G. (1998). Human endplate acetylcholinesterase deficiency caused by mutations in the collagen-like tail subunit

(ColQ) of the asymmetric enzyme. *Proceedings of the National Academy of Sciences of the United States of America*, Vol. 95, No. 16, pp. 9654-9659, ISSN 0027-8424

Ohno, K., Milone, M., Brengman, J. M., LoMonaco, M., Evoli, A., Tonali, P. A. & Engel, A. G. (1998). Slow-channel congenital myasthenic syndrome caused by a novel mutation in the acetylcholine receptor ε subunit. *Neurology*, Vol. 50 (Suppl. 4), No., pp. A432 (abstract), ISSN 0028-3878

Ohno, K., Anlar, B. & Engel, A. G. (1999). Congenital myasthenic syndrome caused by a mutation in the Ets-binding site of the promoter region of the acetylcholine receptor epsilon subunit gene. *Neuromuscular Disorders*, Vol. 9, No. 3, pp. 131-135, ISSN 0960-8966

Ohno, K., Brengman, J. M., Felice, K. J., Cornblath, D. R. & Engel, A. G. (1999). Congenital end-plate acetylcholinesterase deficiency caused by a nonsense mutation and an A-->G splice-donor-site mutation at position +3 of the collagenlike-tail-subunit gene (COLQ): how does G at position +3 result in aberrant splicing? *American Journal of Human Genetics*, Vol. 65, No. 3, pp. 635-644, ISSN 0002-9297

Ohno, K., Engel, A. G., Brengman, J. M., Shen, X.-M., Heidenrich, F. R., Vincent, A., Milone, M., Tan, E., Demirci, M., Walsh, P., Nakano, S. & Akiguchi, I. (2000). The spectrum of mutations causing endplate acetylcholinesterase deficiency. *Annals of Neurology*, Vol. 47, No., pp. 162-170, ISSN 0364-5134

Ohno, K., Tsujino, A., Brengman, J. M., Harper, C. M., Bajzer, Z., Udd, B., Beyring, R., Robb, S., Kirkham, F. J. & Engel, A. G. (2001). Choline acetyltransferase mutations cause myasthenic syndrome associated with episodic apnea in humans. *Proceedings of the National Academy of Sciences of the United States of America*, Vol. 98, No. 4, pp. 2017-2022, ISSN 0027-8424

Ohno, K., Engel, A. G., Shen, X.-M., Selcen, D., Brengman, J., Harper, C. M., Tsujino, A. & Milone, M. (2002). Rapsyn mutations in humans cause endplate acetylcholine-receptor deficiency and myasthenic syndrome. *American Journal of Human Genetics*, Vol. 70, No. 4, pp. 875-885, ISSN 0002-9297

Ohno, K., Sadeh, M., Blatt, I., Brengman, J. M. & Engel, A. G. (2003). E-box mutations in the *RAPSN* promoter region in eight cases with congenital myasthenic syndrome. *Human Molecular Genetics*, Vol. 12, No. 7, pp. 739-748, ISSN 0964-6906

Ohno, K. & Engel, A. G. (2004). Lack of founder haplotype for the rapsyn N88K mutation: N88K is an ancient founder mutation or arises from multiple founders. *Journal of Medical Genetics*, Vol. 41, No. 1, pp. e8, ISSN 0022-2593

Okada, K., Inoue, A., Okada, M., Murata, Y., Kakuta, S., Jigami, T., Kubo, S., Shiraishi, H., Eguchi, K., Motomura, M., Akiyama, T., Iwakura, Y., Higuchi, O. & Yamanashi, Y. (2006). The muscle protein Dok-7 is essential for neuromuscular synaptogenesis. *Science*, Vol. 312, No. 5781, pp. 1802-1805, ISSN 0036-8075

Okuda, T., Haga, T., Kanai, Y., Endou, H., Ishihara, T. & Katsura, I. (2000). Identification and characterization of the high-affinity choline transporter. *Nature Neuroscience*, Vol. 3, No. 2, pp. 120-125, ISSN 1097-6256

Patton, B. L., Chiu, A. Y. & Sanes, J. R. (1998). Synaptic laminin prevents glial entry into the synaptic cleft. *Nature*, Vol. 393, No. 6686, pp. 698-701, ISSN 0028-0836

Peng, H. B., Xie, H., Rossi, S. G. & Rotundo, R. L. (1999). Acetylcholinesterase clustering at the neuromuscular junction involves perlecan and dystroglycan. *Journal of Cell Biology*, Vol. 145, No., pp. 911-921, ISSN 0021-9525

Ptacek, L. J., George, A. L., Jr., Griggs, R. C., Tawil, R., Kallen, R. G., Barchi, R. L., Robertson, M. & Leppert, M. F. (1991). Identification of a mutation in the gene causing hyperkalemic periodic paralysis. *Cell*, Vol. 67, No. 5, pp. 1021-1027, ISSN 0092-8674

Ptacek, L. J., George, A. L., Jr., Barchi, R. L., Griggs, R. C., Riggs, J. E., Robertson, M. & Leppert, M. F. (1992). Mutations in an S4 segment of the adult skeletal muscle sodium channel cause paramyotonia congenita. *Neuron*, Vol. 8, No. 5, pp. 891-897, ISSN 0896-6273

Ramarao, M. K., Bianchetta, M. J., Lanken, J. & Cohen, J. B. (2001). Role of rapsyn tetratricopeptide repeat and coiled-coil domains in self-association and nicotinic acetylcholine receptor clustering. *Journal of Biological Chemistry*, Vol. 276, No. 10, pp. 7475-7483, ISSN 0021-9258

Ramarao, N. K. & Cohen, J. B. (1998). Mechanism of nicotinic acetylcholine receptor cluster formation by rapsyn. *Proceedings of the National Academy of Sciences of the United States of America*, Vol. 95, No. 7, pp. 4007-4012, ISSN 0027-8424

Reimer, R. J., Fon, E. A. & Edwards, R. H. (1998). Vesicular neurotransmitter transport and the presynaptic regulation of quantal size. *Current Opinion in Neurobiology*, Vol. 8, No. 3, pp. 405-412, ISSN 0959-4388

Richard, P., Gaudon, K., Andreux, F., Yasaki, E., Prioleau, C., S, B., Barois, A., Ioos, C., Mayer, M., Routon, M. C., Mokhtari, M., Leroy, J. P., Fournier, E., Hainque, B., Koenig, J., Fardeau, M., Eymard, B. & D, H. (2003). Possible founder effect of rapsyn N88K mutation and identification of novel rapsyn mutations in congenital myasthenic syndromes. *Journal of Medical Genetics*, Vol. 40, No. 6, pp. 81e, ISSN 0022-2593

Sanes, J. R. (1997). Genetic analysis of postsynaptic differentiation at the vertebrate neuromuscular junction. *Current Opinion in Neurobiology*, Vol. 7, No. 1, pp. 93-100, ISSN 0959-4388

Schara, U., Christen, H. J., Durmus, H., Hietala, M., Krabetz, K., Rodolico, C., Schreiber, G., Topaloglu, H., Talim, B., Voss, W., Pihko, H., Abicht, A., Muller, J. S. & Lochmuller, H. (2010). Long-term follow-up in patients with congenital myasthenic syndrome due to *CHAT* mutations. *Eur J Paediatr Neurol*, Vol. 14, No. 4, pp. 326-333, ISSN 1090-3798

Schmidt, C., Abicht, A., Krampfl, K., Voss, W., Stucka, R., Mildner, G., Petrova, S., Schara, U., Mortier, W., Bufler, J., Huebner, A. & Lochmuller, H. (2003). Congenital myasthenic syndrome due to a novel missense mutation in the gene encoding choline acetyltransferase. *Neuromuscular Disorders*, Vol. 13, No. 3, pp. 245-251, ISSN 0960-8966

Selcen, D., Milone, M., Shen, X. M., Harper, C. M., Stans, A. A., Wieben, E. D. & Engel, A. G. (2008). Dok-7 myasthenia: phenotypic and molecular genetic studies in 16 patients. *Annals of Neurology*, Vol. 64, No. 1, pp. 71-87, ISSN 0364-5134

Selcen, D., Juel, V. C., Hobson-Webb, L. D., Smith, E. C., Stickler, D. E., Bite, A. V., Ohno, K. & Engel, A. G. (2011). Myasthenic syndrome caused by plectinopathy. *Neurology*, Vol. 76, No. 4, pp. 327-336, ISSN 0028-3878

Senderek, J., Muller, J. S., Dusl, M., Strom, T. M., Guergueltcheva, V., Diepolder, I., Laval, S. H., Maxwell, S., Cossins, J., Krause, S., Muelas, N., Vilchez, J. J., Colomer, J., Mallebrera, C. J., Nascimento, A., Nafissi, S., Kariminejad, A., Nilipour, Y., Bozorgmehr, B., Najmabadi, H., Rodolico, C., Sieb, J. P., Steinlein, O. K., Schlotter,

B., Schoser, B., Kirschner, J., Herrmann, R., Voit, T., Oldfors, A., Lindbergh, C., Urtizberea, A., von der Hagen, M., Hubner, A., Palace, J., Bushby, K., Straub, V., Beeson, D., Abicht, A. & Lochmuller, H. (2011). Hexosamine biosynthetic pathway mutations cause neuromuscular transmission defect. *American Journal of Human Genetics*, Vol. 88, No. 2, pp. 162-172, ISSN 0002-9297

Shen, X.-M., Ohno, K., Sine, S. M. & Engel, A. G. (2005). Subunit-specific contribution to agonist binding and channel gating revealed by inherited mutation in muscle acetylcholine receptor M3-M4 linker. *Brain*, Vol. 128, No., pp. 345-355, ISSN 0006-8950

Shen, X. M., Ohno, K., Milone, M., Brengman, J. M., Tsujino, A. & Engel, A. G. (2003). Effect of residue side-chain mass on channel kinetics in second transmembrane domain of muscle AChR. *Molecular Biology of the Cell*, Vol. 14 (Suppl), No., pp. 223a (abstract), ISSN 1059-1524

Sine, S. M., Ohno, K., Bouzat, C., Auerbach, A., Milone, M., Pruitt, J. N. & Engel, A. G. (1995). Mutation of the acetylcholine receptor alpha subunit causes a slow-channel myasthenic syndrome by enhancing agonist binding affinity. *Neuron*, Vol. 15, No. 1, pp. 229-239, ISSN 0896-6273

Smith, F. J., Eady, R. A., Leigh, I. M., McMillan, J. R., Rugg, E. L., Kelsell, D. P., Bryant, S. P., Spurr, N. K., Geddes, J. F., Kirtschig, G., Milana, G., de Bono, A. G., Owaribe, K., Wiche, G., Pulkkinen, L., Uitto, J., McLean, W. H. & Lane, E. B. (1996). Plectin deficiency results in muscular dystrophy with epidermolysis bullosa. *Nature Genetics*, Vol. 13, No. 4, pp. 450-457, ISSN 1061-4036

Tsujino, A., Maertens, C., Ohno, K., Shen, X.-M., Fukuda, T., Harper, C. M., Cannon, S. C. & Engel, A. G. (2003). Myasthenic syndrome caused by mutation of the SCN4A sodium channel. *Proceedings of the National Academy of Sciences of the United States of America*, Vol. 100, No., pp. 7377-7382, ISSN 0027-8424

Valenzuela, D. M., Stitt, T. N., DiStefano, P. S., Rojas, E., Mattsson, K., Compton, D. L., Nunez, L., Park, J. S., Stark, J. L., Gies, D. R. & et al. (1995). Receptor tyrosine kinase specific for the skeletal muscle lineage: expression in embryonic muscle, at the neuromuscular junction, and after injury. *Neuron*, Vol. 15, No. 3, pp. 573-584, ISSN 0896-6273

Vogt, J., Morgan, N. V., Marton, T., Maxwell, S., Harrison, B. J., Beeson, D. & Maher, E. R. (2009). Germline mutation in DOK7 associated with fetal akinesia deformation sequence. *Journal of Medical Genetics*, Vol. 46, No. 5, pp. 338-340, ISSN 0022-2593

Wang, H.-L., Auerbach, A., Bren, N., Ohno, K., Engel, A. G. & Sine, S. M. (1997). Mutation in the M1 domain of the acetylcholine receptor alpha subunit decreases the rate of agonist dissociation. *Journal of General Physiology*, Vol. 109, No. 6, pp. 757-766, ISSN 0022-1295

Wang, H.-L., Milone, M., Ohno, K., Shen, X.-M., Tsujino, A., Batocchi, A. P., Tonali, P., Brengman, J., Engel, A. G. & Sine, S. M. (1999). Acetylcholine receptor M3 domain: stereochemical and volume contributions to channel gating. *Nature Neuroscience*, Vol. 2, No. 3, pp. 226-233, ISSN 1097-6256

Wang, H.-L., Ohno, K., Milone, M., Brengman, J. M., Evoli, A., Batocchi, A. P., Middleton, L. T., Christodoulou, K., Engel, A. G. & Sine, S. M. (2000). Fundamental gating mechanism of nicotinic receptor channel revealed by mutation causing a congenital myasthenic syndrome. *Journal of General Physiology*, Vol. 116, No. 3, pp. 449-462, ISSN 0022-1295

Wells, L., Vosseller, K. & Hart, G. W. (2001). Glycosylation of nucleocytoplasmic proteins: signal transduction and O-GlcNAc. *Science*, Vol. 291, No. 5512, pp. 2376-2378, ISSN 0036-8075

Wirtz, P. W., Titulaer, M. J., Gerven, J. M. & Verschuuren, J. J. (2010). 3,4-diaminopyridine for the treatment of Lambert-Eaton myasthenic syndrome. *Expert Rev Clin Immunol*, Vol. 6, No. 6, pp. 867-874, ISSN 1744-666X

Wu, H., Xiong, W. C. & Mei, L. (2010). To build a synapse: signaling pathways in neuromuscular junction assembly. *Development*, Vol. 137, No. 7, pp. 1017-1033, ISSN 0950-1991

Yasaki, E., Prioleau, C., Barbier, J., Richard, P., Andreux, F., Leroy, J. P., Dartevelle, P., Koenig, J., Molgo, J., Fardeau, M., Eymard, B. & Hantai, D. (2004). Electrophysiological and morphological characterization of a case of autosomal recessive congenital myasthenic syndrome with acetylcholine receptor deficiency due to a N88K rapsyn homozygous mutation. *Neuromuscular Disorders*, Vol. 14, No. 1, pp. 24-32, ISSN 0960-8966

Yeung, W. L., Lam, C. W., Fung, L. W., Hon, K. L. & Ng, P. C. (2009). Severe congenital myasthenia gravis of the presynaptic type with choline acetyltransferase mutation in a Chinese infant with respiratory failure. *Neonatology*, Vol. 95, No. 2, pp. 183-186, ISSN 1661-7800

Zenker, M., Aigner, T., Wendler, O., Tralau, T., Muntefering, H., Fenski, R., Pitz, S., Schumacher, V., Royer-Pokora, B., Wuhl, E., Cochat, P., Bouvier, R., Kraus, C., Mark, K., Madlon, H., Dotsch, J., Rascher, W., Maruniak-Chudek, I., Lennert, T., Neumann, L. M. & Reis, A. (2004). Human laminin beta2 deficiency causes congenital nephrosis with mesangial sclerosis and distinct eye abnormalities. *Human Molecular Genetics*, Vol. 13, No. 21, pp. 2625-2632, ISSN 0964-6906

Zhang, B., Luo, S., Wang, Q., Suzuki, T., Xiong, W. C. & Mei, L. (2008). LRP4 serves as a coreceptor of agrin. *Neuron*, Vol. 60, No. 2, pp. 285-297, ISSN 0896-6273

11

Motor Neuron Disease

Hamdy N. El Tallawy
Assiut University
Egypt

1. Introduction

Neurologists in the 19th century recognized that muscle weakness could be due to primary disorders of muscle or secondary to loss of neuromuscular integrity, as happens when peripheral nerves are cut or when motor neurons degenerate. Furthermore, it was observed that there are forms of motor neuron degeneration which selectively affect upper motor neurons or lower motor neurons. A combination of upper and lower motor neuron dysfunction was named amyotrophic lateral sclerosis (ALS) by Charcot and Joffroy (Ringel, et al 1993). Jean-Martin Charcot first characterized the disease in 1874, naming the illness Amyotrophic lateral sclerosis (ALS) (Swash, 2001). In USA, ALS or Lou Gehrig's disease are terms used to describe all forms of the disease, whatever the combination of upper and lower motor neuron involvement (Ringel, et al 1993). ALS is now a term which classifies the most common form of the illness and is often used synonymously with MND (Swash, 2001). In the UK the umbrella term motor neuron disease (MND) is more common. MND is a disease of middle to late life with a mean age of onset of 58 years, (Ringel, et al 1993).

Actually, motor neuron diseases (MND) are a group of degenerative disorders that selectively affect motor neurons in the brain and spinal cord. Two groups of motor neurons are involved, lower motor neurons located in ventral horns of the spinal cord and brainstem motor nuclei, and upper motor neurons located in the cerebral cortex together with pyramidal tracts in spinal cord. The term MND is a broad spectrum term including amyotrophic lateral sclerosis.

2. Definitions and terminology of motor neuron disease (MND)

MND is a group of incurable progressive neurodegenerative disorders in which degeneration involves upper and lower motor neurons in different body regions, resulting in progressive weakness of bulbar, limbs and respiratory musculature, in different combination.

MND is an adult onset neurodegenerative disease which leads inexorably via weakness of limb, bulbar and respiratory muscles to death from respiratory failure three to five years later. (Allum and Shaw 2010).

3. Epidemiology of motor neuron disease

The prevalence of MND is 4-6 per 100,000 in most parts of the world, except the Western Pacific foci, (Leigh, 1991). However, its annual incidence is between 1.5 and 2/100,000 and males are more commonly affected than females (1.4:1). The incidence increases with age with a mean age of onset of 63 years, (Ringel, et al 1993). It ranks as the third most common neurological degenerative disorder after Alzheimer's and Parkinson's disease (Talbot 2002).

In Guam, the incidence of MND has fallen from 87/100,000 in 1962 to 5/100,000 in 1985, (Rodgers-Johanson, et al. 1986).

Within the Caucasian population of Europe and North America, where most of the studies have been conducted, the lowest reported incidence of MND was 0.6 per 100.000 person – years in Italy,(De Domenice, et al. 1988) and the highest reported was 2.4 per 100.000 person-years in Finland(Murros and Fogelholm.1983). However, a lower incidence rate of 0.3/100,000 person-years was reported among Asian population, in China, (Fong, et al. 1996).

In the only well-conducted study of MND incidence among black African population, the incidence of MND was noted to be 0.9 per 100,000 person-years in Libya, (Radhakrishnan, et al. 1986).

The incidence of MND is said to be increasing, but this is probably the result of improved diagnosis, better awareness of the disease and an aging population, (Leigh and Ray-Chaudhuri.1994). The incidence increases after the age of 40 years, peaks in the late 60s and early 70s, and declines rapidly after that, (Logroscino, et al. 2008).

4. Aetiology, pathology and pathogenesis of motor neuron disease

MND is one of the complex and misunderstood diseases that health care professionals may encounter for various different reasons: (1) there are multiple different forms of the disease (Strong and Rosenfeld.2003), (2) the pathogenesis is not fully delineated (Wijesekera and Leigh.2009), (3) diagnosis can occur only by exclusion, (4) there exists only FDA approved medication, riluzole, for the treatment of ALS[2] (Washington.2007), and despite this, (5) there is no cure for this disease.

Environmental exposures during the Gulf war have been proposed as the explanation for an increased incidence of ALS among Gulf War veterans (Haley 2003, Horner et al, 2003).

4.1 Neuropathological findings in MND

Gross changes were frontotemporal atrophy, which was usually mild to moderate, neither circumscribed nor of a 'Knife-blade' type, and atrophy of the anterior roots in the cervicothoracic spinal cord, which was seen in cases with definite lower motor neuron involvement. Cortical atrophy was marked in the limbic system including the temporal pole, parahippocampus and amygdala but usually spared the hippocampus in typical ALS - Dementia (ALS-D) cases. (Yoshida 2004).

Histological changes included neuronal loss and gliosis with sponginess in layers II and III of frontotemporal cortices with predominant involvement of the limbic system including the anterior cingulated gyrus, anterior temporal and insular lobes, parahippocampus, subiculum and amygdale in typical cases. (Yoshida 2004).

The full pathogenesis of ALS is not well understood as it has not been fully elucidated by medical research. However, several key factors can be noted including: (1) Genetics, (2)

Excitotoxicity, (3) Oxidative stress, (4) Mitochondrial dysfunction, (5) Impaired axonal transport, (6) Neurofilament aggregation, (7) Protein aggregation, (8) Inflammatory dysfunction and contribution of non-neuronal cells, (9) Deficits of neurotrophic factors and dysfunction of signaling pathways, and (10) Apoptosis, (Wijesekera and Leigh.2009 and Shaw. 2005).

4.2 Genetics

Up to 90% of all ALS cases, occurs without family history, (sporadic ALS) and about 10% of cases are familial ALS (FALS). SALS is clinically indistinguishable from FALS, but the average age of onset in FALS is somewhat earlier, (Celveland and Rothstein (2001). Enteroviral infections and mutations of superoxide dismutase 1gene (SOD1) have been implicated in the pathogenesis of MND (oluwale et al 2001). About 25% of ALS cases, (Celveland and Rothstein (2001), and 2% of the sporadic cases, are linked to mutations in the gene encoding copper/zinc superoxide dismutase (SOD1). It is Known that there may be as many as six gene loci that code for the ALS phenotype, but only three have been identified. Several other mutations have also been documented to possibly take part in the pathogenesis of ALS, (Wijesekera and Leigh, 2009). Since the link between SOD1 and FALS was first established, >90 FALS-linked SOD1 mutations have been discovered, (Celveland and Rothstein (2001). Most of these mutations are point missense mutations, (Anderson, et al. 2003). Most of the genetics are transmitted via the autosomal dominant route, though some are autosomal recessive and others may be sex-linked, (Wijesekera and Leigh.2009).

4.3 Excitotoxicity

Excitotoxicity is a term used to signify the damage that occurs to neuronal cells that are characterized by overstimulated glutamate receptors, as glutamate is the major excitatory neurotransmitter in the human central nervous system (Riluzol monograph. 2011). As SOD1 codes for the major reuptake protein of glutamate, a mutation limits the concentration levels of that reuptake protein, allowing an excessive amount of glutamate to be present in the neuronal synapse. It is also postulated that glutamatergic toxicity plays a direct role in the destruction of neuronal cells in patients with ALS.(Shaw. 2005).

4.4 Oxidative stress

Oxidative stress is of particular interest to researchers due to the fact that the SOD1 gene mutation that is known to cause ALS, normally codes for an anti-oxidant protein. (Riluzol momgraph. 2011)

4.5 Mitochondrial dysfunction

There are many new data which supports the theory that mitochondrial dysfunction plays an important role in the pathogenesis of ALS. Multiple cases of dysfunctional mitochondria have been noted in post-mortem analyses of ALS patients. (Wijesekera and Leigh.2009) Dysfunctional mitochondria have also been linked to the SOD1 gene mutation in mice models. (Shaw. 2005)

4.6 Impaired axonal transport

The theory that axonal transport is a key to ALS pathogenesis stems from SOD1 transgenic mice models. Mice from these models often show slowed anterograde and retrograde axonal transport. Although no human ALS patient has presented with this problem, yet it is known to occur in several other neuromuscular disorders of the human body. (Wijesekera and Leigh.2009)

4.7 Neurofilament aggregation

Abnormal neuronal assembly, including accumulation of neurofilaments, are often seen in ALS patients. Neurofilaments can combine with a toxic form of peripherin, an intermediate filament protein, and become toxic to neurons even at modest concentration levels. This combination has been found in the spinal cord of ALS patients and not in controls. This evidence points to neurofilament aggregation as being a part of ALS pathogenesis. (Wijesekera and Leigh.2009)

4.8 Protein aggregation

Long debates as to whether protein aggregation take a part in disease pathogenesis have been occurred. It is possible that these inclusions may simply be innocent bystanders, or even beneficial to the cells. (Wijesekera and Leigh.2009)

4.9 Inflammatory dysfunction and contribution of non-neuronal cells

It has been recently discovered that SOD1 mutations alone are insufficient to cause ALS in transgenic mice, making the case that non-neuronal cells, as microglial and dendritic cells, may play a part in ALS pathogenesis (Shaw, 2005). ALS patients commonly experience activation of the non-neuronal microglial and dendritic cells. This activation has been shown to produce inflammatory cytokines such as interleukins and tumor necrosis factor (TNF). However, recent trials have yet to see success in utilizing immunomodulatory drug therapies to curve the progression of ALS. (Wijesekera and Leigh.2009).

4.10 Deficits of neurotrophic factors and dysfunction of signaling pathways

Lowered levels of neurotrophic factors have been noticed in post-mortem analysis of several ALS patients. In addition, three mutations in the Vascular Endothelial Growth Factors (VEGF) gene were thought to be associated with an increased risk for developing ALS. However, recently these finding have come under scrutiny due to an inability to replicate research results. (Wijesekera and Leigh.2009)

4.11 Apoptosis

Current research also skews towards examining if ALS motor neuron destruction occurs via a programmed cell death, or apoptosis. Several studies have shown that cell death due to ALS often occurs because of this programmed apoptosis, yet these findings are still being reviewed and discussed heavily. (Shaw. 2005).

5. Clinical presentation of motor neurone disease

Dilemmas of symptoms and signs are described for diagnosis of MND and its subtypes. Motor symptoms of both upper and lower motor neuron dysfunction can occur in any muscle group, including limbs, and, or bulbar regions. Combinations of the previous motor symptoms is not characteristic for MND and can be observed in many diseases, known as "MND Mimic Disorders" such as, Kennedy's diseases, multifocal motor neuropathy, brainstem lesions (syrinx, stroke,.......... etc)

Meticulous evaluation by thorough history and examination by two or more specialists of neurology are required for diagnosis of MND. Special investigations are required for diagnosis of MND and differentiation from MND mimics.

Preclinical stage	Diagnosis stage	Progression stage	Terminal stage
• Long duration (months or even years • Disease spread through motor system • Usually Asymptomatic	• Selective involvement of motor neurons in the anterior horns of the spinal cord early and late in the disease (Swash et al. 1986) • corticospinal pathways in the cord are similarly, asymmetrically affected (Ingram and Swash 1987) • Onuf"s sacral nucleus (innervate anal and urinary sphincter muscles) are always spared (Schroder, and Reske Nelson 1984) • Ocular motor nuclei are also relatively resistant (Mulder 1982)	• weakness of one leg followed by other leg and patient will require a wheelchair to assist him • Swallowing Problems • Respiratory muscle weakness and dyspnea • All these symptoms are observed in different combinations according to different subtypes of MND	• Respiratory insufficiency symptoms orthopnea, excessive daytime sleepiness, poor concentration, memory and appetite and signs of tachypnea, tachycardia, syncope and confusion, (Radunovic et al 2007.) • Nursed and care for 24 hours • Medication, Diet, Hygiene and special attention for respiration.

Table 1. Stages of Motor Neuron Disease (MND)

6. Bad prognostic factors for MND

1. Late age of onset.
2. Severe and early presentations of bulbar symptoms.
3. Respiratory complications.

The classical concept that MND only affects the motor system is obsolete. MND is considered to be a multisystem neurodegenerative disease. There is increasing clinical evidence for autonomic dysfunction (Baltadzhieva, et al 2006 and Takeda, et al, 1994), sensory abnormalities (Takeda et al, 1994) (Pugdahl et al, 2007) and ophthalmoplegia

(Takeda, et al, 1994) in MND. On the other hand, there are good pathological accounts of the involvement of sympathetic and parasympathetic neurons, (Takeda, et al, 1994), Onuf's nucleus (which innervates the pelvic floor sphincteric muscles), (Takeda, et al, 1994) peripheral sensory nerves, (Isaacs, et al. 2007) and oculomotor nuclei. (Takeda, et al, 1994). However, in practical terms, the presence of prominent ophthalmoplegia, sensory signs or sphincter dysfunction should raise doubts regarding the diagnosis of MND, unless there are a clear alternative explanation. Death usually results from ventilatory muscle weakness causing respiratory failure.

7. Motor neuron disease presenting to non neurological specialists

Respiratory: Progressive respiratory Failure

Ear, nose, and throat: Dysphagia.

Orthopaedics/ neurosurgery: Foot drop or other symptoms suggestive of compressive radiculopathy

Elderly care: Difficulty walking. (Talbot 2002).

	ALS	PMA	PLS	PBP
1. Age of onset	50-70 years		40 – 60 years	
2. Percent of Frequency (Leigh et al 2003)	60 – 70 %	10 %	1 %	20%
3. Incidence (Strong and Rosenfeld, 2003)	1,2-1,8/100,000	-----	1/1000,000- Brugman and wokkle 2004	-----
4. Prevalence (van der, Graaff, 2004)	5-9/100,000	-----	10-20/1000,000- Brugman and wokkle 2004	-----
5. Male to female Ratio (Leigh et al 2003)	3:2	3:4	3:1 (Talbot 2002)	1:1
6. Anatomical localization	Cortical & spinal	spinal cord	Limb, Bulbar (Pseudo bulbar)	Bulbar, Speech and limb
7. Upper Motor Neuron manifestations	Present	Absent	Present	Absent
8. Lower Motor Neuron manifestation	Present	Present in Limb muscles	absent	Present in bulbar muscles
9. Cognitive impairment	Present and some group of ALS without cognitive impairment	Present	Usually absent (Raaphorst et al 2010)	Absent

10. Bulbar symptoms	Present	Absent	Present	Promiment
11. Mimic syndromes	-Compressive myeloradiculopathy, -Paraneoplastic syndrome, -Encephalo-myelitis with anterion horn cell involvement	-Inflammatory Myopathy -Multifocal motor neuropathy with conduction block -Myasthenia Gravis -Toxic Neuropathies -Post polio Progressive muscular atrophy	-Primary progressive multiple sclerosis, -vit. B12 deficiency -Hereditay spastic Paraparesis, -Rarely small vessel cerebrovascular diseases -cervical Spondylotic myelopathy	Posterior inferior cerebellar artery occlusion
12. Emotional lability	May be Present	Present	Prominent	Absent
13. Investigotions a. EMG&CV	Positive- lower motor neuron manifestations	Positive- lower motor neuron manifestations	Normal	Fibrillation and Positive sharp waves.
b. MRI brain When Bulbar manifestations are isolated symptoms and signs	Normal	Normal	Normal	Normal
c. MRI spinal cord All Limb onset without bulbar symptoms	Normal	----	Normal	----
14. Prognosis Median Survival (Leigh et al 2003)	3-4 years	5 years, more long survivors (>10 years)	20 years and More	2-3years

Table 2. Clinical Subtypes of Motor Neuron Disease

8. Cognitive function impairment in motor neuron disease

Cognitive impairment is increasingly being recognized in MND. Subtle subclinical cognitive defects and frontal lobe dysfunction may be demonstrated in up to half of MND patients with detailed neuropsychological testing (Ringholz, et al. 2005). Several genetic mutations of MND have been identified in association with frontotemporal dementia and/or parkinsonism (Valdmanis and Rouleau. 2008). It is well recognized that MND is a multisystem disorder (Geser, et al, 2008) with compromise of regions beyond the motor system, including cortical areas which are consistently involved in FTD. It comes as no surprise, therefore, that a proportion of patients presenting with MND manifest cognitive and/or behavioural changes which may be severe enough in some instances to reach criteria for frank FTD.(Irwin, et al, 2007).

8.1 Amyotrophic lateral sclerosis and frontotemporal dementia (ALS-FTD)

There is icreasing clinical, imaging and neurophysiological evidence that ALS represents a multisystem neurodegerative disease. Neurodegeneration is not restricted to motor neurons, but also includes parts of the brain other than the motor cortex, especially the preforntal and/or anterior temporal lobe, that contribute to the clinical syndrome. In some cases an evident dementia that resembles frontotemporal degeneration (FTD) was observed. It is now suggested that ALS and FTD are closely related conditions with overlapping clinical, pathological, radiological, and genetic characteristics. The presence of a frontal dementia in ALS has also crucial practical consequences for management of the patients, whose disorder requires critical life decisions for enteral nutrition and respiratory complications. (Zago, et al. 2010).

8.2 The new classification of cognitive and behavioral disorder in ALS

In 2009, Strong and colleagues articulated new guidelines to direct ongoing investigations of cognitive and behavioral syndromes in ALS (Strong et al., 2009). To define the

Domain	Test
Executive measure	Wisconsin Card Sorting Test, Controlled Oral Word Association, FAS, D Words, Animal fluency, Written Word Fluency Design Fluency, California Card Sorting Test, Stroop Colour-Word Interference Test, Trail Making Test
Memory/Learning	Rey Auditory Verbal Learning Test, California Verbal Learning Test II, Warrington Recognition Memory Test, Wechsler Logical Memory and Visual Reproduction, Wechsler Paired Associate Learning. Kndrik Object Learning Test
Attention/Concentration	Verbal Serial Attention Test, Consonant trigrams Test, Symbol Digit Modit Modality Test, Paced Auditory Serial Addition Task, Digit Span
Language	Boston Naming Test, Graded Naming Test, Pyramid and palm Trees, Peabody Picture Vocabulary Test, British Picture Vocabulary Test, Test for the Reception of grammar
Visual/Spatial	Judgement of line Orientation, Benton Facial Recognition Test, Block Design, Motor-Free Visual Perception Test-Revised, Visual Object and Space Perception Battery
Emotional/ Behavioral functioning	Neuropsychiatric inventory, frontal Behavoural Inventory, Frontal Systems Behavioural Scale

Table 3. Neuropsychological test for the evaluation of cognitive/behavioral impairment in ALS (modifed from Strong et al. 2009), with permission.

neuropsychological status of ALS patients a framework was based on four different axes. Axis I is based on the EL Escorial criteria proposed in 1998, that includes possible, probable, and definite ALS clinical subtypes. This multidimensional approach incorporates several criteria (Brooks et al, 2000). The novelty of the classification lies primarily in Axis II with the proposal of five categories which classify ALS patients along a continuum: (1) ALS patients cognitively and behaviorally intact: (2) ALS patients with mild cognitive impairments; (3) ALS patients with mild behavioral impairment; (4) ALS with a full-fledged fronto-temporal dementia; (5) ALS with other non FTD-forms of dementia.

Axis III indicates the presence, in addition to frontotemporal impairments, of additional non-motoneuronal disease manifestations such as extrapyramidal signs, cerebellar degenerations, autonomic dysfunctions, sensory impairments, and ocular motility abnormalities. The absence of the above indicates a "pure form," while their presence defines "complicated forms" with additional pathological motor aspects. Axis IV, instead, provides the search for factors which could modify the course of the disease. Several disease modifiers have been reported in literature associated with longer survival, age at symptom onset (< 45 years), gender (male/sex), and site of the disease onset (bulbar or limb).

9. Language

Language deficits are occasionally found in the early stages of the disease. (Abrahams, et al. 2004).

The spectrum of language impairment in MND is wider than simply a problem in speech production due to dysarthria, but it is yet to be fully characterized. Reduced verbal output (adynamism) evolving into mutism has been reported, as well as echolalia. Perseverations, stereotypical expressions, (Bak and Hodges. 2004), true non-fluent aphasia with phonological and/or syntactic deficits and comprehension impairment have been reported in isolated cases. (Tsuchiya, et al. 2000)

MND has also been associated with apraxia of speech, in which there is breakdown in articulatroy planning, producing slowed, effortful and dysprosodic speech with problems repeating multisyllabic words. Apraxia of speech is often accompanied by orobuccal apraxia but not necessarily with aphasia.(Duffy, et al ,2007).

10. Memory

It has been difficult to categorize the pattern of memory impairment, but current evidence suggests that memory problems are related to abnormalities in retrieval of the information secondary to frontal dysfunction. (Neary, et al. 2000). Memory problems involve primarily immediate recall, (Phukan. et al. 2007) but impairment of visual memory also has been implicated,(Kew, et al.1993)

Frontal, temporal and thalamic hypoperfusion on SPECT has been shown to correlate with the severity of memory impairment. (Montovan, et al. 2003).

Most strikingly, learning and memory were found to be significantly improved in patients in the later stages of the disease, (Lakerveld et al, 2008).

Definite ALS	Upper and lower motor neuron signs in at least three body regions (upper limb, lower limb, bulbar, thoracic).
Clinically probable ALS	Upper and lower motor neuron signs in at least two regions, with some upper motor neuron signs necessarily rostoral to the lower motor neuron signs
Clinically probable ALS: Laboratory-supported ALS	Clinical signs of upper and lower motor neuron dysfunction in only one region, or when upper motor neuron signs alone are present in one region and lower motor neuron signs defined by electromyographic criteria are present in at least two limbs, with proper application of neuroimaging and clinical laboratory protocols to exclude other causes.
Clinically possible ALS	Clinical signs of upper and lower motor neuron dysfunction are together in only one region, or upper motor neuron signs are found alone in two or more regions, or lower motor neuron signs are found rostral to upper motor neuron signs and the diagnosis of clinically probable: laboratory-supported ALS cannot be proven by evidence on clinical grounds in conjunction with electrodiagnostic, neurophysiological, neuroimaging or clinical laboratory studies. Other diagnoses must have been excluded

* (Brooks, 1994 and Brooks, et al. 2000)
** Als: amyotrophic lateral sclerosis

Table 4. Revised El Escorial criteria for the diagnosis of ALS.*

11. Diagnostic criteria for motor neuron disease (amyotrophic lateral sclerosis, ALS) by** Leigh and Ray – Chaudhuri 1994

The diagnosis of ALS requires the presence of:

- LMN signs (including EMG features in clinically normal muscles)
- UMN signs
- Progression of the disorder

11.1 Diagnostic categories

- **Definite ALS**: UMN plus LMN signs in three regions**
- **Probable ALS:** UMN plus LMN signs in two regions with UMN signs rostral to LMN signs
- **Possible ALS**: UMN plus LMN signs in one region, or UMN signs in two or three regions, such as in monomelic ALS, progressive bulbar palsy, and primary lateral sclerosis
- **Suspected ALS**: LMN signs in two or three regions, such as in progressive muscular atrophy, and other motor syndromes.

11.2 The diagnosis of ALS requires the absence of

- Sensory signs
- Sphincter disturbances
- Visual disturbances
- Autonomic dysfunction
- Parkinson's disease
- Alzheimer-type dementia
- ALS "mimic" syndromes

11.3 The diagnosis of ALS is supported by

- Fasciculation in one or more regions
- Neurogenic change in EMG studies
- Normal motor and sensory nerve conduction (distal motor latencies may be increased)
- Absence of conduction block

Regions are defined as follows: brainstem, brachial, thorax and trunk, crural. UMN= Upper motor neuron; LMN= lower motor neuron.

12. Management of motor neuron disease (MND)

12.1 Investigations

There are no specific investigations for MND. Till now there are no specific biochemical or pathological markers of MND. The aim of Elctrophysiological, Imaging and laboratory investigations is to exclude MND mimics and/ or to support clinical signs presented by the patients.

Allum and Shaw (2010) clarified that investigations are important adjuncts to the clinical diagnosis of MND. Properly used they can provide supportive evidence of the clinical findings and help delineate the extent of disease. Investigations are also important to identify benign or treatable MND mimics.

12.2 Treatment plan of motor neuron disease

Although MND is still incurable disease up till now, in the last two decades MND management has evolved rapidly. Symptomatic treatment of MND still had the upper hand of management plan, especially for respiratory and bulbar complications. A team of work including neurologist, highly qualified nurses, ICU specialist in respiratory complications, psychologist, dietition, physiotherapy and speech therapist must be involved for management plan and follow up of MND patients, table (5).

Thus treatment strategy of MND was aimed towards;

1. Delay Progression of the disease and prevent further loss of motor neurons especially in the early stage of the disease
2. Symptomatomatic treatment to alleviate symptoms of the disease aiming to maintain quality of life

Types of investigatory Tools	Aim	Findings
I- Electrophysiology • Electromyography	Identification of LMN loss help in diagnosis of ALS by establishing the Presence of subclinical LMN involvement (Eisen and Swash. 2001)	• Active denervation (positive sharp waves, fibrillation potentials, Fasciculation Potentials) • Chronic denervation evidenced by large motor unit potentials (Allum and Shaw 2010)
• Single fibre EMG, macro EMG and central motor conduction using magnatic stimulation	Reflect early reinnervation and collateral sprouting and may provide evidence of A.H.C. damage in normal muscles (Leigh Ray - chaudhuri 1994)	Abnormal Jitter and blocking of neuromuscular trans -mission (Leig Ray – chaudhuri 1994)
Nerve conduction studies **Motor conduction Velocity**	To exclude disorders that mimic ALS	• Normal in early stages of ALS. • In advanced disease the compound muscle action potential amplitude becomes reduced, indicating denervation (Daube. 2000)
Sensory conduction velocity	Differentiating ALS From demyelinating neuropathies (Eisen. 2001)	• Typically normal • Abnormal SCV should raise suspicion of an alternative diagnosis (Eisen. 2001)
II-Imaging • MRI spine for Limb onset ALS without bulbar manifestation	To exclude cord and root compression	Normal
• MRI brain for ALS presented by bulbar manifestation	To exclude infiltrative lesion of tongue and pharynx (Turner, et al, 2009)	Normal
III- laboratory investigations • Routine investigations (complete blood count, liver, kidney and thyroid function tests, Blood sugar curve electrolyte, calcium, CK----- etc	To exclude MND minics as - Thyrotoxicosis - lymphomas - Paraneoplastic syndrome - Diabetic amyotrophy.	According to diagnosed neurological disorders

Table 5. Investigatory Tools for MND

Neurologist	Diagnosis, disclosure of diagnosis, treatment and symptom management, initation of respiratory and nutritional interventions, unbiased information regarding research developments
Family Doctor	Symptom control, drug monitoring, liaison with other teams
ALS Specialist Nurse	Liaison with medical team and coordination of care, home visits, practical advice regarding accessing support services, patient advocacy
Speech & Language Therapist	Evaluation and monitoring of dysphagia and aspiration, speech therapy and counseling regarding communication devices
Occupational Therapist	Optimization of the patient's environment. Advice regarding safety awareness, adaptive and splinting devices, activity modification, driving, energy conservation, home modification
Dietitian/Nutritionist	Evaluation of nutritional status and the need for tube feeding, management of dysphagia, management of enteral feeding
Physiotherapist	Evaluation of muscle strength and function, advice regarding walking aids and orthoses, safety awareness
Social Worker	Advice and control, pain management, maintenance of quality of life, preservation of dignity
Psychiatry and Neuropsychology	Evaluation and management of cognitive impairment/ dementia, adjustment disorders, anxiety and depression
Respiratory Physician	Assessment of respiratory dysfunction, initiation of non-invasive ventilation

* (phukan and Hardiman, 2009)

Table 6. Roles of the multidisciplinary team* with permission

12.3 Different types of treatment

1. pharmacological
2. symptomatic and
3. treatment of complications

12.3.1 Pharmacological treatment

Riluzole (2-amino-6-(trifluoromethoxy) benzothiazole, RP 54274) is the only drug licensed to treat ALS. Although the drug reduces glutamate-induced excitotoxicity, its précis mechanism in ALS is unknown. A Cochrane Library meta-analysis (including three double-blind randomized placebo controlled trials by (Miller, 2002) suggests that riluzole provides a 9% gain in the probability of surviving one year and adds approximately 2 months to patient survival.

Riluzole, exerts the following pharmacologic effects:

- An inhibitory effect on glutamate release.
- Inactivation of Voltage - dependent sodium channels.
- Ability to interfere with intracellular events that follow transmitter binding at excitatory amino acid receptor (Riluzole monograph 2011).

- **Dosage** 50mg twice daily
- **Side Effects** Nausea and vomiting, Asthenia, somnolence Headache, dizziness, and vertigo
- Serious Adverse Effects
  - Elevation in liver transaminases. Regular monitoring of liver function is advised (every month for 3 months, every 3 months for a further nine months then annually thereafter).
  - Rare cases of neutropenia have been reported. White cell count must be checked in the case of febrile illness

Contraindications-Renal and hepatic impairment Pregnancy and breast-feeding (Brockington and Shaw, 2003)

12.3.2 Symptomatic treatment

Symptom	Cause	Drugs	Other treatment
Cramps	Changes in motor function	Carbamazepine Phenytion Magnesium (Miller, et al, 1999; Andersen, et al, 2005)	Physiotherapy Physical exercise Massage Hydrotherapy (Miller, et al, 1999; Andersen, et al, 2005)
Spasticity	Corticospinal tract damage	Baclofen Tizanidine Dantrolene Botulinum toxin type A (Wnterholler et al,2002 ; Restivo et al, 2002)	Physiotherapy (Millul et al, 2005) Hydrotherapy Cryotherapy
Exessive watery Saliva	Bulbar weakness	Atropine Hyoscine hydrobromide (Miller, et al, 1999; Andersen, et al, 2005) Amitriptyline (Bradley et al, 2001)	Home suction device Nebulisation (Andersen, et al, 2005) injections of botulinum toxin into parotid glands (Giess et al, 2000/ Winterholler et al, 2001) irradiation of the salivary glands (Iannaccone et al, 1996; Stalpers and Moser, 2002)
Persistent saliva and bronchial secretions	-Bulbar weakness - Respiratory complications	Carbocisteine Propranolol Metoprolol (Newall, et al, 1996)	Home suction device hydrobromide (Miller, et al, 1999/Andersen, et al, 2005) Reduced intake of diary products, alcohol, and caffeine.

Excessive or violent yawning	Corticospinal tract damage (pseudobulbar syndrome)	Baclofen	
Laryngospasm	Pharyngeal sensitivity	Lorazepam	Reassurance
Pain	Immobility, stiffness	- Simple analgesics - Non-steroidal anti-inflammatory drugs - Opioids	Comfort (seating, sleeping, day and night care)
Emotional lability	Pseudobulbar syndrome	Tricyclic antidepressant Selective serotonin-reuptake inhibitors (Iannaccone and Ferini, 1996) Levodopa Dextrometorphan and quinidien (Brooks, et al, 2004)	
Communication difficulties			Speaking techniques (Murphy, 2004) Voice amplifiers Brain-computer interfaces (Kübler et al, 2005)
Constipation	Immobility; opiates, Dehydration	Lactulose Senna	Hydration Increased fiber intake
Depression	- Hopelessness; - Inability to communicate; and frustration	Amitriptyline Citalopram	Psychological support counseling
Insomnia	Discomfort, pain, depression; (consider respiratory insufficiency)	Amitriptyline Zolpidem	Comfort, analgesia
Anxiety	Many Factors	- Lorazepam - Midazolam - Diazepam suppositories	Psychological support, counseling
Fatigue	- Muscle weakness - Anxiety - Depression		Modafinil (Bradly et al 2001)

Table 7. Symptomatic treatment of Motor Neuron Disease. Modified From Radunovic et al 2007 and leigh et al 2003

12.3.3 Treatment of complication

a. Respiratory complications

Respiratory impairment is common in MND and may develop because of respiratory muscle weakness, impaired bulbar function causing aspiration or obstructive sleep apnea, or defects in central control. Dyspnea may be due to infection, pulmonary embolus, or airway obstruction from mucous plug or inhaled pharyngeal contents. (Howard and Wiles,1989).

Symptoms of respiratory insufficiency may be subtle and develop insidiously. Patients may report dyspnea, orthopnea, sleep fragmentation due to hypoventilation, morning headaches, daytime somnolence and fatigue, poor concentration/memory and nocturia. Others may be asymptomatic. Respiratory muscle weakness is an in dependent predictor of quality of life.(Bourke, et al, 2001) and respiratory failure is the most common cause of death in ALS patients. Assessment of respiratory insufficiency includes history, physical examination, rarly morning arterial blood gas, and overnight pulse oximetry.

Nocturnal hypoventilation may present as daytime hypersomnolence, lethargy, morning headaches, poor concentration, depression, anxiety, and irritability, while obstructive sleep apnea is characterized by snoring and restless sleep with abnormal movements. (Howard and orrell 2002).

Types of mechanical ventilation

There are several types of ventilatory aids. These are broadly classified in terms of invasive versus noninvasive.

As its name suggests, invasive techniques require an endotracheal tube or more commonly a tracheostomy. For patients in advanced respiratory failure (ie, no respiratory muscle function), invasive ventilators can assume complete control of ventilation. (Simonds. 2003).

Non- invasive ventilatory aids can be divided into two groups, negative or positive pressure ventilators. Negative pressure is exerted to the chest or abdominal wall mechanically to assist inspiration. Positive pressure devices can be set to deliver variable inspiratory and expiratory pressures, triggered by spontaneous effort (Simonds. 2003).

b. Management of Dysphagia

Management of Dysphagia includes modification of food and fluid consistency, postural advice (e.g. chin tuck: flexing the neck forward on swallowing to protect the airway), and parenteral feeding.

A percutaneous endoscopic gastrostomy (PEG) placement is indicated for those who have symptomatic dysphagia or significant weight loss. (Miller, et al. 2002). Patients and their families should be suitably counseled regarding the benefits and risks of the procedure.

13. Conclusion

Motor neuron disease is of the most common neurodegenerative disorders of unknown etiology, and had no specific treatment. ALS is the commonest type, and in most literatures is used as a synonym for motor neuron disease. Diagnosis is still clinical, mainly, and the investigatory tools have a definite role for diagnosis of other motor neuron mimics. Once motor neuron disease is diagnosed, the prognosis is usually bad, especially when bulbar, and respiratory complications are evident.

14. References

Abrahams S., Goldstein L.H., Simmons A., et al. (2004). World retrieval in amyotrophic lateral sclerosis: a functional magnetic resonance imaging study. Brain;127:1507-17

Allum C.W,& Shaw P. (2010). Motor neurone disease: a practical update on diagnosis and management. Clinical Medicine, Vol 10. No 3: 252-8

Andersen P.M., Borasio G.D., Dengler R., et al. (2005). EFNS task force on management of amyotrophic lateral sclerosis: guidelines for diagnosing and clinical care of patients and relatives. Eur J Neurol;12:921-38.

Andersen P.M., Sims Xin W.W., et al. (2003). Sixteen novel mutations in the Cu/Zn superoxide dismutase gene in amyotrophic lateral sclerosis: a decade of discoveries, defects and disputes. Amyotroph Lateral Scler Other Motor Neuron Disorders;4:62-73.

Bak T.H.,& Hodges J.R.& (2004). The effects of motor neuron disease on language: further evidence. Brain Lang;89:354-61.

Baltadzhieva R., Gurevich T.,& Korezyn A.D. (2006). Autonomic impairment in amyotrophic lateral sclerosis. Curr Opin Neurol;18:487-93.

Bourke S.C., Shaw P.J.,& Gibson G.J. (2001). Respiratory function vs sleep-disorderd breathing as predictors of Qol in ALS. Neurology 57:2040-2044.

Bradley W.G., Anderson F., Bromberg M., et al. (2001). Current management of ALS: comparison of the ALS CARE Database and the AAN Practice Parameter. Neurology;57:500-04.

Brockington A.,& Shaw P. (2003). Developments in the treatment of Motor Neurone Disease. Acnr. Vol 3 N 5 November/December.

Brooks B.R. (1994). EL Escorial World Federation of Neurology criteria for the diagnosis of amyotrophic lateral sclerosis. Subcommittee on Motor Neuron Disease/Amyotrophic Lateral Sclerosis of the World Federation of Neurology Research Group on Neuromuscular Disease and El Escorial " Clinical limits of amyotrophic lateral sclerosis" workshop contributors. J Neurol Sci 124:96-107.

Brooks B.R., Miller R.G., Swash M. & Munsat T.L. (2000). World Federation of Neurology Research Group on Motor Neuron Disease: El Escorial revisited: revised criteria for the diagnosis of amyotrophic lateral sclerosis. Amyotrophic Lateral Scler. Other Motor Neuron Disord, 1:293-239.

Brooks B.R., Thisted R.A., Appel S.H., et al. (2004). Treatment of pseudobulbar affect in ALS with dextromethorphan/quinidine, Neurology;63:1363-70.

Brugman F., & Wokkle J.H.J. (2004). Primary Lateral Sclerosis. Orphanet Encyclopedia. April, http://www.orpha.net/data/patho/GB/uk-PLS.bdf.

Carter G.T., Weiss M.D., Lou J.S., et al. (2005). Modafinil to treat fatigue in amyotrophic lateral sclerosis: an open label pilot study. Am J Hosp Palliat Care;22:55-59.

Cleveland D.W.& Rothstein. J.D. (2001). Nat. Rev Neurosci 11,806-819.

Daube J.R. (2000). Electrodiagnostic studies in amyotrophic lateral sclerosis and other motor neuron disorders. Muscle Nerue; 23:1488-502.

De Domenice P., Malara C.E., Marabello L., et al.(1988). Amyotrophic lateral sclerosis; an epidemiological study in the Province of Messina, Italy, 1976-1985. Neuroepidemiology;7:152-8.

Duffy J.R., Peach R.K., & Strand E.A. (2007). Progressive apraxia of speech as a sign of motor neuron disease. Am J Neuroradial;16:198-208.

Eisen A. (2001). Clinical electrophysiology of the upper and lower motor neuron in amyotrophic lateral sclerosis. Sem Neurol;21:141-54.

Eisen A., & Swash M. (2001). Clinical neurophysiology of ALS. Clin Neurophysiol;112:2190-201.

Fong K.Y., Yu Y.L., Chan Y.W., et al. (1996). Motor neuron disease in Hong Kong Chinese: epidemiology and clinical picture. Neuroepidemiology;15:239-45.

Geser F., Brandmeir N.J., Kwong L.K., et al. (2008). Evidence of multisystem disorder in whole - brain map of pathological TDP-43 in amyotrophic lateral sclerosis. Arch Neurol;65:636-41.

Giess R., Naumann M., Werner E., et al. (2000). Injections of botulinum toxin A into the salivary glands improve sialorrhoea in amyotrophic lateral sclerosis. J Neurol Neurosurg Psychiatry;69:121-23.

Haley R.W. (2003). Excess incidence of ALS in young Gulf War veterans. Neurology;61:750-6.

Horner R.D., Kamins K.G., Feussner J.R. et al. (2003). Occurrence of amyotrophic lateral sclerosis among Gulf War veterans. Neurology;61:742-9.

Howard R.S., Wiles C.M., & Loh L. (1989). Respiratory complications and their management in motor neurone disease. Brain;112:1155-70.

Howard R.S.,& Orrell R.W. (2002). Management of motor neuron disease, Postgrad Med J; 78:736-741.

Iannaccone S.,& Ferini-Strambi L. (1996). Pharmacological treatment of emotional lability. Clin Neuropharmacol;19:532-35.

Ingram D.A.,& Swash M. (1987). Central motor conduction is abnormal in motor neuron disease. J Nerol Neurosurg Psychiatry;50:159-66

Irwin D., Lippa C.F., Swearer J.M. (2007). Cognition and amyotrophic lateral sclerosis (ALS). Am J Alzheimer Dis Other Demen;22:300-12.

Isaacs J.D., Dean A.F., Shaw C.E., et al. (2007). Amyotrophic lateral sclerosis with sensory neuropathy: part of a multisystem disorders? J Neurol Neurosurg Psychiatry; 78:750-3.

Kew J.J.M., Goldstein L.H., Leigh P.N., et al. (1993). The relationship between abnormalities of cognitive function and cerebral activation in amyotrophic lateral sclerosis: a neuropsychological and positron emission tomography study. Brain;116:1399-423.

Kübler A., Nijboer F., Mellinger J., et al. (2005). Patients with ALS can use sensorimotor rhythms to operate a brain-computer interface. Neurology;64:1775-77.

Lakerveld J., Kotchoubey B.,& Kubler A. (2008). Cognitive function in patients with late stage amyotrophic lateral sclerosis. J Neurol Neurosurg Psychiatry;79:25-29. doi:10.1136/jnnp.2007.116178.

Leigh P.N. (1991). Amyotrophic lateral sclerosis and other motor neuron disorders. Curr Opin Neurol Neurosurg;4:586-96.

Leigh P.N., Abrahams S., Al-Chalabi A., Ampong M.-A., Goldstein L.H., Johnson J., et al. (2003). King's MND Care and Research Team. The management of motor neurone disease. J Neurol Neurosurg Psychiatry;74: iv 32-47.

Leigh P.N., & Ray-Chaudhuri K. (1994). Motor neuron disease. J Neurol Neurosurg Psychiatry;57:886-96.

Logroscino G., Traynor B.J., Hardiman O., et al. (2008). Descriptive epidemiology of amyotrophic lateral sclerosis: new evidence and unsolved issues. J Neurol Neurosurg Psychiatry;79:6-11.

Miller R.G., Mitchell J.D., Lyon M.,& Moore D.H. (2002). Riluzole for amyotrophic lateral sclerosis (ALS)/ motor neuron disease (MND). Cochrane Database Syst Rev; CD001447.

Miller R.G., Rosenberg J.A., Gelinas D.F., et al. (1999). Practice parameter: the care of the patient with amyotrophic lateral sclerosis (an evidence-based review): report of the Quality Standards Subcommittee of the American American Academy of Neurology. Neurology;52:1311-23.

Millul A., Beghi E., Logroscino G., Micheli A., Vielli E.,& Zardi A. (2005). Survival of patients with amyotrophic lateral sclerosis in a population-based registry. Neuroepidemiology;25:114-19.

Montovan M.C., Baggio L., Dalla Barba G., et al. (2003). Memory deficits and retrieval processes in ALS. Eur J Neurol;10:221-7.

Mulder D.W. (1982). Clinical limits of amyotrophic lateral sclerosis. In Rowtand LP (ed). Human Motor Neuron Diseases. New York: Raven Press:15-22

Murphy J. (2004). Communication strategies of people with ALS and their partners. Amyotroph Lateral Scler Other Motor Disord;5:121-26.

Murros K. &, Fogelholm R. (1983). Amyotrophic lateral sclerosis in Middle-Finland: an epidemiological study. Acta Neurol Scand;67:41-7.

Neary D., Snowden J.S., & Mann D.M.A. (2000); Cognitive change in motor neurone disease/ amyotrophic lateral sclerosis (MND/ALS). J Neurol Sci;180:15-20.

Newall A.R., & Orser R. (1996). Hunt M. The control of oral secretions in bulbar ALS/MND. J Neurol Sci;139:43-44.

Oluwole O.S.A., Conradi S., Kristensson K.,& Karlsson H. (2004). Human Endogenous Retrovirus W and Motor Neurone Disease. Annals of badan Post graduate Medicine. Vol. 2No 2dec.

Phukan J., Pender N.P, & Hardiman O. (2007). Cognitive impairment in amyotrophic lateral Sclerosis. Lancet Neurol;6:994-1003.

Phukan J., & Hardiman O (2009). The management of amyotrophic lateral. J Neurol. DOI 10.1007/s00415-0090142-9.

Pugdahl K., Fuglsang-Frederiksen A., de Carvalho M., et al. (2007). Generalised sensory system abnormalities in amyotrophic lateral sclerosis: a European multicentre study. J Neurol Neurosurg Psychiatry;78:746-9.

Raaphorst J., de Visser M., Linssen W.H., de Haan R.,J., & Schmand B. (2010). The cognitive profile of amyotrophic lateral sclerosis: A meta-analysis. Amyotroph. Lateral Scler., 11:27-37.

Radhakrishnan K., Ashok P.P., Sridharan R., Mousa M.E. (1986). Descriptive epidemiology of motor neuron disease in Benghazi, Libya. Neuroepidemiology;5:47-54.

Radunovic A., Mitsumoto H.,& Leigh P.N. (2007). Clinical Care of Patients with Amyotrophic Lateral Sclerosis. Lancet Neurology.; 10:931-25.

Restivo D.A., Lanza S., Marchese-Ragona R.,& Plameri A. (2002). Improvement of masseter spasticity by botulinum toxin facilitates PEG placement in amyotrophic lateral sclerosis. Gasreoenterology;123:1749-50.

Riluzole monograph. Facts and comparisons online. [cited 2011 Feb 19] Available at: http://online.factsandcomparisons.com.

Ringel S.P., Murphy J.R., Alderson MK, et al.(1993). The natural history of amyotrophic lateral sclerosis. Neurology;43:1316-22.

Ringholz G.M. Appel S.H, Bradshaw M., et al. (2005). Prevalence and patterns of cognitive impairment in sporadic ALS. Neurology;65:586-90.

Rodgers-Johanson P., Garruto R.M., Yanagihara R., Chen K.M., Gajdusek D.C.,& Gibbs C.J. (1986). Amyotrophic lateral sclerosis and parkinsonism-dementia on Guam: a 30 year evaluation and neuropathologic trends. Neurology;36:7-13.

Schroder H.D.,& Reske-Nielsen E. (1984). Preservation of the nucleus – pelvic floor motor system in amyorophic lateral sclerosis. Clin Neuropathol;3:210-6

Shaw PJ. (2005). Molecular and cellular pathways of neurodegeneration in motor neuron disease. J Neurol Neurosurg Psychiatry; 76:1046-1057.

Simonds A.K. (2003). Home ventitation. Eur Respir J; 22:38s-46s.

Stalpers L.J., & Moser E.C. (2002). Results of radiotherapy for drooling in amyotrophic lateral sclerosis. Neurology;58:1308.

Strong M., & Rosenfeld J. (2003). Amyotrophic lateral sclerosis: a review of current concepts. ALS and other motor neuron disorders;4:136-143

Strong M.J., Grace G.M., Freedman M., Lomen-Hoerth C, Woolley S, Goldstein L.H. Murphy J. ,Shoesmith C., Rosenfeld J., Leigh P.N., Bruijn L., Ince P.,& Figlewiez D. (2009). Consensus criteria for the diagnosis of front-otemporal cognitive and behavioral syndromes in amyotrophic lateral sclerosis. Amyotroph. Lateral Scler. 10:131-146,.

Swash M. (2001). Amyotrophic lateral sclerosis: current understanding. J Neurosci Nurs;33:245-53.

Swash M., Leader M., Browen A.,& Swettenhan K. (1986). Focal loss of anterior horn cells in the cervical cord in motor neuron disease. Brain;109:939-52

Takeda S., Yamada M., Kawasaki K., et al. (1994). Motor neuron disease with multi-system involvement presenting as tetraparesis, ophthalmoplegia and sensori-autonomic dysfunction. Acta Neuropathol;88:193-200.

Talbot K. (2002). Motor neurone disease, Postgrad Med J.;78:513-519.

Tsuchiya K., Ozawa E., Fukushima J., et al. (2000). Rapidly progressive aphasia and motor neuron disease: a clinical, radiological, and pathological study of an autopsy case with circumscribed lobar atrophy. Acta Neuropathol;99:81-7.

Turner M.R., Kiernan M.C, Leigh P.N., & Talbot K. (2009). Biomarkers in amyotrophic lateral sclerosis. Lancet Neurol;8:94-109.

Valdmanis P.N., & Rouleau G.A. (2008). Genetics of familial amyotrophic lateral sclerosis. Neurology;70:144-52.

Van der Graaff M. (2004). Amyotrophic lateral sclerosis. Orphanet Encyclopedia. September. http://www.prpha.net/data/patho/GB/uk-ALS.pdf.

Washington, D.C. (c2007). The ALS Association; [updated 2008 Oct; cited 2011.Feb 17]. Available from http://www.alsa.org/.

Wijesekera L.C. & Leigh P.N. (2009). Amyotrophic lateral sclerosis. Orphanet Journal of Rare Diseases [cited 2011 Feb 17] ; 4(3) [about 22p.]. Avalilable from: http://www.ojrd.com/content/4/1/3.

Winterholler M.G., Erbguth F.J., Wolf S.,& Kat S. (2001). Botulinum toxin for the treatment of sialorrhoea in ALS: serious side effects of a transductal approach. J Neurol Neurosurg Psychiatry;70:417-18.

Winterholler M.G., Heckmann J.G. Hecht M. & Erbguth F.J. (2002). Recurrent trismus and stridor in an ALS patient: successful treatment with botulinum toxin. Neurology;58:502-03.

Yoshida M. (2004). Amyotrophic lateral sclerosis with dementia: The clinicopothological spectrum, Neuropathology;24:87-102.

Zago S., Poletti B., Morelli C., Doretti A., & Silani V. (2010). Archives italiennes de Biologie, 149;39:56,.

12

Spinal Muscular Atrophy

Yasser Salem
[1]University of North Texas Health Science Center,
[2]Cairo University, Faculty of Physiotherapy,
[1]USA
[2]Egypt

1. Introduction

1.1 Overview and incidence

Spinal muscular atrophy (SMA) is a neuromuscular disorder characterized by degeneration of alpha motor neurons resulting in hypotonia, progressive muscular weakness and atrophy.[30] Spinal muscular atrophy is one of the leading hereditary causes of infant mortality,[31] it comprises the second most common fatal progressive diseases after cystic fibrosis.[28] Spinal muscular atrophy is the most common neuromuscular disease in childhood after Duchenne muscular dystrophy with an estimated incidence of 1 per 5,000 to 10,000 live births.[4,11]

2. Pathogenesis

Spinal muscular atrophy is known to be genetic disorder that is inherited as an autosomal recessive disorder but some dominant or X-linked traits are reported. The pathological basis of SMA is abnormality of the large anterior horn cells in the spinal cord caused by deletion or mutation of the Survival Motor Neuron-1 (SMN1) gene located at chromosome region 5q.[1] Absence of all or part of the SMN has been detected in 98% of patients with SMA[18] and results in reduction of the full length protein necessary for proper function of the anterior horn cells.[10,13] The decreased level of the SMN protein results in selective death of spinal motor neurons,[31] with the severity of the disease being inversely proportional to the amount of the SMN in the anterior horn cells.[1]The severity of SMA ranges from total paralysis and need for ventilatory support to relatively mild muscle weakness.[1, 32]

3. Clinical manifestation and classification

SMA is manifested by various clinical features that cause a variety of debilitating symptoms. Muscle weakness is a hallmark feature of SMA and patients with SMA are among the weakest and most hypotonic seen in any muscle clinic.[13] Clinically, the disease is characterized by progressive symmetrical muscle weakness, which starts proximally and moves distally, with the proximal muscles being more affected than the distal muscles.[5] Muscle weakness is associated with muscle atrophy, hypotonia, absence or marked decrease of deep tendon reflexes, fasciculation of the tongue, and tremors of the hand.[5,20] Patients with SMA have normal intellectual function. Contractures and spinal deformity have been reported to be common impairments. Pulmonary infections and restrictive lung disease are the most serious complications in SMA.[12] In general, the clinical course of SMA is highly variable, and it is more of a continuous spectrum with the age of onset from birth to adulthood, and the age of death from infancy to normal life expectancy. The severity of the diseases and clinical manifestations show a continuous range from the very severe to very mild forms of the disease.[20] With age, muscle weakness increases, and the symptoms progress and patients lose their functions over time.[25] The progression of the disease process varies both between and within types.[21] Current evidence suggests that maximum function achieved is more closely related to life expectancy than age at onset.[24] Based on the age at onset, clinical presentation, and the maximum functional level achieved, SMA is usually classified into the following broad types.

3.1 Type I SMA (Werdnig-Hoffmann disease)

Type I SMA is the most severe form of SMA, it is also known as Werdnig-Hoffman disease. The age of onset is typically from birth or in the first 6 months of life and the child never developing independent sitting. Werdnig-Hoffmann disease is characterized by severe generalized muscle weakness and hypotonia.[20] Infants typically have significant wasting, and weakness in the limbs and trunk and present with decreased movements, especially against gravity. Most infants present with lack of head control and are never able to roll from supine or to pull to sitting.[13] Significant oral motor weakness results in difficulties in sucking and swallowing and makes feeding progressively more difficult. Weakness of the intercostal muscles results in limited respiratory function, and breathing is usually entirely diaphragmatic resulting in development of abnormal breathing patterns and respiratory complications. The severity of respiratory complications is generally proportional to the weakness.[24] Early morbidity and mortality are commonly associated with pulmonary complications,[30] and death occurs during the first 2 to 3 years of life.

3.2 Type II SMA (Intermediate form)

Children with the intermediate form have an onset between 6 and 18 months of age.[17] They are able to sit and may develop ability to stand but they are unable to walk independently.[21,30] Some of the less involved children are able to walk with braces or assistive devices at some point of their life.[8] Children with type II exhibit symptoms of weakness similar to type I SMA but with much less severe degree. Distal muscle weakness is less severe than proximal muscle weakness and starts later in the course of the disease. There is a delay in the acquisition of motor skills, with the majority of those children sit at the age of 12 months of age. As the disease progresses, children exhibit more weakness and regressed gross motor development. Feeding and swallowing are not difficult. Contractures are common including scoliosis or kyphoscoliosis. Early onset and rapidly progressing scoliosis is uniformly present; severity of scoliosis increases as the disease progresses and may require bracing and/or spinal fusion. Pulmonary complications are pervasive especially with scoliosis and as the disease progresses. Ventilatory assistance is common in later stages of the disease.

3.3 Type III SMA (Kugelberg-Welander disease)

Type III SMA, often referred to as Kugelberg-Welander disease or Juvenile-onset SMA, is the mild form of the disease. Children with type III SMA have an onset age typically after 18 months. This form is more variable in age of onset, although most diagnosis prior to age 3 years is typical, weakness in other mild cases may not be noticeable until late childhood. Patients are able to achieve independent walking and whilst some children may lose this ability in childhood, others maintain walking until adolescence or adulthood.[30] Early motor milestones are often normal, including ability to walk, which is achieved at the normal age or slightly late. Although they are able to ambulate, they may show difficulty with walking at some point in their clinical course secondary to proximal muscle weakness. Walking is characterized by lack of balance, falls, increased lumbar lordosis, hyperextended knees or genu recurvatum, and excessive waddling. Muscle weakness mainly affects proximal muscles of the lower extremities and is less severe than types I and II SMA. Proximal muscle weakness often results in difficulty in stairs climbing, hopping, running and jumping. Gower's' maneuver may be present when getting up off the floor. Scoliosis and pulmonary complications are common in patients with type III SMA but less frequent and not severe as in patients with type II SMA. The incidence and severity of complications including scoliosis and pulmonary complications are related to the degree of muscle weakness and the functional status. Many patients with type III lose the ability to functionally ambulate as they get weaker during adulthood. Individuals with type III SMA usually have normal life expectancy.

3.4 SMA type IV (Adult-onset form)

Adult-onset SMA is a rare type. The onset of the disease is in the adulthood, typically in the third or fourth decades. The signs and symptoms are similar to those of type III SMA but the impairments and degree of disability are often mild. Life expectancy is normal.

3.5 Other forms of SMA

There are other very rare types of SMA disorders with similar symptoms but they are caused by different genes other than SMN1 and genetic mutation. Other forms of SMA include *distal spinal muscular atrophy*, characterized by distal muscle weakness; *X-linked spinal and bulbar muscular atrophy (Kennedy disease*), an X-linked adult onset form of SMA; *childhood bulbar SMA (Fazio-londe disease), a progressive bulbar palsy; Hexosaminidase a deficiency,* with variable neurologic findings, including progressive dystonia, spinocerebellar degeneration, and lower motor neuron disease; and *Monomelic muscular atrophy,* a cervical form of spinal muscular atrophy.[24]

4. Diagnosis

Diagnosis of SMA is suspected on the bases of the clinical picture, muscle biopsy and electromyography. Genetic testing is the only definitive diagnostic test for patients with SMA. With the use of genetic testing, the role of EMG and muscle biopsy in confirming the diagnosis of SMA is limited. They can be used for the diagnosis of patients with SMA who present without homozygous deletion of the SMN gene.[32] Genetic testing of SMA shows a deletion of the SMN gene on the fifth chromosome. EMG findings usually show a pattern of denervation including fibrillation potentials, positive sharp waves, and large amplitude, short duration actions potentials. Sensory nerve conduction velocities are normal with no marked decrease of motor nerve conduction velocities. Muscle biopsy provides evidence of muscle denervation with groups of small atrophic fibers with large hypertrophic fibers.

5. Prognosis

The course of SMA is relentlessly progressive. Prognosis varies according to the age of onset, type of SMA, and the maximum function achieved. The age at the time of the onset has the strongest relationship to prognosis. It appears that the earlier the onset of the disease, the faster the progression and the poorer the prognosis. The current prognosis for children with type I SMA is very poor, with the death usually occurs in the first two years of life as a result of respiratory failure caused by respiratory complications. Some children with SMA type I can survive beyond two years of age with the use of ventilator assistance.[1] The prognosis of type II SMA is extremely variable. Patients with type II SMA have short life span; survival into adulthood is possible with aggressive respiratory care. Majority of patients with type III SMA remain independent in ambulation throughout adult life. Patients with Type III SMA are expected to have normal life expectancy. Patients with the onset begins before two years of age continue to ambulate until an average of twelve years of age. Patients with the onset after two years of age continue to ambulate throughout the adult life.[25]

6. Assessment

Since assessment is important for guiding clinical management and for evaluating therapeutic outcomes, thorough assessment of patients with SMA is essential. Assessment should include regular assessment pertinent to children with neuromuscular disorders such as assessment of posture, muscle strength, performance, range of motion, gait assessment, respiratory assessment, and quality of life measures. Assessment of functional status and level of disability using standardized outcome measures should be also included.

6.1 Joint integrity, range of motion and muscle flexibility

Active and passive joint range of motion can be assessed using goniometry. Functional range of motion, muscle length, and soft tissue flexibility should be assessed using standard methods. Assessment of joint integrity, range of motion and muscle flexibility should be done periodically to monitor development of contractures, particularly when the patient loses ability to ambulate.

6.2 Assessment of posture

Routine posture examination should be performed on a regular basis. Posture examination includes examination of resting posture and changes in posture that occur with movement. Examination for the presence of scoliosis is essential especially for patients who are wheelchair dependent.

6.3 Muscle strength

Assessing muscle strength in children can be difficult, because the results depend on the patient's effort.[15] Strength deficits in children with SMA can be assessed using manual muscle testing (MMT) or hand-held dynamometer. Manual muscle testing is the most widely method to assess muscle strength in clinical practice. It is a reasonably easy and inexpensive in measuring muscle strength in patients with SMA, but it does not allow grading small changes in muscle strength. A handheld dynamometer can be used to quantify muscle strength. Using a dynamometer is easy and comfortable and allows for measuring small changes in strength over a continuous range.[19]

6.4 Respiratory function

Pulmonary function tests are parts of the regular assessment in patients with SMA to monitor changes in respiratory status. Routine assessment of respiratory function includes complete pulmonary function tests, including sprirometery, lung volumes, and respiratory muscle function tests.[30] Assessments of cough effectiveness and breathing pattern are important for the non-ambulatory patients or patients who are too weak or too young to perform pulmonary function testing.[30]

6.5 Gait

No disease-specific gait test or measure exists for patients with SMA. Description of gait deviations and safety and stability during walking should be included as part of routine gait analysis. The 10-Meter Walk test can be used to measure gait speed. The Six Minute Walk Test or the Two Minute Walk Test can be used to measure endurance during gait.

6.6 Measurement of functional status and quality of life

Examination of functional status including examination of functional mobility skills and activities of daily living is an important consideration. Several clinical outcome measures can be used to measure functional outcomes in patients with SMA including generic measures and disease-specific measures. Generic outcome measures commonly used in patients with SMA include the Gross Motor Function Measure, the Test of Infant Motor Performance, the Alberta Infant Motor Scale, the Wee Functional Independence Measure, the Motor Function Measure, and the EgenKlassifikation Scale. Disease-specific outcome measures include the Hammersmith Functional Motor Scale, the Modified Hammersmith Functional Motor Scale, the Expanded Hammersmith Functional Motor Scale, the Children's Hospital of Philadelphia Test of Strength in spinal muscular atrophy, the Infant Test for Neuromuscular Disease, and the Spinal Muscular Atrophy Functional Rating Scale. Selection of the outcome measures to be used is based on age of the patient, patient's functional level, aspects of function being measured, ease of administration, and burden imposed on the patient. The Pediatric Quality of Life Inventory (PedsQL) instrument can be used to measure quality of life.

7. Management

No specific therapy is currently available for SMA. Treatment is usually supportive, and may include physical therapy, occupational therapy, nutrition, orthotic management, and possibly surgical intervention. Appropriate recommendations are made on the basis of each patient's presentation and functional level.[15] The most important goal in the management of the patients is to achieve maximal independent living with maximized mobility, and to prevent the development of complications.[2,9,13,15,30] Treatment focuses on prevention of complications of severe weakness including restrictive lung disease, orthopedic deformities, immobility, and psychosocial problems.

The multidisciplinary approach is important to assess and address the needs of the patient/family. The multidisciplinary team might consist of neurologist, pediatrician, physiatrist, physical therapist, occupational therapist, speech therapist, nutritionist, pulmonary specialist, orthotist, genetic counselor, social worker, and psychologist. Family education and patient/family centered care are important parts in the management of patients with SMA. Education should include the disease process, associated impairments and complications, physical limitations, functional abilities, prognosis, and expected outcomes.

7.1 Therapeutic exercises and strength training

The overall therapeutic goals are to achieve maximal independence in mobility,[15] and to prevent and delay progression of complications. Exercise programs may help to improve and maintain range of motion, maintain mobility, and prevent or slow the progression of contractures, orthopedic deformities and respiratory failure.

Strengthening exercises have been shown to be effective to slow the deterioration of muscle weakness in patients with neuromuscular disorders. Strengthening exercises may prolong ambulation and delay dependence on wheelchair for mobility in patients with neuromuscular disorders including children with Duchenne muscular dystrophy. Strengthening exercises may be used to slow the deterioration in muscle strength. The role of strengthening exercises in SMA is not well established due to lack of clinical trials on the effects of exercise programs and lack of trials critical data to support appropriate exercise prescription. Appropriate exercise recommendations in SMA are based on the patient's presentations and functional status, and therapists' experience with similar neuromuscular conditions. Recommendations regarding strengthening of patients with SMA include precautions and guidelines from other degenerative muscle diseases.[7]

In patients with neuromuscular diseases, excessive strengthening exercises may contribute to deterioration in muscle strength by increasing muscle degeneration.[7] Therefore, excessively strenuous strengthening such as excessive resistive exercises, eccentric exercises, and maximal aerobic training should be avoided. Excessive fatigue and overwork weakness should be avoided, frequent rests and self-initiated rests should be given frequently especially for the weaker patients and patients with decreased respiratory functions. Positioning and support can be used to maximize biomechanical advantage and minimize the effects of gravity. Monitoring with oximetry is recommended particularly for patients with compromised respiratory functions. It is important to monitor responses to exercises such as fatigue, pain, and muscle soreness.

Strengthening exercises for SMA may include low-intensity strengthening exercises, and submaximal aerobic exercise. Since there is no evidence to support traditional strength training for patients with SMA, practicing functional activities and tasks of activities of daily living may be good recommendation for those individuals. These exercises and activities should be designed based on the age, developmental stage, and functional level.

Exercise strategies for young children and infants may include practicing developmental skills. This includes activities to facilitate head and trunk control; floor mobility skills such as rolling and creeping; facilitation of weight shift and weight bearing and transitions between positions; and facilitations of upright positions and skills such as sitting, standing and walking as appropriate.[3] For the less involved and older individuals, exercise strategies include practice functional activities such as standing and walking, and gentle aerobic programs.

7.2 Participation in physical activities

Weakness and difficulty in moving independently in patients with SMA contribute to physical inactivity and limited participation in exercise programs. The consequences of physical inactivity are particularly detrimental, could contribute to secondary impairments and may lead to additional decline in functional status. Recent evidence suggests that engagement in physical activities helps improve physical functioning in children with disability. Participation in physical activities may promote physical functioning, quality of life, health, and well-being.

Participation in physical activity may include participation in recreational and sports activities. Recreational programs that can be beneficial include swimming, cycling, and riding when appropriate.[6] Activities should be selected carefully with the goal of improving functional performance and daily activities, promoting aerobic fitness and preventing complications of inactivity. Activities should be selected based on the age, developmental skills, and functional abilities.

7.3 Aquatic exercises

Aquatic therapy or hydrotherapy is being used on an increasing basis and has been shown to be beneficial for children with SMA.[26] The use of aquatic therapy in SMA may be related to the physical properties of water. The properties of water provide weight relief and postural support, facilitate antigravity movements allowing more freedom of movement, and provide an opportunity to perform activities that may be too difficult to accomplish on land.[26] Aquatic exercises provide low-intensity strength training, walking and balance exercises, and aerobic training without the fear of fatigue or overwork.

7.4 Feeding and nutrition

Infants with type I SMA have poor oral motor control with sucking and chewing and tendency to get fatigued easily during feeding and swallowing. Lack of head control and head support may also affect swallowing. Those children may have difficulty getting enough nutrition and are at risk of aspiration. Some infants may require indwelling nasogastric tube to supplement oral feeding. Gastrostomy may be an option for some children to improve carer satisfaction and quality of life,[23] and to avoid aspiration.

7.5 Management of contractures

Muscle contractures and orthopedic deformities are common complications among patients with SMA. Contractures and orthopedic deformities occur primarily in type II and type III patients who have longer periods of muscle weakness. Contractures develop secondary to muscle weakness, muscle imbalance, lack of mobility, and poor posture and positioning. Development and severity of contractures are related to the severity of muscle weakness, the duration of muscle weakness, and immobility. Muscle contractures are common in muscles that cross two joints or more. Classic contractures are seen in iliotibial band, hip flexors, knee flexors and plantar flexors.

Prevention and treatment of contractures are important issues in the management of patients with SMA. Management of contractures should begin before the contractures exist. Management of contractures includes combination of consistent program of range of motion exercises, positioning, regular stretching, and splinting. Muscle groups that are at risk of developing contractures should be targeted for stretching. Range of motion and stretching exercises can be used to preserve and increase flexibility. Active range of motion and stretching exercises can be used to maintain flexibility and prevent contractures in the ambulatory patients. In the non-ambulatory patients, regular range of motion program and passive stretching are used to prevent development and slow progression of contractures. Ankle foot orthoses and night splints can be used to maintain flexibility and range of motion. Positioning devices and custom fitted equipment can be used for positioning to provide low-intensity prolonged stretching. A tilt in space or recliner chairs can be used to allow easy positioning changes. Standing program provides low-intensity prolonged stretch that can be used for the non-ambulatory children.

7.6 Adaptive equipment and assistive devices

Patients with SMA frequently benefit from use of assistive and adaptive devices, with changing needs as their condition progresses. Adaptive equipment and assistive devices can be used to provide positioning, control contractures and deformities, and support function. The choice of assistive devices for patients with SMA is based on individual clinical decisions due to lack of definite intervention trials. The decision to use an assistive device should be a collaborative decision between the patient, family, orthopedic surgeon, physiatrist, and therapist.

7.6.1 Orthotics

Ankle foot orthoses (AFO) or night splint can be used to provide prolonged stretch to control the progression of plantar flexion contractures. Knee splints may be used to control hamstring flexibility and knee flexion contractures. Thigh binders can be used to control iliotibial band contractures. Assistive devices including braces, taping, AFO, knee-ankle-foot orthoses (KAFO), and hip-knee-ankle-foot orthoses (HKAFO) can be used to provide support and maintain joints alignments. Assistive devices may be used to facilitate stability, weight bearing and upright posture during standing and ambulation.

7.6.2 Positioning devices

Positioning devices can be used to provide support, and control contractures and deformities. Positioning devices can be custom fitted, special foam, or cushions. They allow easy positioning and stretching, and provide support. Head and trunk lateral support can be used to accommodate for weak neck and trunk muscles and lack of head and trunk control, they can be used to assist in positioning and to maintain upright head and trunk during sitting.

7.6.3 Standing devices

Non-ambulatory patients with SMA may benefit from a standing program using standing frames or swivel walkers. Standing programs are used for non-ambulatory patients to prevent or reduce secondary impairments by maintaining muscle extensibility, preventing muscle and soft tissue contracture, promoting optimal musculoskeletal development, and to address the issue of reduced bone mineral density.[27,29]

7.6.4 Wheelchairs and seating systems

Because of the progressive weakness associated with SMA, many patients benefit from a wheeled mobility device as the primary means of locomotion. Wheelchair seating system deserves special considerations since many patients require a full-time use of the wheeled mobility device. The course and progression of the disease, presenting symptoms, degree of spinal deformity, and whether the patient is using mechanical ventilation should be taken into considerations when deciding on a mobility device. Manual wheelchairs allow the patients to maintain upper body strength and cardiovascular endurance. A power wheelchair should be considered when impairments prevent manual propulsion. Power wheelchairs enable patients to maintain a level of independence while moving within their environment and to compensate for mobility limitations.[14] For young children who are not ambulatory, power mobility may be used to provide independent mobility at appropriate developmental age.[25] Children as young as two years can independently propel wheelchair.[14, 25]

7.7 Management of scoliosis

Progressive weakness and reduced mobility associated with SMA place the patients at risk of contractures and scoliosis. Scoliosis is the most serious orthopedic problem seen in patients with SMA. Scoliosis develops earlier and progresses faster in non-ambulatory children than ambulatory children, scoliosis is seen in almost all children with type II SMA and majority of patients with type III, with the severity is less in type III SMA as compared to type II SMA. The incidence and severity of scoliosis increase with age and severity of muscle weakness, with the severity and progression of scoliosis increase once patients lose ambulation and become dependent on wheelchair for ambulation. Reduced respiratory function is common in patients with scoliosis. As muscle weakness progresses, the degree of scoliosis increases causing more discomfort and difficulty in positioning and respiration. Presence and degree of spinal deformity should be monitored periodically by examination and routine radiography, particularly for the non-ambulatory patients or as patient loses ambulation. Spinal x-rays are indicated once there is clinically detected scoliosis.[32] Range of motion program and spinal positioning are important to provide comfort and slow the progression of spinal deformities. Adequate trunk supports on a wheelchair, and wheelchair modifications such as custom molding, gel or air cushions may be needed to provide maximum support, and comfort and may minimize the progression of spinal deformity. As scoliosis progresses, external bracing such as thoraco-lumbo-sacral orthosis can be used to provide support and to apply forces to realign the vertebral column. External bracing is used to reduce, prevent, or slow the progression of scoliosis.[16] Surgical correction of scoliosis is required for patients to stop the progression of scoliosis and to maintain function and respiratory reserve.[22] The decision and timing of surgical intervention are based on degree of scoliosis, curve progression, pulmonary function, and bony maturity.[30] Surgical correction of spinal fusion is indicated to prevent further progression and deterioration of scoliosis and respiratory function. The outcomes of spinal stabilization include improved sitting balance, endurance and cosmetics[30] and slowed pulmonary progression. Intensive preoperative and postoperative physical therapy is required to prevent respiratory complications, and loss of strength or function after spinal fusion.[13] Orthotic intervention, new wheelchair or wheelchair modification are likely to be required after the surgeries and should be included in the preoperative plan of care.

7.8 Management of respiratory complications

Lung diseases resulting from weakness associated with SMA are the most common and most serious complications of SMA.[12] Respiratory impairments place the patient at risk for respiratory tract infections, and pulmonary insufficiency/failure, and are the major causes of morbidity and mortality.

The key respiratory problems in SMA are impaired cough with poor clearance of lower airway secretions; hypoventilation; chest wall and lung underdevelopment; and recurrent infections.[30] Sleep-disordered breathing resulting from hypoventilation is common in SMA.

Cardiopulmonary endurance reduces markedly once the child becomes wheelchair dependent. Increased weakness, decreased mobility level, and development of scoliosis are important factors to consider when assessing the respiratory function and progression of respiratory complications.

Patients with SMA should be evaluated by a respiratory care specialist. Routine evaluation of respiratory function including pulmonary function testing should be done on a regular bases. Pulmonary function testing with forced vital capacity can be used as a baseline and as a predictor of respiratory reserve. Pulse oximeters can be used at home as to indicate when the child is not ventilating properly.[12]

Providing information about respiratory care and anticipated future needs is crucial to respiratory management of SMA.[30] Patients with SMA and their families should learn how to monitor the respiratory function. Signs of respiratory insufficiency include deceased alertness, confusion, headache, pallor, and night-time restlessness.

Chest infections should be treated with antibiotics, postural drainage, chest physical therapy, and when appropriate, assisted ventilation. Patients and families should be educated on how to perform postural drainage techniques, assisted coughing, and breathing exercises.

Respiratory care for patients with SMA includes airway clearance techniques, respiratory exercises, chest physical therapy, and noninvasive ventilation, including intermittent positive pressure ventilation, bilevel positive airway pressure ventilation, and negative pressure ventilation. Ventilatory assistance might be used for patients with respiratory failure.

7.9 Genetic counseling

Genetic counseling for patients or parents who wish to have another child is extremely important. SMA genetic testing can be used for carrier detection and detection of an affected fetus.

7.10 Vocational counseling

Some patients with SMA are limited to occupations that do not require physical demands. Vocational counseling and planning may be beneficial early during high school years to facilitate transition from school to postsecondary education. Vocational counseling may be necessary to help adjustment to work settings.

7.11 Psychological support

Counseling and psychological support are important strategies in the management of SMA. Anxiety and depression can greatly impact patients and families' quality of life and their abilities to cope with the diseases and progressive changes in function and abilities. Formal counseling and psychological support should be available to assist patients and families coping with the severity and progression of the disease. Patients and families should be educated regarding the disease process and expectations and making sure that families are having the appropriate expectations for mobility and function.

8. Summary

Spinal muscular atrophy, a neuromuscular disorder, is one of the leading genetic causes of infant mortality. The disease is caused by deletion or mutation of the SMN1 gene and a reduction in the levels of functional SMN, resulting in selective death of spinal motor neurons. The type of SMA (I, II, III, or IV) is determined by the age of onset, the severity of symptoms, and the maximum function achieved. There are other rare types of SMA disorders with similar symptoms but they are caused by different genes other than SMN1 and genetic mutation. Spinal muscular atrophy is characterized by severe progressive muscle weakness, atrophy and hypotonia. Complications of muscle weakness include decreased mobility function, restrictive lung disease, contractures, orthopedic deformities and psychosocial problems. There is no cure for SMA. Treatment is usually supportive and focuses on management of the symptoms and preventing complications of muscle weakness. Pulmonary complication is a hallmark of the disease and is the main cause of death especially in type I and type II SMA. The prognosis and clinical course of SMA are highly variable, and they are more of a continuous spectrum with the age of death from infancy to normal life expectancy.

9. References

Bach, J., Baird, S., Plosky, D., Navado, J., & Weaver, B. (2002). Spinal muscular atrophy type 1: management and outcomes. *Pediatric Pulmonology*, Vol. 34, pp. 16-22.

Burnett, B., Crawford, T., & Summer, C. (2009). Emerging treatment options for spinal muscular atrophy. *Current Treatment Options Neurology,* Vol. 11, pp. 90-101.

Case, L., & Kishnani, P. (2006). Physical therapy management of Pompe disease. *Genetics In Medicine,* Vol. 8, pp. 318-327.

Chung, B., Wong, V., & Ip, P. (2004). Spinal muscular atrophy: survival pattern and functional status. *Pediatrics,* Vol. 114, pp. e548-e553.

Cifuentes-Diaz, C., Frugier, T., & Melki, J. (2002). Spinal muscular atrophy.*Seminars in Pediatric Neurology,* Vol. 9, pp. 145-150.

Eagle, M. (2002). Report on the Muscular Dystrophy Campaign workshop: exercise in neuromuscular diseases. *Neuromuscular Disorders,* Vol. 12, pp. 975-983.

Fowler, W. (2002). Role of physical activity and exercise training in neuromuscular diseases.*American Journal of Physical Medicine and Rehabilitation,* Vol. 81, pp. S187–S195.

Granta, C., Cornelio, F., Bonfiglioli, S., Mattutini, P., & Merlini, L. (1987). Promotion of ambulation of patients with spinal muscular atrophy by early fitting of knee-ankle-foot orthoses. *Developmental Medicine and Child Neurology,* Vol. 29, pp. 221-224.

Grondard, C., Biondi, O., Armand, A., Lécolle, S., Gaspera, B., Pariset, C., Li, H., Gallien, C., Vidal, P., Chanoine, C., & Charbonnier, F. (2005). Regular exercise prolongs survival in a type 2 spinal muscular atrophy model mouse. *The Journal of Neuroscience,* Vol. 25, pp. 7615-7622.

Hirtz, D., Innaccone, S., Heemskerk, J., Gwinn-Hardy, K., Moxley, R., & Rowland, L. (2005). Challenges and opportunities in clinical trials of spinal muscular atrophy. *Neurology,* Vol. 65, pp. 1352-1357.

Iannaccone, S. (1998). Spinal muscular atrophy.*Seminars in Neurology,* Vol. 18, pp 19-26.

Iannaccone, S. (2007). Modern Management of Spinal Muscular Atrophy.*Journal of Child Neurology,* Vol. 22, pp. 974-978.

Iannaccone, S., Smith, S., & Simard L. (2004). Spinal muscular atrophy.*Current Neurology and Neuroscience Reports,* Vol. 4, pp. 74-80.

Jones, M., McEwen, I., & Hansen, L. (2003). Use of power mobility for a young child with spinal muscular atrophy. *Physical Therapy,* Vol. 83, pp. 253-262.

Kostova, F., Williams, V., Heemskerk, J., Iannaccone, S., DiDonato, C., Swoboda, K., & Maria B. (2007). Spinal Muscular Atrophy: Classification, diagnosis, management, pathogenesis, and future research directions. *Journal of Child Neurology,* Vol. 22, pp. 926-945.

Kotwicki, T., & Jozwiak, M. (2008). Conservative management of neuromuscular scoliosis: personal experience and review of literature. *Disability and Rehabilitation,* Vol. 30, pp. 792–98.

Kroksmark, A., Beckung, E., & Tulinius, M. (2001). Muscle strength and motor function in children and adolescents with spinal muscular atrophy II and III. *European Journal of Paediatric Neurology,* Vol. 5, pp. 191-198.

Lefebvre, S., Bürglen, L., Reboullet, S. Clermont, O., Burlet, P., Viollet, L., Benochou, B., Cruaud, C., Millasseau, P., Zeviani, M., Le Paslier, D., Frézal, J., Cohen, D.,

Weissenbach, J., Munnich, A., & Melki, J. (1995). Identification and characterization of a spinal muscular atrophy determining gene. *Cell,* Vol. 80, pp. 155-165.

Montes, J., Gordon A.,Pandya, S., De Vivo, D., & Kaufmann, P. (2009). Clinical outcome measures in spinal muscular atrophy. *Journal of Child Neurology,* Vol. 24, pp. 968-978.

Nicole, S., Diaz, C., Frugier, T., & Melki, J. (2002). Spinal muscular atrophy: recent advances and future prospects. *Muscle and Nerve,* Vol. 26, pp. 4-13.

O'Hagen, J., Glanzman, A., McDermott, M., Ryan, P., Flickinger, J., Quigley, J., Riley, S., Sanborn, E., Irvine, C., Martens, W., Annis, C., Tawil, R., Oskoui, M., Darras, B., Finkel, R., & De Vivo, D. (2007). An expanded version of the Hammersmith Functional Motor Scale for SMA II and III patients.*Neuromuscular Disorders,* Vo. 17, pp. 693-697.

Oskoui, M., & Kaufmann, P. (2008). Spinal Muscular Atrophy. *Neurotherapeutic,* Vol. 5, pp. 499–506.

Roper, H., & Quinlivan, R. (2010). Implementation of "the consensus statement for the standard of care in spinal muscular atrophy" when applied to infants with severe type 1 SMA in the UK. *Archives of Diseases in Childhood,* Vol. 95, pp.845-849.

Russman, B. (2007). Spinal Muscular Atrophy: Clinical Classification and Disease Heterogeneity. *Journal of Child Neurology,* Vol. 22, pp. 946-951.

Russman, B., Bucher, C., White, M., Samaha, F., & Iannaccone, S. (1996). Function changes in spinal muscular atrophy II and III. *Neurology,* Vol. 47, pp. 973-976.

Salem, Y., & Gropack, S.J. (2010). Aquatic therapy for a child with type III spinal muscular atrophy: a case report. *Physical and Occupational Therapy in Pediatrics,* Vol. 30, pp. 313-324.

Salem, Y., Lovelace-Chandler, V., Zabel, R. & Grossman, A. (2010). Effects of prolonged standing on gait in children with spastic cerebral palsy. *Physical and Occupational Therapy in Pediatrics,* Vol. 30, pp. 54-65.

Semprini, L., Tacconelli, A., Capon, F., Brancati, F., Dallapiccola, B., & Novelli, C. (2001). A single strand conformation polymorphoism-based carrier test for spinal muscular atrophy. *Genetic Testing,* Vol. 5, pp. 33-37.

Stuberg, W.A. (1992). Considerations related to weight-bearing programs in children with developmental disabilities. *Physical Therapy,* Vol, 72, 35-40.

Wang, C., Finkel, R., Bertini, E., Schroth, M., Simonds, A., Wong, B., Aloysius, A., Morrison, L., Main, M., Crawford, T., Trela, A., & Participants of the International Conference on SMA Standard of Care. (2007). Consensus statement for standard of care in spinal muscular atrophy. *Journal of Child Neurology,* Vol. 22, pp. 1027-1049.

Whitehead, S., Jones, K., Zhang, X., Cheng, X., Terns, R., & Terns, M. (2002). Determinants of the interaction of the spinal muscular atrophy disease protein SMN with the demathylarginine-modified box H/ACA small nucleolarribonucleoprotein GAR1. *The Journal of Biological Chemistry,* Vol. 277, pp. 48087-48093.

Wong, B. (2006). Management of the child with weakness. *Seminars in Pediatric Neurology*, Vol.13, pp. 271-278.

13

Respiratory Muscle Aids in the Management of Neuromuscular Respiratory Impairment to Prevent Respiratory Failure and Need for Tracheostomy

A. J. Hon and J. R. Bach
Department of Physical Medicine and Rehabilitation,
UMDNJ-New Jersey Medical School
USA

1. Introduction

Respiratory impairment results from primary disease of the lungs / airways or from impairment of the respiratory muscles. The proper identification of the respiratory impairment allows for proper management to decrease morbidity and mortality. Patients with neuromuscular impairment typically have hypoventilation or ventilator insufficiency/failure resulting in hypercapnia, hypoxia and an ineffective cough. In contrast, lung and airway diseases are characterized by hypoxia with eucapnia or hypocapnia, which often occur during an exacerbation resulting in acute respiratory failure (ARF). Often physicians evaluate and treat both as respiratory insufficiency/failure.

Historically and even currently, when neuromuscular patients develop respiratory failure the traditional paradigm has been resorting to tracheostomy, resulting in increasing weakness of inspiratory muscles and loss of ventilator free breathing ability. In contrast, we and others with neuromuscular patient populations, successfully use a new management paradigm including noninvasive interfaces for intermittent positive pressure ventilation (NIV) in place of tracheostomy (TIV) to maintain not only life but also quality of life (Bach, 2010). It has been noted previously that patient populations prefer NIV over TIV both overall and specifically with regards to comfort, convenience, speech, swallowing, cosmesis, and safety (Bach, 1993).

NIV can provide from intermittent up to continuous ventilatory support for patients with advanced neuromuscular disease who have normal lung tissue but respiratory muscle weakness. These concepts and techniques can be used for any patient with respiratory muscle weakness, for example high level traumatic spinal cord injury and polio patients (Bach, 1991; Bach & Alba, 1990; Bach et al., 1989). Even in patients with severely dysfunctional expiratory muscles with little to no vital capacity or maximum expiratory pressures, noninvasive pressure aids can provide effective cough flows. The inability to cough up secretions, due to an ineffective cough, often results in mucous plugging of the airways, but when using noninvasive ventilatory muscle aids, a cough can be augmented for effective and sufficient secretion removal.

Inspiratory and expiratory muscle aids, including devices and manual assisted techniques, result in intermittent pressure changes to assist inspiratory and expiratory muscles in their natural function. Noninvasive inspiratory and expiratory muscle aids are used to maintain lung and chest wall compliance, maintain normal alveolar ventilation, and to maximize cough peak flows (CPF) thus preventing episodes of acute respiratory failure, especially during intercurrent chest infections. This allows for decreased hospitalizations and prolongs survival without tracheostomy for patients with Duchenne muscular dystrophy (DMD), Spinal Muscular Atrophy including type 1 (SMA), amyotrophic lateral sclerosis (ALS), and others.

2. Pathophysiology

Respiratory muscle groups include inspiratory muscles (predominately the diaphragm), expiratory muscles (predominately abdominal and chest wall muscles used for coughing) and bulbar-innervated muscles (used to protect the airway). Many patients with ventilatory insufficiency manage for years without ventilator use but at the cost of orthopnea and hypercapnia which can result in compensatory metabolic alkalosis which depresses central ventilatory drive. As a result the brain becomes accustomed to the hypercapnia without obvious symptoms of ventilatory failure. Patients not introduced to NIV are oftentimes prescribed supplemental oxygen which exacerbates hypercapnia and eventually results in the coma of carbon dioxide narcosis and ventilatory arrest.

Patients with inspiratory and expiratory muscle weakness can be sustained using NIV. Ventilatory insufficiency/failure spans the spectrum from those with only diaphragm dysfunction (resulting in nocturnal ventilatory insufficiency/failure when in bed) to complete inspiratory muscle failure. Patients with complete inspiratory and expiratory muscle failure (with as little as 0 mL of vital capacity) can be completely supported using NIV for over 50 years without tracheostomy (Bach, 2004). Some of them use only nocturnal ventilatory aids and use glossopharyngeal breathing (GPB) to maintain ventilation during the day (Bach, 2004).

3. Evaluating a patient

On initial presentation, ambulatory patients with hypercapnic ventilatory insufficiency often initially report exertional dyspnea and later morning headaches, fatigue, sleep disturbances and hypersomnolence (Bach & Alba, 1990). On the other hand wheelchair users may report wheelchair users may report very few symptoms, e.g., anxiety, dyspnea, and difficulty with sleep, except during a respiratory infection. Physical signs of tachypnea, paradoxical breathing, hypophonia, nasal flaring, accessory respiratory muscle use, cyanosis, flushing, pallor and airway secretion and congestion are signs of increasing carbon dioxide levels. Lethargy and confusion are indicative of carbon dioxide narcosis, which can be reversed with proper management through NIV.

Evaluation can include obtaining a vital capacity (VC), cough peak flows (CPF), capnography/oximetry and a polysomnogram. VC is measured in the supine and sitting positions. The VC supine is a superior indicator of ventilatory dysfunction as hypoventilation begins and is worse during sleep. The difference between the two should be less than 7 percent, while a value greater than 20 percent indicates need for nocturnal NIV. If the patient wears a thoracolumbar brace, a VC should be recorded with and without the brace as the fit can improve or worsen the VC.

Spirometry is also used for monitoring the maximum insufflation capacity (MIC), that is, the ability to "air stack". The ability to air stack is holding with the glottis a maximal volume by holding consecutively delivered volumes of air delivered from a manual resuscitator or volume cycling ventilator. Interfaces that can be used for air stacking include a simple mouthpiece or when the lips are too weak for this, a nasal interface or lipseal. In patients who have learned glossopharyngeal breathing (GPB) techniques, this enables them to approach or attain the MIC independently.

Cough Peak Flow (CPF), measured with a peak flow meter, is an indicator of the patient's cough effectiveness. A CPF of 160 L/m is the minimum needed for sufficiently effective coughing and airway clearance to reliably permit safe extubation (Bach & Saporito, 1996). This is also the best indicator for tracheostomy removal, regardless of pulmonary function, that is, the status of the inspiratory and expiratory muscles. Patients with a VC of less than 1,500 mL should have an assisted CPF measured using a maximal lung volume by air stacking and an abdominal thrust for a manually assisted cough. The abdominal thrust should be delivered simultaneously to the opening of the glottis.

In patients without significant intrinsic lung disease, arterial blood gas sampling is unnecessary. Many patients (25%) tend to hyperventilate due to discomfort or anxiety from the procedure (Currie et al., 1986), so accurate results can be difficult to obtain. Oximetry monitoring and capnography, which is the measurement of end tidal pCO_2, provide more useful information. Most conveniently they can be performed in the home.

Patients with questionable symptoms, multiple hourly nocturnal oxyhemoglobin desaturations to below 95%, and elevated nocturnal $PaCO_2$ should undergo a trial of nocturnal NIV. If the questionably symptomatic patient finds nocturnal NIV to be more burdensome than the symptoms of ventilatory insufficiency, the patient can discontinue NIV and should be reevaluated in 3 to 6 months.

In symptomatic patients with a normal VC, no carbon dioxide retention and no clear pattern of oxyhemoglobin desaturation, a polysomnogram is warranted to evaluate for sleep disordered breathing (Williams et al., 1991). Patients with obesity-hypoventilation also should be treated with NIV or pressure or volume control ventilation and not CPAP. Neuromuscular disease NMD patients with decreased VC have no indication for undergoing polysomnography as the device is programmed to interpret each apnea and hypopnea as having a central nervous system or obstructive etiology rather than being due to inspiratory muscle weakness. Treatment of asymptomatic NMD patients based solely on polysomnographic abnormalities with continuous positive airway pressure (CPAP) or low spans of bi-level PAP is ineffective or at the least, suboptimal.

4. Lung expansion therapy

Lung expansion therapy often results in increasing VC, increasing CPF, maintaining or increasing pulmonary compliance, decreasing atelectasis and facilitating introduction of NIV. Various devices and techniques have been developed to prolong survival without tracheotomy through maintaining pulmonary compliance, and augmenting inspiratory and expiratory muscle function. For example, researchers have found that Duchenne muscular dystrophy patients requiring up to continuous ventilator dependence as NIV, can avoid hospitalizations, pulmonary morbidity and mortality for decades and tracheotomy indefinitely when properly managed with respiratory muscle aids (Gomez-Merino & Bach, 2002). Forty percent of ALS patients can survive for almost a year on average and up to 8 years without a tracheostomy tube despite continuous ventilator dependence supplied via NIV (Bach et al., 2004).

4.1 Maintaining pulmonary compliance

Maintaining pulmonary (chest wall and lung) compliance, constantly and consistently maintaining normal alveolar ventilation, and maximizing cough peak flows are essential to preventing episodes of ARF, avoiding hospitalizations and prolonging survival without tracheotomy. Particularly for children, maintaining chest wall/lung compliance promotes more normal lung and chest wall growth. Regular lung and chest wall mobilization is done by air stacking, receiving deep insufflations, or using nocturnal NIV for small children who cannot cooperate with air stacking (Bach et al., 2000). With increasing respiratory muscle weakness, the patient cannot expand the lungs to the predicted inspiratory capacity. This results in chest wall contractures and lung restriction (decreased pulmonary compliance).

Regular mobilization through deep insufflations, air stacking or NIV can result in an increase in VC and CPF. The degree to which the MIC exceeds the VC (MIC-VC) indicates glottis/bulbar innervated muscle integrity and correlates with the ability to use NIV rather than require tracheotomy. The Lung Insufflation Capacity (LIC) is the maximum passive insufflation volume using the assistance of a device (Bach & Kang, 2000).

In patients with inability to close the glottis, insufflation can be achieved passively through the use of a Cough Assist™, pressure cycling ventilator with pressures 40 to 70 cm H_2O, or using a manual resuscitator with the exhalation valve blocked to air stack (Figure 1). Patients are instructed to air stack at least 10 to 15 times, 2 to 3 times a day once the VC is found to have decreased below 80% of predicted normal. For NIV users, volume cycling is preferable to pressure cycling as it enables air stacking and this allows for increased volume of voice (Bach et al., 2008). In patients with primarily ventilatory impairment, CPAP is not useful since it does not aid inspiratory or expiratory muscles.

In addition, patients who are able to air stack are also able to use NIV. If at any point the patient is intubated, he or she can more easily be extubated directly to NIV regardless of ventilator free breathing ability (VFBA). Proper instruction is essential as the extubation of inexperienced patients without VFBA to NIV can at times result in panic, ventilator dyssynchrony, asphyxia or even reintubation.

In patients, such as infants, who can not cooperate with active insufflation therapy, that is, who are unable to air stack, oral-nasal interfaces are used for deep passive insufflations. Infants with spinal muscular atrophy (SMA) of any type or any neuromuscular disease with paradoxical chest wall movement require nocturnal NIV to promote normal chest wall/lung growth, prevent pectus excavatum, as well as possibly for ventilatory assistance (Bach et al., 2002). Often by 14 to 30 months children can become cooperative with deep insufflation therapy.

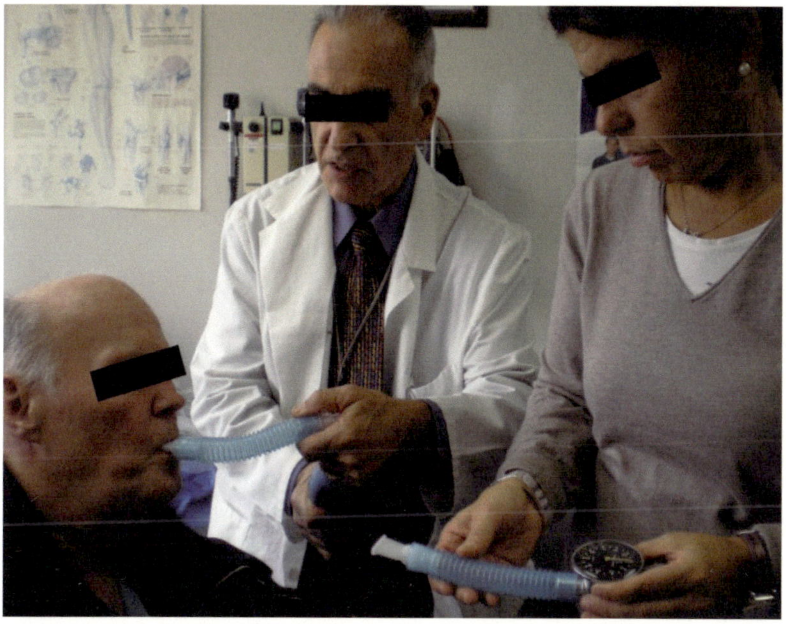

Fig. 1. Patient demonstrating air stacking using a manual resuscitator.

4.2 Inspiratory muscle assistance

Historically, negative pressure body ventilators have been used to apply pressure to the body for ventilatory support, but this is less effective than NIV as they can cause obstructive apneas and are decreasingly efficacious with increasing age and decreasing pulmonary compliance (Bach et al, 1989). In figure 2, the intermittent abdominal pressure ventilator (IAPV) or "Exsufflation Belt" is a body ventilator that can augment tidal volumes from 300 to 1,200 mL. The intermittent inflation of the elastic air sac worn in a corset or belt under the patient's clothing moves the diaphragm upward to assist in expiration. With bladder deflation, passive inspiration occurs with the diaphragm and abdominal contents returning to resting position with gravity. For effective use the trunk must be 30 degrees or more from the horizontal. Patients with inspiratory capacity or ability to glossopharyngeal breathe can add volumes of air to those mechanically taken in. Patients with less than one hour of breathing tolerance usually prefer it to NIV during daytime hours (Bach & Alba, 1991).

Inspiratory muscles can be assisted using NIV. There are no contraindications to long term use of NIV other than uncontrollable seizures. Multiple interfaces can be used and they can be introduced to the patients in a clinic or home setting. They include 15 mm angled mouth pieces, lipseals, and nasal and oral-nasal interfaces. Open NIV systems include mouthpiece *or* nasal NIV which rely on central nervous system reflexes to prevent insufflation air leakage during sleeping (Bach &Alba, 1990; Bach et al., 1955). A closed system, such as by using a lipseal-nasal prong system, can avoid excessive leakage by delivering air via mouth *and* nose during sleep (Figure 3). In addition to minimizing insufflation leakage, they maximize skin comfort. Using nocturnal NIV improves daytime O_2 and CO_2. Supplemental O_2 and sedatives should be avoided to maintain maximal nocturnal NIV effectiveness.

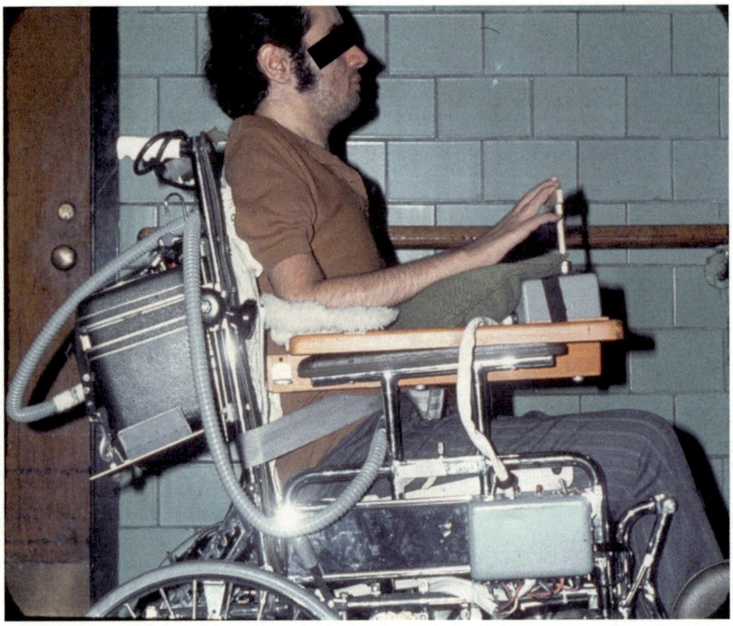

Fig. 2. High level spinal cord injured patient with no measurable vital capacity or ventilator-free breathing ability using an intermittent abdominal pressure ventilator for daytime ventilatory assistance (Exsufflation Belt™, Philips-Respironics International Inc., Murrysville, PA) and using a lipseal for nocturnal support for 15 years.

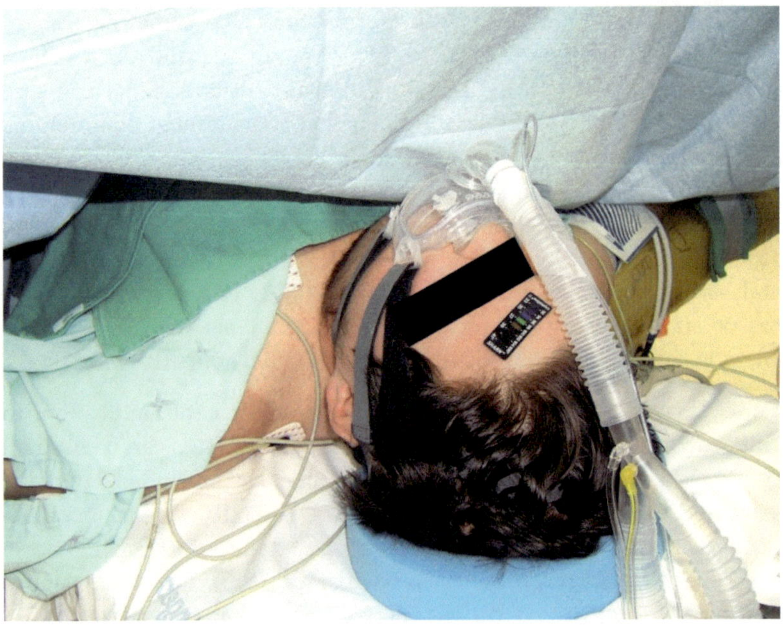

Fig. 3. Duchenne muscular dystrophy patient using an interface that includes nasal prongs with lip covering to provide a closed system of ventilatory support during sleep, here seen using it during surgery with general anesthesia.

In patients with some neck movement and lip function, the 15 mm angled mouthpiece interface is the most useful, and is able to be used by some patients all day (Ishikawa, 2005). Often times patients can keep the mouthpiece near the mouth with a metal clamp attached to the wheelchair or affixed onto the motorized wheelchair controls, most commonly the sip and puff, chin or tongue controls. The patient can grab the mouthpiece for supplemental air or full breath support, as demonstrated in Figure 4.

The volume ventilator is set for large tidal volumes, commonly 800 to 1500 mL. Therefore, the patient can control the volume of air obtained and can use air stacking to cough, increase speech volumes, and maintain pulmonary compliance. To use mouthpiece NIV a patient must be able to move the soft palate posteriocranially to seal off the nasopharynx, open the glottis and vocal cords, and maintain hypopharynx and airway patency. These movements quickly become reflexive. They must and usually can be quickly relearned by patients who have been ventilated via tracheostomy and have lost them (Bach et al., 1993).

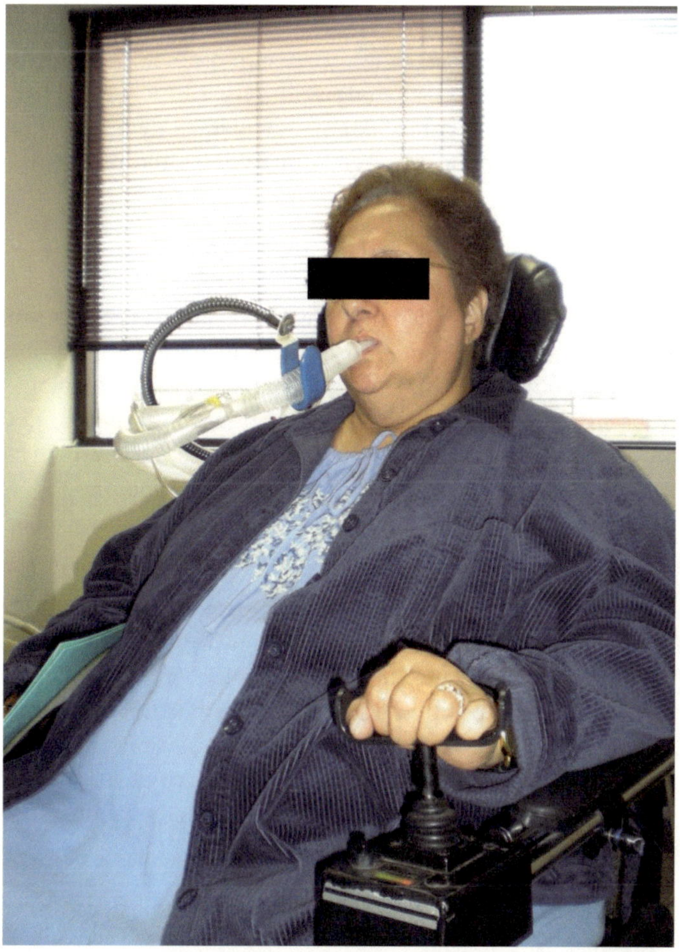

Fig. 4. A 66 year old woman with multiple sclerosis and continuous ventilator dependence using a 15 mm angled mouth piece for daytime support for 27 years despite having only 30 mL of vital capacity.

For those who are unable to grab or maintain a tight seal on a mouthpiece for daytime NIV, such as infants, nasal NIV using small nasal prong systems can be ideal and can be used continuously as a viable alternative to tracheostomy (Bach & Alba, 1990). To prevent oral insufflation leakage during nasal NIV, patients learn to close the mouth or seal the oropharynx with the soft palate and tongue. Humidifying the air is essential for nocturnal mouthpiece/lipseal ventilation but infrequently for nocturnal nasal NIV. Suboptimal humidification results in dry, irritated mucous membranes and increased airflow resistance to up to 8 cm H_2O (Richards et al., 1996). The air can be warmed to body temperature and humidified using a hot water bath humidifier to decrease irritation of nasal membranes (Richards et al., 1996).

Complications from NIV are few. At times abdominal distension can occur sporadically. The air usually passes as flatus when the patient is mobilized in the morning. If severe, it can increase ventilator dependence and result in necessary placement of a gastrostomy or nasogastric tube to burp out the air or a rectal tube to decompress the colon. In 1000 NIV users there was noted to be one case of pneumothorax despite aggressive lung mobilization and expansion three times daily with NIV support for most and, indeed for over 50 years in many cases (Suri et al., 2008). Often mistakenly noted to be a complication or limiting aspect of NIV, secretion management remains the most important aspect of noninvasive management.

4.3 Cough Augmentation: Expiratory muscle assistance

Cough Augmentation is essential in maintaining the health of patients with a poor cough due to weak expiratory muscles. Essential techniques include manually assisted coughing, mechanically assisted coughing (MAC), glossopharyngeal breathing, and oximetry monitoring to guide in airway clearance when using these techniques. Routine suctioning through the upper airway or indwelling airway tubes misses the left main stem bronchus 90 percent of the time (Fishburn et al., 1990). Manually assisted coughing is the application of an abdominal thrust timed to glottis opening after filling the lungs maximally with air, usually through air stacking, Figure 5A and Figure 5B.

The air stacking is important for patients with less than 1500 mL VC. With air stacking, manually assisted coughing has produced air flows of 4.3 ± 1.7 L/sec compared to 2.5 ± 2.0 L/sec unassisted (Kang & Bach, 2000). In our population of 364 NMD patient able to air stack the mean VC in the sitting position was 996.9 mL, while the mean MIC by air stacking was 1647.6 mL. Upper airway obstruction, often due to severe bulbar-innervated muscle dysfunction, is indicated by the inability to generate 160 L/m of assisted CPF with a VC or MIC greater than 1 L. With CPF this low, the airway should be evaluated by laryngoscopy and reversible lesions corrected surgically.

Mechanical insufflation-exsufflation (CoughAssist™) augments or substitutes for inspiratory and expiratory muscles. Both mechanical and manually assisted cough techniques provide effective exsufflation flows in the left and right airways, allowing for their use in place of deep suctioning. Patients prefer MAC compared with suctioning for comfort and effectiveness, in addition to finding it less tiring (Gastang et al., 2000).

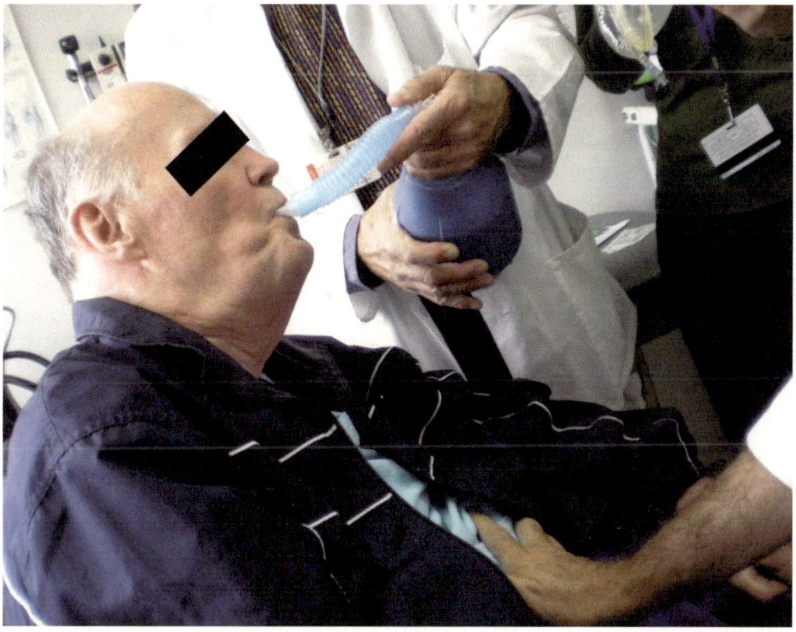

Fig. 5.A. Manually assisted coughing with abdominal thrust applied concomittant with glottic opening following air stacking with flows to be measured by peak flow meter.

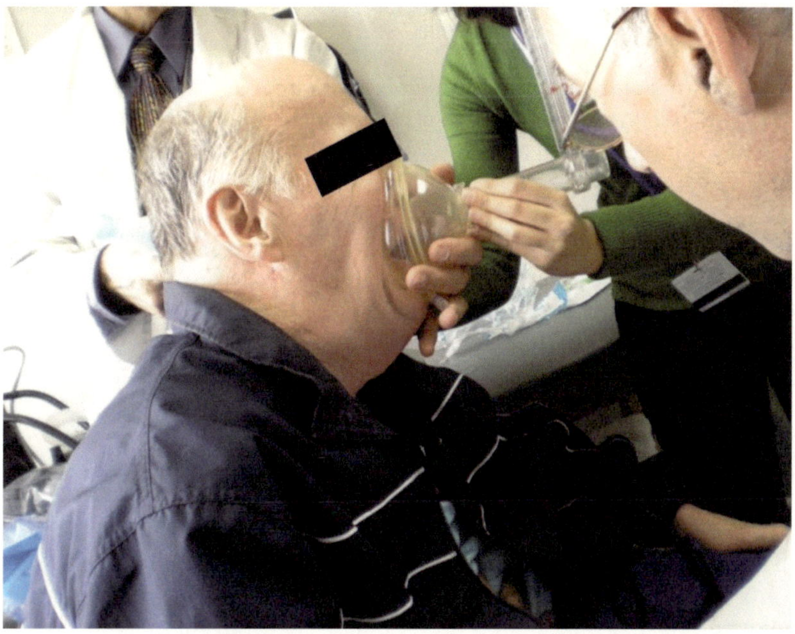

Fig. 5.B. Assisted cough peak flow measured by peak flow meter.

4.3.1 Mechanically assisted coughing

Mechanically assisted coughing (MAC) combines mechanical insufflation-exsufflation with an exsufflation-timed abdominal thrust to increase CPF. The CoughAssist™ can be manually or automatically cycled with the deep insufflations followed immediately by deep exsufflations, ideally with pressures of 40 to 60 alternating with -40 to -60 cm H_2O. Interfaces for MAC include oral-nasal masks, a simple mouthpiece, or translaryngeal or tracheostomy tubes. With use via a tracheostomy tube, the cuff, if present, should be inflated. Manual cycling allows caregiver-patient coordination during inspiration and expiration with the insufflation and exsufflation.

Treatments can be as frequent as up to every 30 minutes during respiratory infections and post-extubation. One treatment set includes about five cycles of MAC followed by a short period of normal breathing or ventilator use to avoid hyperventilation. When patients cannot cooperate with MAC, the timing of the insufflation and exsufflation is adjusted to the patient's breathing to provide maximum chest expansion and rapid lung emptying, in general 2 to 4 seconds for adults but much more quickly for small children. Treatments continue until no further secretions are able to be removed and oxyhemoglobin desaturation due to mucus plugging is reversed. The abdominal thrust is also important for infants. By 2.5 to 5 years of age, children become accustomed to coughing simultaneously with the insufflation-exsufflation.

With the elimination of airway secretions and mucus using MAC, vital capacity, abnormal pulmonary flow rates and oxyhemoglobin saturation can improve immediately (Bach et al., 1993). Fifteen percent to 42 percent increase in VC was noted immediately following MAC for 67 patients with "obstructive dyspnea" and a 55 percent increase in VC was noted in patients with neuromuscular conditions (Barach, 1954). In ventilator assisted neuromuscular disease patients with chest infections, a 15 to 400 percent (200 to 800 mL) increase was noted following secretion removal with MAC (Bach, 1993).

Although MAC can augment and even substitute for the inspiratory and expiratory muscles, if bulbar innervated muscles, which prevent airway collapse and protect against food and saliva aspiration, are inadequately functioning, tracheotomy becomes indicated. However, this is generally only observed in advanced bulbar ALS patients. Patients with intact bulbar muscle function can usually air stack to volumes of 3 L or more, and, unless very scoliotic or obese, a properly delivered abdominal thrust can result in assisted CPF of 6 to 9 L/s, which is sufficient to clear secretions and prevent pneumonia and ARF without requiring MAC. Those with moderately impaired bulbar muscle function, e.g., non-ALS neuromuscular disease patients like those with Duchenne muscular dystrophy, that limits assisted CPF to less than 300 L/m benefit the most from MAC (Gomez-Merino, 2002).

4.3.2 Glossopharyngeal Breathing

Glossopharyngeal Breathing (GPB) is a technique that involves "gulping" boluses of air into the lungs using the glottis to add to the inspiratory effort. Six to 9 gulps (40 mL to 200 mL) total a full breath. The technique can be taught, to assist inspiratory and indirectly expiratory muscle function in patients with good bulbar-innervated musculature (Bach et al., 1987), allowing for discontinuation of ventilator use from minutes up to a whole day. Initial training can be supplemented with a training manual and videos (Dail et al., 1979;

Dail & Affeldt, 1954). The patient's developing proficiency can be monitored using spirometry to measure the milliliter of air per gulp, gulps per breath and the breaths per minute as seen in Figure 6.

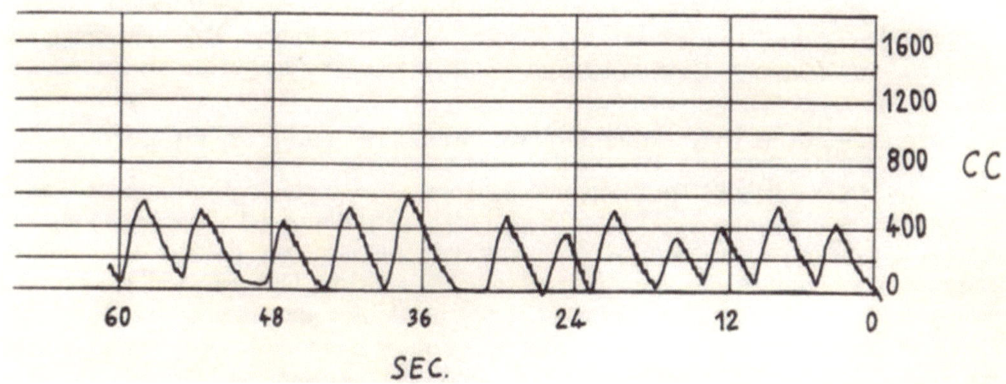

Fig. 6. Glossopharyngeal breathing used for 6 liters of minute ventilation in "gulps" of 60 to 90 mL or 6 to 8 gulps per breath, 12 breaths per minute, for autonomous respiration despite having 0 mL of vital capacity for 52 years (Bach et al., 1987).

Normal minute ventilation and normal alveolar ventilation can be maintained by glossopharyngeal breathing for individuals with little to no measurable vital capacity. Autonomous breathing is possible from minutes to up to all day by using it. It has been noted that 60% of ventilator users with no autonomous ability to breathe and sufficient bulbar muscle function can use GPB for ventilator-free breathing (Bach et al., 1987; Bach & Alba, 1990). This technique is ideal in the event of ventilator failure or disconnection during the day or night (Bach et al., 1987; Bach, 1991). The versatility and safety afforded by GPB are safeguards that make noninvasive management safer than support via tracheostomy. Although severe oropharyngeal muscle weakness can limit the effectiveness of GPB, 13 Duchenne muscular dystrophy patients with no breathing tolerance could be maintained solely with GPB (Bach et al. 2007).

4.3.3 Oximetry monitoring

Oximetry monitoring, through the use of a pulse oximeter, is essential in managing patients with NMD using respiratory muscle aids. A SpO_2 alarm set at 94% alerts the patient to take deeper breaths to maintain SpO_2 consistently over 94% all day (Gomez-Marino & Bach, 2002), and when tiring, to take ventilator assisted breaths usually via a mouthpiece. Thus, SpO_2 feedback provides a method to monitor a hypercapnic patient with desaturation due to chronic alveolar hypoventilation and during transition from tracheostomy ventilation. If the patient is unable to independently maintain a sufficient level of at least SpO_2 of 94%, mouthpiece or nasal NIV should be initiated for increasing periods to maintain normal SpO_2 which helps to reset central ventilatory drive. Thereby, oximetry feedback facilitates the introduction and indicates the extent of daytime need for mouthpiece and/or nasal NIV. In addition, oximetry monitoring is especially useful during episodes of respiratory tract infection as an indicator to use MAC to prevent cold triggered pneumonias and acute respiratory failure, usually due to mucus plugging in the NIV patient population. Proper instruction of NIV and MAC, and rapid access to MAC during the onset of a chest cold may be all that is necessary to avert pneumonia, ARF and subsequent hospitalizations.

Especially in infants and small children, with often inadequate cough to prevent chest colds from triggering pneumonia and ARF, MAC should be used for any desaturation below 95 percent. In continuous NIV users, desaturations are usually due to bronchial mucus plugging, which can develop into atelectasis and pneumonia if the secretions are not quickly cleared.

5. Contraindications to noninvasive aids: Invasive ventilatory support

Certain patient populations are better managed with tracheostomy. Contraindications to noninvasive aid include ventilator dependence with depressed cognitive function, orthopedic conditions interfering with noninvasive interface use, restrictive pulmonary syndrome along with severe pulmonary disease necessitating high FiO_2, or uncontrolled seizures or substance abuse (Waldhornet al., 1990). In addition, the presence of a nasogastric tube can hamper the fitting of a nasal interface and the use of mouthpiece or nasal NIV by limiting soft palate closure of the pharynx and the necessary seal at the nose. For neuromuscular disease patients, only those with severe bulbar dysfunction, as observed with severe bulbar ALS resulting in the inability for protect the airway, require tracheotomy (Bach et al., 2004). Other than for the occasional spinal muscular atrophy type 1 patient, tracheotomy is rarely if ever indicated for Duchenne muscular dystrophy or any other neuromuscular disease (Bach et al., 2009). Although tracheostomy ventilation can support alveolar ventilation and extend survival for many NMD patients (Bach, 1996), morbidity and mortality outcomes are not as favorable as by noninvasive approaches (Bach et al., 1998; Toussaint et al., 2006).

6. Long term outcomes

A number of centers have reported up to continuous NIV dependence to maintain patients with neuromuscular disease. One hundred and one of our nocturnal only NIV users became continuously NIV dependent for 7.6 ± 6.1 years to 30.1 ± 6.1 years of age with 56 patients still living. Twenty six became continuously dependent on NIV without requiring hospitalization, while eight continuous tracheostomy ventilation users were decanulated to noninvasive NIV. Using the above described techniques for the DMD patient population, we have extubated 31 "unweanable" intubated patients consecutively to NIV/MAC without resort to tracheotomy (Bach & Martinez, 2001). Also reported by Kohler et al., continuous NIV can prolong life in DMD. Seven of our DMD patients have lived to over 40 years of age requiring continuous NIV for 20 years or more.

Of our 71 SMA type 1 patients sustained with NIV, (mean age 86.1 months (range 13–196) with only 13 deaths at 52.3 months (range 13-111)), fifteen SMA-1 patients are over age 10 and 6 over age 15 without tracheostomy tubes and despite requiring continuous NIV in most cases (Bach et al., 2009). Sixty seven of the patient population could verbally communicate. Schroth also reported use of continuous NIV for SMA type 1 patients (2009). Of seventeen SMA type 1 patients using tracheostomy ventilation with mean age 78.2 months (range 65–179), 25 of 27 lost all autonomous breathing ability immediately upon tracheotomy. Those who had not developed verbalization prior to tracheotomy did not develop vocalization following the procedure. Two brothers with SMA-1 are pictured initially at age 4 then at age 14 and 16 with no VC sustained entirely with NIV (Figure 7 and Figure 8).

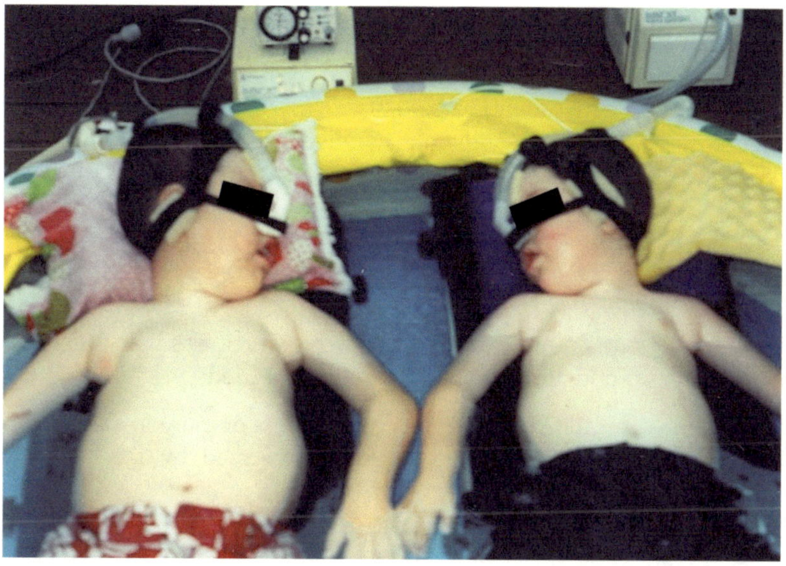

Fig. 7. Two brothers with spinal muscular atrophy type 1 and continuous ventilator dependence since 4 months of age.

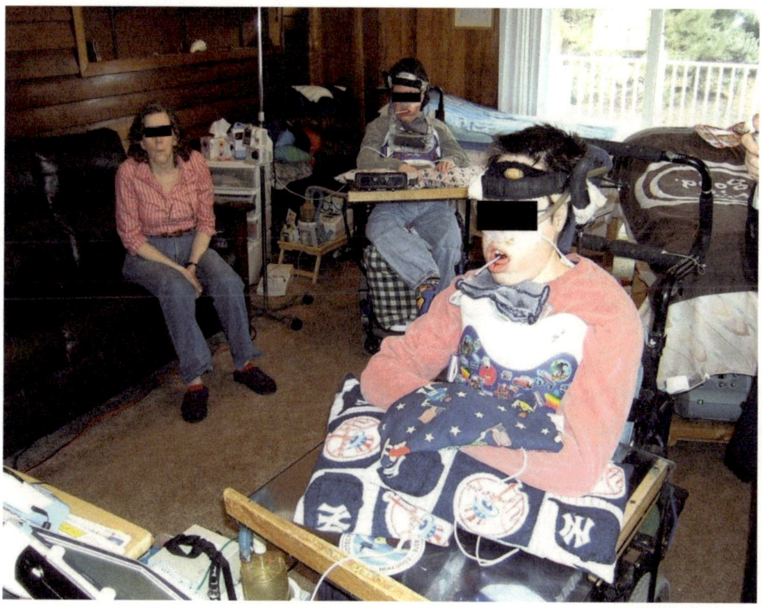

Fig. 8. The same brothers as in Figure 7, now 16 and 14 years of age and with no measurable vital capacity.

In our 176 ALS patients using nocturnal NIV, 42 percent (109 ALS patients) progressed to requiring continuous NIV due to progression of disease, developing severe bulbar innervated muscle impairment that would eventually lead to requiring tracheotomy. Significant aspiration, resulting in consistent baseline SpO_2 desaturations to below 95%, due to the weakness of bulbar innervated muscles is the sole indication for tracheotomy in NMD.

7. Extubation of "unweanable" patient

Using new NMD specific extubation criteria and protocol, including MAC and pulse oximetry monitoring, "unweanable" patients with DMD, SMA, ALS, and other neuromuscular diseases, e.g., SCI and polio, were successfully extubated to NIV (Bach, 2010).

Extubation Criteria for Unweanable Ventilator Dependent Patients
1. Afebrile and normal white blood cell count
2. $PaCO_2$ 40 mm Hg or less at peak inspiratory pressures less than 30 cm H_2O on full ventilatory support and normal breathing rate, as needed
3. Oxyhemoglobin saturation (SpO_2) ≥ 95% for 12 hours or more in ambient air
4. All oxyhemoglobin desaturations below 95% reversed by mechanically assisted coughing and suctioning via translaryngeal tube
5. Fully alert and cooperative, receiving no sedative medications
6. Chest radiograph abnormalities cleared or clearing
7. Air leakage via upper airway sufficient for vocalization upon cuff deflation

Table 1. Adapted from Bach, J.R. (2010). Extubation of Patients With Neuromuscular Weakness. *Chest, 137(5), 1033-1039*

The extubation criteria and protocol have been developed for the neuromuscular disease specific patient population. Instead of spontaneous breathing trials which patients typically undergo prior to extubation attempts, once a NMD patient meets the criteria cited in Table 1, he or she can be directly extubated to nasal NIV, assist control 800 to 1500 mL and rate 10-14 breaths/minute in ambient air, with aggressive MAC. Ideally the orogastric or nasogastic tube should be removed to facilitate proper fitting of the NIV interface which can be nasal, oro-nasal and/or mouthpiece interfaces.

As the patient receives full volume support via NIV, the assisted CPF, or CPF obtained by abdominal thrust following air stacking, is measured within 3 hours of extubation. Patients with sufficient neck movement and lip function used the 15 mm angled mouthpiece and weaned themselves as tolerated by taking fewer and fewer positive pressure ventilations. For those unable to effectively use the 15 mm mouth piece, diurnal nasal NIV was used via nasal prongs, with a nasal or oronasal interface used for nocturnal ventilation. Patients were educated and trained in air stacking and manually assisted coughing and assisted and unassisted CPF were measured.

For SpO_2<95%, ventilator positive inspiratory pressure (PIP), interface or tubing air leakage, CO_2 retention, ventilator settings, and MAC were considered. Therapists, nurses, and especially family and personal care attendants were trained and provided with a CoughAssist™ to use MAC via oro-nasal interfaces up to every 30 min until airway secretions cleared and SpO_2 could be maintained consistently above 94 percent. Open gastrostomies were performed under local anesthesia using NIV without complication in 7 patients with unsafe post-extubation oral intake.

One hundred and fifty seven consecutive "unweanable" patients were treated including 25 with SMA, 20 with DMD, 16 with ALS, 17 with spinal cord injury, 11 with postpolio syndrome, and 68 with other NMD. Eighty three of these were transferred from other hospitals after refusing tracheostomy after inability to pass spontaneous breathing trials. They were successfully extubated to NIV and MAC despite being unable to pass spontaneous breathing trials before or after extubation. Not requiring re-intubation during the hospitalization defined extubation success. Prior to hospitalization 96 (61%) patients had no experience with NIV, 41 (26%) used it part-time, and 20 (13%) were continuously NIV dependent.

There was an extubation success rate of 95% (149 patients) on first attempt. On patients with assisted CPF ≥ 160 L/m, all 98 extubations were successful. Six of 8 patients who had assisted CPF less than 160 L/m initially failed extubation but succeeded on subsequent attempts (Bach et al, 2010). Only two bulbar ALS patients with no measurable assisted CPF underwent tracheotomy (Bach et al., 2010). Multiple centers now routinely extubate DMD patients to NIV directly to avoid tracheotomy.

8. "Unweanable" patient decannulation

In 1996 we initially reported the decannulation of 50 unweanable patients with neuromuscular weakness (Bach & Saporito, 1996). Any ventilator dependent patient with sufficient bulbar-innervated musculature to prevent significant secretion aspiration is a candidate for decannulation to NIV. This is ideal as decanulation facilitates speech and swallowing. The basic principles for decannulation are essentially identical to those for extubation. Patients with tracheostomy tubes and with no VFBA, possessing VC of 250 mL or greater developed VFBA subsequent to decannulation. Within 3 weeks of decannulation, most weaned to only nocturnal NIV.

9. Conclusion

The ability to decannulate and maintain survival of neuromuscular disease patients using NIV in place of tracheostomies is indeed possible, and in fact preferable regarding aspects of convenience, speech, swallowing, cosmesis, comfort, safety, and is preferred overall (Bach, 1993). The extubation criteria set forth is a simple evaluation of patients with NMD (ventilatory muscle weakness) compared with the extensive "ventilator weaning parameters" used as criteria along with spontaneous breathing trials considered for the extubation of patients with intrinsic/obstructive lung diseases before extubating them.

To maintain a sufficient SpO_2 of greater than 94 percent, inspiratory and expiratory muscle aid is used to prevent and manage desaturations and hypercapnia instead of supplemental oxygen. "Unweanable" patients, with sufficient glottic function to prevent significant aspiration of secretions, can be extubated to NIV and maintained on NIV for many years, averting tracheostomy. In the NMD patient population, with primarily ventilatory muscle weakness rather than intrinsic lung disease, this alternative paradigm provides optimal management and quality of life.

10. References

Bach, J.R. (1991). New approaches in the rehabilitation of the traumatic high level quadriplegic. *Am J Phys Med Rehabil*, 70:13-20

Bach, J.R. (1993). A comparison of long-term ventilatory support alternatives from the perspective of the patient and care giver. *Chest*, 104:1702-1706

Bach, J.R. (1993). Mechanical insufflation-exsufflation: comparison of peak expiratory flows with manually assisted and unassisted coughing techniques. *Chest*, 104:1553-1562

Bach, J.R. (1996). Conventional approaches to managing neuromuscular ventilatory failure. In: *Pulmonary rehabilitation: the obstructive and paralytic conditions.* Bach JR, ed. Philadelphia: Hanley & Belfus, 285-301

Bach, J.R. (2004). Management of patients with neuromuscular disease. Philadelphia: Hanley & Belfus

Bach, J.R. & Alba, A.S. (1990). Management of chronic alveolar hypoventilation by nasal ventilation. *Chest*, 97:52-57

Bach, J.R. & Alba, A.S. (1991). Intermittent abdominal pressure ventilator in a regimen of noninvasive ventilatory support. *Chest*, 99:630-636

Bach, J.R. & Alba, A.S. (1990). Noninvasive options for ventilatory support of the traumatic high level quadriplegic. *Chest*, 98:613-619

Bach, J.R., Alba, A.S., Bodofsky, E., Curran, FJ & Schultheiss, M. (1987). Glossopharyngeal breathing and noninvasive aids in the management of post-polio respiratory insufficiency. *Birth Defects*, 23:99-113

Bach, J.R., Alba, A.S. & Saporito, L.R. (1993). Intermittent positive pressure ventilation via the mouth as an alternative to tracheostomy for 257 ventilator users. *Chest*, 103:174-182

Bach, J.R., Alba, A.S. & Shin, D. (1989). Management alternatives for post-polio respiratory insufficiency: assisted ventilation by nasal or oral-nasal interface. *Am J Phys Med Rehabil*, 68:264-271

Bach, J.R., Baird, J.S., Plosky, D., Navado, J & Weaver, B. (2002). Spinal muscular atrophy type 1: management and outcomes. *Pediatr Pulmonol*, 34:16-22

Bach, J.R., Bianchi, C. & Aufiero, E. (2004). Oximetry and indications for tracheotomy in amyotrophic lateral sclerosis. *Chest*, 126:1502-07

Bach, J.R., Bianchi, C., Finder. J., Fragasso, T., Goncalves, M.R., Ishikawa, Y., Ramlall, A.K., McKim, D., Servera, E., Vianello, A., Villanova, M. & Winck, J.C. (2007). Tracheostomy tubes are not needed for Duchenne muscular dystrophy. *Eur Respir J.*, 30:179-180

Bach, J.R., Bianchi, C., Vidigal-Lopes, M., Turi, S. & Felisari, G. (2007). Lung inflation by glossopharyngeal breathing and "air stacking" in Duchenne muscular dystrophy. *Am J Phys Med Rehabil*, 86:295-300

Bach, J.R., Gonçalves, M.R., Hamdani, I. & Winck, J.C. (2010). Extubation of unweanable patients with neuromuscular weakness: a new management paradigm. *Chest*, 137:1033-1039

Bach, J.R., Gupta, K., Reyna, M. & Hon, A. (2009). Spinal muscular atrophy type 1: prolongation of survival by noninvasive respiratory aids. *Pediatric Asthma, Allergy & Immunology*, 22:151-162

Bach, J.R. & Kang, S.W. (2000). Disorders of ventilation: weakness, stiffness, and mobilization. *Chest,* 117:301-303

Bach, J.R., Mahajan, K., Lipa, B., Saporito, L. & Komaroff, E. (2008). Lung insufflation capacity in neuromuscular disease. *Am J Phys Med Rehabil,* 87:720-725

Bach, J.R. & Martinez, D. (2011). Duchenne muscular dystrophy: continuous noninvasive ventilatory support prolongs survival. Respir Care, 56:744-750

Bach, J.R., Rajaraman, R., Ballanger, F., Tzeng, A.C., Ishikawa, Y., Kulessa, R. & Bansal, T. (1998). Neuromuscular ventilatory insufficiency: the effect of home mechanical ventilator use vs. oxygen therapy on pneumonia and hospitalization rates. *Am J Phys Med Rehabil,* 77:8-19

Bach, J.R., Robert, D., Leger, P. & Langevin, B. (1995). Sleep fragmentation in kyphoscoliotic individuals with alveolar hypoventilation treated by nasal IPPV. *Chest,* 107:1552-1558

Bach, J.R. & Saporito, L.R. (1996). Criteria for extubation and tracheostomy tube removal for patients with ventilatory failure. A different approach to weaning. *Chest,* 110:1566-1571

Bach, J.R., Smith, W.H., Michaels, J., Saporito, L., Alba, A.S., Dayal, R. & Pan, J. (1993). Airway secretion clearance by mechanical exsufflation for post-poliomyelitis ventilator assisted individuals. *Arch Phys Med Rehabil,* 74:170-177

Barach, A.L. & Beck, G.J. (1954). Exsufflation with negative pressure: physiologic and clinical studies in poliomyelitis, bronchial asthma, pulmonary emphysema and bronchiectasis. *Arch Intern Med,* 93:825-841

Currie, D.C., Munro, C., Gaskell, D. & Cole PJ. (1986). Practice, problems and compliance with postural drainage: a survey of chronic sputum producers. *Br J Dis Chest,* 80:249-253

Dail, C.W. & Affeldt, J.E. *Glossopharyngeal breathing [video].* Los Angeles: Department of Visual Education, College of Medical Evangelists, 1954

Dail, C., Rodgers, M., Guess, V., et al. *Glossopharyngeal breathing.* Downey, CA: Rancho Los Amigos Department of Physical Therapy, 1979

Fishburn, M.J., Marino, R.J., Ditunno, J.F. Jr. (1990). Atelectasis and pneumonia in acute spinal cord injury. *Arch Phys Med Rehabil,* 71:197-200

Garstang, S.V., Kirshblum, S.C. & Wood, K.E. (2000). Patient preference for in-exsufflation for secretion management with spinal cord injury. *J Spinal Cord Med,* 23:80-85

Gomez-Merino, E. & Bach, J.R. (2002). Duchenne muscular dystrophy: prolongation of life by noninvasive respiratory muscle aids. *Am J Phys Med Rehabil,* 81:411-415

Ishikawa, Y. (2005). Manual for the care of patients using noninvasive ventilation. Japan Planning Center, Matsudo, Japan

Kang, S.W. & Bach, J.R. (2000). Maximum insufflation capacity. *Chest,* 118:61-65

Kohler, M., Clarenbach, C.F., Böni, L., Brack, T., Russi, E.W., Bloch, K.E. (2005). Quality of life, physical disability, and respiratory impairment in Duchenne muscular dystrophy. *Am J Respir Crit Care Med,* 172:1032-1036

McKim, D.A. & LeBlanc, C. (2006). Maintaining an "oral tradition": specific equipment requirements for mouthpiece ventilation instead of tracheostomy for neuromuscular disease. *Respiratory Care,* 51:297-298

Richards, G.N., Cistulli, P.A., Gunnar Ungar, R., Berthon-Jones, M., Sullivan, C.E. (1996). Mouth leak with nasal continuous positive airway pressure increases nasal airway resistance. *Am Respir Crit Care Med*, 154:182-186

Schroth, M.K. (2009). Special considerations in the respiratory management of spinal muscular atrophy. *Pediatrics*, 123:S245-S249

Suri, P., Burns, S.P., Bach, J.R. (2008). Pneumothorax associated with mechanical insufflation-exsufflation and related factors. Am J Phys Med Rehabil, 87:(11)951-955

Toussaint, M., Steens, M., Wasteels, G. & Soudon, P. (2006). Diurnal ventilation via mouthpiece: survival in end-stage Duchenne patients. *Eur Respir J*, 28:549-555

Waldhorn, R.E., Herrick, T.W., Nguyen, M.C., O'Donnell, A.E., Sodero, J. & Potolicchio, S.J. (1990). Long-term compliance with nasal continuous positive airway pressure therapy of obstructive sleep apnea. *Chest*, 97:33-38

Webber, B. & Higgens, J. (1999). Glossopharyngeal breathing: what, when and how? [video] Aslan Studios Ltd., Holbrook, Horsham, West Sussex, England

Williams, A.J., Yu, G., Santiago, S., Stein, M. (1991). Screening for sleep apnea using pulse oximetry and a clinical score. *Chest*, 100:631-635

14

Neuromuscular Diseases in the Context of Psychology and Educational Science

Andrea Pieter and Michael Fröhlich
Institute for Prevention and Public Health,
University of Applied Sciences (DHfPG),
Institute for Sport Science, Saarland University
Germany

1. Introduction

In this chapter, neuromuscular diseases will be examined from both a psychological and an educational science perspective. Neuromuscular diseases are usually accompanied by many types of psychological strain as functional loss due to immobility or pain often corresponds to emotional impairment, such as fear or depression. The restrictions caused by the disease often remain life-long because as far as current knowledge is concerned no cure has been found yet. Patients' experiences have an immediate impact on both their beliefs about whether and how they can influence the course of their disease, and on their individual perception of their quality of life (Lohaus & Schmitt, 1989). A series of experiments showed that health-related control beliefs and individual quality of life of persons suffering from a serious chronic disease can be lower than of healthy persons (Benassi et al., 1988; Kleftaras, 1997). However, there are hardly any empirical findings pertaining to the area of neuromuscular diseases to this effect. Nevertheless, we may presume that health-related control beliefs and individual quality of life differ between patients with neuromuscular diseases and healthy persons. The following will summarize the findings from two studies, examining the extent of how persons with different neuromuscular diseases differ from healthy persons regarding their evaluation of their individual quality of life and health-related control beliefs.

Poverty reports and reports on the correlation between the social situation of people and their health agree that persons with a lower level of education (usually parameterized via the type of graduation achieved) often show a particularly poor state of health, or that they are sicker or die earlier than persons with a higher level of education (Altgeld & Hofrichter, 2000; Jungbauer-Gans & Kriwy, 2003; Richter, 2005; Lambert & Ziese, 2005; Robert Koch Institut & Bundeszentrale für gesundheitliche Aufklärung, 2008). Both health sciences and health politics agree that education by imparting knowledge and promotion of individual disposition and talent support the development of health in childhood and adolescence, and also corresponds to better health in adulthood (Lambert & Ziese, 2005).

Almost all epidemiological studies report on social inequality in the sense of unequal access to life opportunities and life risks. Furthermore, data on individual educational biography is being gathered in almost all international health surveys. Many of the social differences not only map different living conditions, but also result in tangible advantages and disadvantages among the individual members of society (Richter, 2005). Especially during the past two decades, a vast number of publications have shown that a low socio-economic status (defined as a low degree of educational achievement, low-level job, and/or low income) is accompanied by an increased degree of mortality and morbidity (Mielck, 2000). This applies to children, adolescents, adults, men, and women alike.

Why the mortality of someone who has a low income or a low degree of educational achievement, respectively, but who does not have to starve or freeze is higher than the mortality of someone with a higher income or educational level does not seem to be obvious when only seen at a glance. Education, occupational status, and income continue to influence the state of health only indirectly and are transferred with factors associated with social status. The large number of health-relevant living conditions and behaviors makes a complete explanation of status-specific differences in morbidity and mortality almost impossible (Mielck & Helmert, 2006). To date, the focus of scientific discourse has been on the unsolved causal chain of the socio-economic status affecting the state of health and the state of health in turn influencing the socio-economic status (Mielck & Helmert, 2006). The question of the extent to which both may be confounded by a third variable complicates the causal approach even more.

Findings on educational differences in respect of disease frequency and health-related behavior are reported in particular by the Robert Koch Institute (2006) within the framework of a telephone survey on health. Heart attacks, angina pectoris, arthrosis, chronic back pain, and dizziness in men are related to a low educational level. In women, the educational level is related to hypertension, diabetes mellitus type 2, and chronic bronchitis (Lambert & Ziese, 2005). Furthermore, educational differences also become evident in health-related behavior (smoking prevalence, physical activity, etc.), the distribution of overweight and obesity, as well as the usage of information sources referring to health-related topics. It needs to be noted that in this context, the term "education" is often used unidimensionally and current definitions from the area of educational science are neglected.

2. Health-related quality of life in the context of education

2.1 Theoretical approach – Definition

Health-related quality of life is a multidimensional construct that has so far managed to escape a clear definition, which explains why the term is extended, always depending on the definition criteria (Daig & Lehmann, 2007). Another difficulty is finding plausible criteria for a distinct, empirical validation. In principle, this context leads to the question to what extent criteria can be used for explaining the term, with the help of which it is possible to reflect and describe the general state of health regardless of existing diseases, or, on the other hand, whether it would not be preferable to rather base the explanation of the term on disease-specific criteria. With the latter, health would be defined as the degree of disease that allows an individual to perform actions that the individual wants to perform.

Despite the problems described it seems possible to close in to the construct from different perspectives. For example, the WHO sees quality of life as "an individual's perception of his/her position in life in the context of the culture and value systems in which he/she lives, and in relation to his/her goals, expectations, standards and concerns. It is a broad-ranging concept, incorporating in a complex way the person's physical health, mental state, level of independence, social relationships, and their relationship to salient features of their environment" (WHOQOL-Group, 1994, p. 43). The term also includes personal targets, expectations, criteria, and concerns. People are, however, faced with a number of influencing factors: For example, physical health, mental state, social relationships, as well as personal beliefs influence an individual's quality of life (Radoschewski, 2000). The term quality of life is, at the same time, closely connected with happiness, content, and well-being, often even used as synonyms (Daig & Lehmann, 2007).

Health-related quality of life is viewed in the context of the state of health and ability to act of people who suffer from disease or are chronically ill (Bullinger et al., 2000). According to Schumacher et al. (2003), primarily four dimensions play a determining role:

1. disease-related physical discomfort,
2. mental state,
3. disease-related functional restrictions in daily life,
4. quality of social contacts.

Health-related quality of life is a result of many individual, complex evaluation and assessment processes that, in turn, all need to be analyzed based on many dimensions, as well (Daig & Lehmann, 2007). They include, for example, emotional well-being, together with a feeling of security, a stable and predictable environment, positive feedback by others, as well as interpersonal relationships, which means that one feels accepted in a community and works regularly. Moreover, personal development in terms of education, targeted activities, and physical well-being defined by health care, mobility, a sense of wellness, and a healthy diet, play an essential role. Not to be neglected in this context are self-determination, social integration, the right of privacy, and property.

2.2 Quality of life within the framework of neuromuscular diseases

Quality of life comprises the emotional, social, mental, and functional areas of human life (Bullinger & Pöppel, 1988). It cannot be observed from the outside but can only be indirectly derived from various aspects. These aspects mainly include a person's physical well-being, functional capabilities and performance in various areas of life, the number and quality of relationships with other human beings, and physical shape. Especially with long-time chronic diseases, individual quality of life is very important for the patients. Considering all this is essential for the patients' dignity during medical treatment, which particularly applies to long-term treatment and care. Since an evaluation of quality of life is unreliable and variable due to disease, treatment, and impairments it is probably best assessed by patients themselves (Helmchen, 1990). In practice, quality of life is rather still determined by doctors' diagnoses and not by the patients themselves. A number of studies show, however, that there can be significant differences between these two evaluations. When recording quality of life, the postulate of the subject reference of the measurement of quality of life should be taken into account, and indicators of personal and social resources should be integrated in the measurement (Siegrist, 1990).

With neuromuscular disease, functional loss caused by pain or immobility are often so serious that individual quality of life strongly depends on the way the patients cope with and handle their state. To maintain and enforce required lifestyle changes, such as participating in specific movement programs (Koch & Burgunder, 2002), self-regulating mechanisms and support from the social environment (e.g., family, friends, other ill persons, etc.) are decisive factors. In the course of neuromuscular diseases, personal and social resources play a special role in the development and impact of the disease (Koch & Burgunder, 2002).

Interestingly, studies show that compared to a healthy group of persons, patients with chronic, impairing, and progressive diseases express comparable or even better assessments of their subjective quality of life. This phenomenon is usually called the "well-being paradox" or "satisfaction paradox", or adaptation. It means that difficult living conditions do not necessarily have to result in poorer assessments of subjective well-being or quality of life (Daig & Lehmann, 2007). Robbins et al. (2001) showed that the assessment of the quality of life of patients with ALS does not primarily depend on the physical state of health. In a study by Lulé et al. (2008), the average subjective quality of life of ALS patients was 66-72 % and thus in an area that is comparable with healthy control persons. Similar results regarding the fact that many chronically ill people feel "quite well actually" are reported by Raspe (1990). He is of the opinion that ill people obviously differentiate between perception and description of complaints and an evaluation of their overall situation. Even if somatic manifestations of disease and complaints have already led to disorders in the mental and social balance, it is apparent that the afflicted persons do not inevitably connect each disorder with dissatisfaction and negative evaluations. Being ill usually affects the performance and reliability of the body. Physical ability is therefore an important, but not an exclusive component of quality of life. Quality of life indicators are criterion variables that can change in the short and medium term depending on disease characteristics and therapy (Siegrist, 1990). For instance, Diehl et al. (1990) were able to show during their examinations involving tumor patients that the disease brought to light variation and maturing opportunities that had so far been unknown to the persons. They discovered new meanings and values, particularly regarding their relationships with other persons, expectations of life, and their newly obtained ability to set priorities and distinguish between the important and unimportant. This all means that the risk of a possibly drastically reduced lifetime seems to shift life-related preferences.

It has long been known that the educational background of a person corresponds to the subjective assessment of health and disease aspects (Boltanski, 1976). In patients with ALS, Lulé et al. (2008) discovered confounding variables in terms of education and depressive symptomatology: the higher the degree of education, the lower the depression value. Based on these findings, the first study was to elicit the extent to which persons with various neuromuscular diseases differ from healthy persons in their assessment of overall quality of life, and to what extent education is influencing this aspect.

2.3 Study 1 – Quality of life and education in the context of neuromuscular diseases

2.3.1 Methodology

For this study, data of 178 persons was collected. The experimental group comprised 96 persons, 37 men and 59 women with an average age of 50.02 years (SD = 13.22 years). The most frequent disease patterns were muscular dystrophy (22.9 %), muscular atrophy (9.3 %), and ALS (6.2 %). The control group consisted of 82 persons who did not suffer from either neuromuscular or other chronic diseases. This group comprised 37 men and 45 women with an average of 38.67 years (SD = 11.05). The distribution between the sexes did not show any significant differences ($\chi^2 = 0.79$; df = 1; Cramérs V = 0.07). The persons with neuromuscular diseases exhibited a significantly higher age than the control group (F = 37.84; df = 1; $p < 0.05$; $\eta = 0.42$). In terms of education, the test persons were divided into the categories "without advanced technical college entrance qualification" and "with advanced technical college entrance qualification and university entrance qualification". A significant difference became evident insofar as the persons of the control group had a higher educational level ($\chi^2 = 14.81$; df = 3; p = 0.05; Cramérs V = 0.29).

The general overall quality of life was surveyed using the EUROHIS-QOL 8 Item Index questionnaire (Brähler et al., 2007). Within the scope of this survey tool, the psychological, physical, social, and environmental dimensions of the quality of life are recorded based on two items each see Table 1. The index value is calculated by adding the 8-item scale values. The higher the value, the better the quality of life was estimated (Brähler et al., 2007). The individual items are to be answered using a five-step format ("Does not apply at all" to "Applies completely").

Item	Subscale	Factor
How would you rate your quality of life?	Psychological	Endogenous
How satisfied are you with your health?	Psychological	Endogenous
Do you have enough energy for everyday life?	Physiological	Endogenous
How satisfied are you with your ability to perform your daily activities?	Physiological	Endogenous
How satisfied are you with yourself?	Social	Endogenous
How satisfied are you with your personal relationships?	Social	Endogenous
Have you enough money to meet your needs?	Environment	Exogenous
How satisfied are you with the conditions of your living place?	Environment	Exogenous

Table 1. Items of the EUROHIS-QOL 8 Item Index

In addition to the general descriptive methods, such as averages and standard deviations, the inferential statistics check was performed in dependence of the scale level with the corresponding tests for difference checks. The prognostic potential was done via η or η^2, respectively. For internal consistency revision of the items, Cronbach's α was calculated. The significance level was set to $p < 0.05$.

2.3.2 Results and discussion

The overall index (sum of four subscales) as a value for general overall quality of life showed a major difference (F = 36.80; df = 1; $p < 0.05$; $\eta^2 = 0.18$) between the experimental group (26.95 ± 6.02) and the control group (31.68 ± 4.25) in the linear model based on the factors Group (neuromuscular disease vs. no neuromuscular and chronic disease) and

Education (without advanced technical college entrance qualification vs. with advanced technical college entrance qualification or university entrance qualification), as well as the covariate Age. The interaction of Group by Education did not result in any significant differences ($F = 3.16$; $df = 1$; $p = 0.08$; $\eta^2 = 0.02$). When analyzing the individual subscales, major effects became evident in the following dimensions:

Subscale	Experimental group	Control group
Psychological	5.82 ± 1.68	7.72 ± 1.42
Physiological	6.21 ± 2.06	7.87 ± 1.37
Social	7.18 ± 1.84	7.99 ± 1.26
Environment	7.51 ± 2.12	7.91 ± 1.76

Table 2. Significant main effects of subscales (all $p < 0.05$)

Moreover, the physiological subscale showed a significant interaction of Group and Education ($F = 8.00$; $df = 1$; $p < 0.05$; $\eta^2 = 0.05$). Summing up these findings, it is safe to state that persons not suffering from neuromuscular diseases report a higher degree of satisfaction with life than ill persons (Fröhlich et al., 2009). This difference is evident both from the overall index as well as the questionnaire's subscales. Since the age of the persons surveyed can influence the result it was taken into account as a covariate. The analysis of the level of education influencing the satisfaction with life did not show any major connection between education and assessment of the quality of life. This also applies if the persons suffering from neuromuscular diseases and having a higher degree of education degree of education report on the general overall quality of life. In contrast to the findings of Robbins et al. (2001), Lulé et al. (2008), and Raspe (1990), the assessment of overall quality of life within the scope of this survey of persons having a neuromuscular disease is lower than in a comparison sample with persons not suffering from neuromuscular or other chronic diseases.

3. Health-related quality of life in the context of education

3.1 Theoretical approach – Definition

In line with the construct of control beliefs, persons expect to be able to positively influence or control their own health-related behavior (Lohaus, 1992; Petermann & Roth, 2006). This construct is based on the social learning theory by Rotter (1966) and the *locus of control of reinforcement* concept used therein. The center of the concept is that people assume that they can influence events in their life (Krampen, 1988; Ferring & Filipp, 1989). This particularly applies to how they presume that their own state of health may be influenced by their own or other people's actions (e.g. doctors, physical therapists) or even by fate. Other theories related to the concept refer to the model of learned helplessness by Seligman (1975), the cognitive depression model by Beck (1972), and the self-efficacy theory by Bandura (1977).

According to Filipp and Mayer (2005), to perceive oneself as competent and be convinced of the efficacy of one's actions is fundamental human pursuit, which can already be observed in the first year of one's life. The belief to be able to influence and control one's health is usually based on previous knowledge about effects that individuals have learned of during their development, and on the experiences made concerning self-determination and heteronomy in the areas of physical and health-related processes (retrospective behavioral plasticity). Accordingly, control beliefs in this area are understood as the generalized results of previous learning experience (Lohaus & Schmitt, 1989), which are accompanied by divergences if previous knowledge and experiences exist for different forms of disease, which can lead to different expectations of the diseases' controllability.

If persons believe that their actions can lead to or influence specific events they have what is called an internal control belief. If persons think they are not able to bring about certain events through their own actions but are instead convinced that other people's actions or even luck or fate are the cause of events, these persons are said to have social-external or fatalistic-external control beliefs (Levenson, 1972, 1974). In this context, internal control beliefs are evaluated as a personality resource for mental well-being and for coping with health-related issues (Krampen, 1988). Faith in the influence of medical staff (social-internal) can stabilize the patients' well-being if they depend on medical help (Taylor, 1999). Fatalism, however, is deemed dysfunctional for psychological adaptation (Krampen, 1988). Here, aspects of independent and interdependent self-construction come to play an important role, i.e., to what extent persons experience themselves as actively planning and self-determined (Pieter et al., 2010), or to what extent persons define themselves via the association with other persons (Hannover & Kühnen, 2002).

The scope of subjective perception of control options correlates to thinking, feeling, and acting. Often, a low control belief is directly related to depression, anxiety, and low self-esteem (Bandura, 1993, Resetka et al., 1996). Positive control beliefs, however, are accompanied by optimism. Difficult tasks are considered as individual challenges (Caraway et al., 2003; Hintze & Shapiro, 1999). Persons with a high control belief show a higher degree of stamina and recover faster from setbacks when faced with difficult and unpleasant tasks (Bandura, 1999; Jerusalem & Mittag, 1999; Määta et al., 2002). Positive control beliefs are pointed out as predictors or correlates of the ability to handle stress and mental and physical health in a large number of empirical surveys (Flammer, 1990; Kuhl, 2001; Schwarzer & Fuchs, 1996). A subjectively deemed low controllability of the disease can lead to reduced ability to act according to Biebrich and Kuhl (2004). If persons feel helplessly subjected to the disease they can hardly demonstrate intact control during the hard-to-control phases of the disease's development.

A number of studies report that health-related control beliefs cannot be explained exclusively based on the condition of persons and that the connection of health-related control beliefs is moderated beyond the current condition by other variables (summarizing, see Fröhlich et al., 2007). In this context it was shown that a low educational level and/or low income are accompanied more by lower and fatalistic-external control beliefs and less reverting to own capabilities (Ross & Sastry, 1999). Since control beliefs not only depend on existing diseases and complaints, but also on health-related attitudes, perceptions, and comparisons - on the one hand concerning the individual course of the disease and on the other concerning the social reference group - educational differences can have particularly serious effects. The general question arises whether a stronger development of control beliefs is influenced by the educational level, or if the general condition or current state of health has a stronger influence on the subjective control beliefs on health and disease.

3.2 Control beliefs within the framework of neuromuscular diseases

Neuromuscular diseases usually bring many handicaps for the affected, such as physical damage, restricted functionality and activity, and general performance limitations in daily life. These restrictions often correspond to emotional burden, such as fears, depression, low self-esteem, and the endangerment of professional and social participation and integration. The majority of patients must change their lifestyle to adapt to the disease genesis. They must undergo frequent diagnostic examinations, continue to take their medication, and possibly even make use of stationary therapy. The restrictions often remain life-long because as far as current knowledge is concerned no cure has been found yet (Fröhlich et al., 2010; Pieter et al., 2011).

To date, a series of examinations has shown that health-related control beliefs in persons suffering from a major chronic disease can be less than in healthy persons. Krampen (1988), for example, found that depressive patients exhibited a reduced self-concept of their own ability and internality as well as a socially induced externality and significantly increased fatalistic externality. A connection between reduced internal control beliefs and increased fatalistic externality with depressive moods has also been proved in numerous studies (Burger, 1984; Benassi et al., 1988; Kleftaras, 1997; Weinmann et al., 2001). The question whether these control beliefs cause a depressive mood or whether the depressive mood causes the control beliefs remains unanswered at this point.

As stated above, control beliefs associated with health and disease are mostly based on previous knowledge about effects on health and disease, which individuals have attained in the course of their lives, and on the experiences made concerning self-determination and heteronomy in the area of physical processes (Lohaus & Schmitt, 1989). It is an obvious assumption that control beliefs differ between healthy and ill persons. Particularly with diseases occurring multiple times or over a long time, learning experience regarding individual control options (both internal and external control) is likely to exist. Based on these assumptions, the control beliefs of both persons suffering from neuromuscular diseases and healthy persons will be examined and compared in the second study.

3.3 Study 2 – Control beliefs and education in the context of neuromuscular diseases

3.3.1 Methodology

The overall sample of this study consisted of 176 persons (41.2 % men and 58.8 % women) with an average age of 44.67 years (SD = 13.42). The experimental group comprised 94 persons (38.5 % men and 61.5 % women) suffering from a neuromuscular disease diagnosed by a doctor. The average age of this partial sample was 50.02 years (SD = 13.22). The control group represents a random sample of 82 persons who were recruited through direct contact. Precondition for being assigned to this group was, as in Study 1, that the persons had not been diagnosed with neither neuromuscular nor other chronic diseases. These test persons had an average age of 38.32 years (SD = 10.65) and were 45.1 % men and 54.9 % women.

The test persons were asked to evaluate their current general state of health based on a seven-level Likert scale (1 = "very poor" to 7 = "very well") (as to the reliability of this method, please refer to Ravens-Sieberer et al., 2000; Gunzelmann et al., 2006). Persons without neuromuscular disease set their state of health at an average of 5.78 (SD = 0.91), the ones with neuromuscular diseases at 3.74 (SD = 1.26). Their evaluations differed significantly ($F = 111.88$; $df = 1$; $p < 0.05$; $\eta_p^2 = 0.40$). In the control group, one person evaluated themselves as currently not healthy at all, 7 persons experienced themselves as partly healthy, and 78 persons felt completely healthy. In contrast, 38 persons of the experimental group considered themselves as absolutely unhealthy at the point of the survey, 30 persons felt partly healthy, and 20 persons felt completely healthy despite their neuromuscular disease.

Degree of education	**Overall sample (N = 176)**	**Experimental group (N = 94)**	**Control group (N = 82)**
Without advanced technical college/university entrance qualification	73 (41.5 %)	51 (54.2 %)	22 (26.8 %)
With advanced technical college/university entrance qualification	103 (58.5 %)	43 (45.8 %)	60 (73.2 %)

Table 3. Educational level of test persons from Study 2

The questionnaire developed by Lohaus and Schmitt (1989) on recording control beliefs about disease and health was used as a survey tool. The questionnaire includes three subscales that correspond to the control belief dimensions "internality", "social externality", and "fatalistic externality". All items of the measurement tool are formulated as statements that the test participants can process based on a six-level scale. From their answers, a score is calculated that expresses the control belief in the three subscales. All items avoid the terms "health" and "disease", rather pointing to physical states that both healthy and ill persons are familiar with. Lohaus and Schmitt (1989) postulate that therefore, both healthy and ill persons can process the items in the same manner. For statistical review, absolute and percentage frequencies were calculated in addition to average values and standard deviations. To meet the requirement of sufficient cell frequency, the educational level was categorized into the group of test persons with certificate of secondary education/general school-leaving certificate and in the group of test persons with advanced technical college/university entrance qualification. Furthermore, using the median and identical category ranges, the current general state of health was divided into very ill persons, partly healthy, and completely healthy persons. Due to the low degree of cell frequency in the control group (see remarks on sample) this group is not considered in the calculations of the current general state of health.

For the inferential statistics check, variance-analytical procedures were calculated after verifying the corresponding preconditions. To estimate the effect size, eta squared (η^2) or partial eta squared (η_p^2), respectively, were applied. Values for ANOVA calculations of 0.1 and 0.24 are to be viewed as small effects, values of 0.25 and 0.39 as medium, and above 0.4 as large effects (Bortz & Döring 2006). Since there are major differences in the two groups in terms of age ($F = 40.97$; $df = 1$; $p < 0.05$; $\eta_p^2 = 0.19$), the age was taken into account in all calculations as a covariate. The level of significance was $p < 0.05$.

3.3.2 Results and discussion

In the internality subscale, persons with neuromuscular diseases and healthy persons differ significantly ($F = 9.91$; $df = 1$; $p = 0.02$; $\eta_p^2 = 0.06$). The following table illustrates the relevant average values and standard deviations:

	Without advanced technical college/university entrance qualification	With advanced technical college/university entrance qualification
Experimental group	28.22 ± 7.12	25.44 ± 7.54
Control group	22.85 ± 7.81	20.93 ± 5.64

Table 4. Average values and standard deviations for the internality subscale

Concerning the educational level (without advanced technical college/university entrance qualification vs. with advanced technical college/university entrance) no significant differences ($F = 1.10$; $df = 1$; $p = 0.30$) were founded. However, for persons with neuromuscular disease, this subscale exhibited a significant difference ($F = 6.55$; $df = 2$; $p = 0.02$; $\eta_p^2 = 0.13$) between very ill persons and completely healthy persons ($p < 0.05$), as well as between partly healthy and completely healthy persons ($p < 0.05$).

In the social externality subscale, neither group differences ($F = 1.61$, $df = 1$; $p = 0.21$) nor educational differences ($F = 1.51$; $df = 1$; $p = 0.22$) were evident. With persons with neuromuscular disease, no significant differences ($F = 2.64$; $df = 2$; $p = 0.08$) were evident concerning the evaluation of the general state of health. When observing the fatalistic externality subscale, there are no group differences between ill and healthy persons ($F = 1.08$; $df = 1$; $p = 0.30$). However, in terms of education, significant differences between persons without advanced technical college/university entrance qualification and persons with advanced technical college/university entrance qualification came to light ($F = 4.50$; $df = 1$; $p = 0.04$; $\eta_p^2 = 0.03$). The average values and standard deviations are illustrated in the following table:

	Without advanced technical college/university entrance qualification	With advanced technical college/university entrance qualification
Experimental group	29.91 ± 8.25	33.15 ± 6.95
Control group	32.15 ± 5.81	35.25 ± 4.37

Table 5. Average values and standard deviations for the fatalistic externality subscale

For persons with neuromuscular disease, a significant difference ($F = 4.20$; $df = 2$; $p = 0.02$; $\eta_p^2 = 0.09$) is shown in this subscale between completely ill and partly healthy persons ($p < 0.05$).

Persons suffering from neuromuscular diseases are obviously more convinced than healthy persons that their own activities and actions positively influence the course of their disease, which enables them to better cope with health-related burdens. Regarding their health, they experience themselves as actively planning and acting in a self-determined way. All this is evidence for optimism in this group and the conviction that difficult tasks represent a challenge and can be solved. In all, this finding is in favor of the mental health of the examined persons with neuromuscular somatic disease. The lower values in the group of healthy persons could be based on the fact that previous knowledge and experience with severe diseases are lacking or only very rare and thus lead to different expectations of the individual scope of actions than is the case with ill persons. Ill persons seem to be able to anticipate and assess the future impact of their own behavior based on their existing experience with diseases. In contrast, healthy persons can align their behavior only with mentally represented states of disease (Goschke, 2004).

Even if persons with neuromuscular diseases are objectively seen ill they still estimate their current general state of health as rather well. A large number of the persons surveyed even feel completely healthy. When looking at the diagnoses of these persons with a view to their subjective control beliefs it becomes evident that the three subgroups differ significantly in their internality. Those persons who assessed themselves as partly healthy at the time of the survey have the highest degree of internality, followed by the completely ill and the completely healthy. The diagnoses in these cases again speak for a learning effect or, respectively, can be interpreted as a clue that the terms health and sickness are indeed social constructs. Considerably more partly healthy persons than completely sick persons consider luck and coincidence to be strongly influencing their disease, i.e. completely sick persons will more likely actively fight their disease using their own means or asking others for help.

With respect to education, there was only a significant difference when it came to fatalistic externality. Persons with a higher level of education (with advanced technical college/university entrance qualification) are more convinced that health and sickness depend on coincidence and fate. This conviction, however, can turn out to be dysfunctional for psychological adaptation within the framework of coping with a disease. This seems to be strange to the group of those with a higher level of education and contradicts the findings of Ross and Sastry (1999). At first glance, the result is surprising and requires more detailed verification in further surveys. At large, however, the low effect size and the fact that the test persons of the experimental group generally have a lower level of education need to be considered here, as well (Fröhlich & Pieter, 2009).

4. Conclusion

Persons suffering from neuromuscular diseases are more convinced than healthy persons that their own activities and actions positively influence the course of their disease. They use this personality resource to a higher degree, which enables them to better cope with their personal health-related problems. They experience themselves as actively planning and self-determined with respect to their health. This is evidence of optimism in this group and the conviction that difficult tasks represent a challenge and can be solved. Overall, these findings all points toward the mental health of the persons examined here with a neuromuscular somatic disease. The lower values of the healthy persons may result from their lack of or very little previous knowledge and experience with severe diseases and that they therefore have different expectations of their individual ability to act than ill persons. Ill persons seem to be able to anticipate and assess the future impact of their own behavior based on their existing experience with diseases. In contrast, healthy persons can align their behavior only with mentally represented states of disease (effect anticipation and determination sensu Goschke 2004). The anticipation is thus directly associated with the individual learning history of the person. Therefore, it seems easier for persons with neuromuscular disease to establish preventive goals that are not based on the current needs, but rather geared to the satisfaction of future requirements. This type of suppression of current needs in favor of future needs requires a certain measure of willpower in an individual (cf. Goschke, 2004; Pieter et al., 2010).

Even if persons with neuromuscular diseases are objectively seen ill they still estimate their current general state of health as rather well. A large number of the persons surveyed even feel completely healthy. Considerably more partly healthy persons than completely sick persons consider luck and coincidence to be strongly influencing their disease, i.e. completely sick persons will more likely actively fight their disease using their own means or asking others for help.

With respect to education, there was only a significant difference when it came to fatalistic externality. Persons with a higher level of education (with advanced technical college/university entrance qualification) are more convinced that health and sickness depend on coincidence and fate. This means that these persons turn out to be less persistent in difficult and uncomfortable health-related situations, that their ability to act is reduced and that they process setbacks slower. This may be explained by an inability to anticipate and assess the future impact of their behavior. Being convinced of the fact that a disease depends on coincidence and fate is accompanied by the feeling of being helplessly exposed to the disease. According to Tausch (2008), feelings such as helplessness or powerlessness are further promoted by not understanding external processes and subsequently recognizing pointlessness.

In addition to the fact that it is difficult to compare educational levels within age groups, it is also difficult to suitably record education and learning processes in general (Reinmann, 2010). Therefore, the question arises whether the operationalization of the construct of education (in the sense of educational level achieved) selected in this context may not be sufficiently exhaustive as an explanatory variable in the context of health, and whether education as a health resource should rather be a combination of many more factors than mere education in the sense of educational level achieved. In this context, an operationalization of education via competence seems to be more plausible even though a definition of the term is difficult because it has multiple connotations in both informal and scientific speech (Hartig, 2009). In educational research, the comprehension of competences as learnable, context-specific cognitive performance dispositions has been proven (Hartig, 2009). In health research, they should also include motivational orientations, attitudes, tendencies, and expectations sensu Weinert (1999). Instead of operationalizing general education via school education, an approach taken from positive psychology (see Seligman, 2010) and the resulting deliberations on the meaning of the so-called "wisdom competences" seem to be more productive in the area of health (see also Baumann & Linden, 2008) and more suitable in connection with coping with the stresses of life. When considering the assumptions by Erikson (1976) about the central development task in adolescence being to master one's one life and fate, this presumes a certain degree of "mature thinking" in an individual (Baumann & Linden, 2008, p. 32). This mature thinking can be described as relativizing, dialectic, complementary, and closely corresponding with learning processes, but not necessarily with the level of education achieved. In its highest form, this type of thinking is called "wisdom" in psychological development research (Baltes & Smith, 1990; Staudinger & Baltes, 1996), represents - according to current knowledge - an important resource in terms of positively coping with critical life events (Baumann & Linden, 2008), and could therefore be utilized in health research. In this context, wisdom can be defined as skill or expertise in a specific context, with the thoughts on this being based on philosophic, implicit, and explicit wisdom theories (for an overview, see Baumann & Linden, 2008). From these theories, a ten-dimensional model of wisdom competencies has been derived, comprising cognitive, emotional, and motivational competencies. Furthermore, it is to analyze what are the differences between the neuromuscular disorders and other chronic disorders causing disability in the context of psychology and educational science and what are the effects of the therapy of different neuromuscular disorders in this context. The low degrees of cell frequency in the present studies not allow these conclusions. Further studies could shed a more detailed light on this area of research.

5. Summary

It was examined to what extent persons with various neuromuscular diseases differ in terms of their evaluation of their individual quality of life and health-related control beliefs in from a comparison sample. As expected, healthy persons reported a higher degree of satisfaction with life. In contrast, persons with neuromuscular disease display a higher degree of internal and a lower degree of fatalistic control beliefs.

According to these findings, education is ascribed only a limited, explanatory value in association with health-related control beliefs. It is recommended that further studies extend the concept of education to include health sciences based on current findings from educational research. One option is a diagnostic on wisdom competencies carried out using established measurement methodology and linked with health-specific knowledge, skills, and strategies.

6. References

Altgeld, T. & Hofrichter, P. (2000). *Reiches Land – Kranke Kinder? Gesundheitliche Folgen von Armut bei Kindern und Jugendlichen.* Mabuse. ISBN 978-3-93305-021-2, Frankfurt a. M., Germany

Baltes, P.B. & Smith, J. (1990). Weisheit und Weisheitsentwicklung: Prolegomena zu einer psychologischen Weisheitstherapie. *Zeitschrift für Entwicklungspsychologie und Pädagogische Psychologie,* Vol. 22, No. 2, (June 1990), pp. 95-135, ISSN 0049-8637

Bandura, A. (1977). Self-efficacy: Toward a unifying theory of behavioral change. *Psychological Review,* Vol. 84, No. 2, (June 1977), pp. 191-215, ISSN 0033-295X

Bandura, A. (1993). Perceived self-efficacy in cognitive development and functioning. *Educational Psychologist,* Vol. 28, No. 2, (June 1993), pp. 117-148, ISSN 0144-3410

Bandura, A. (1999). Exercises of personal and collective self-efficacy in changing societies. In: *Self-efficacy in changing societys,* A. Bandura, pp. 1-45, Cambridge University Press, ISBN 978-0-52158-696-2, Cambridge, USA

Baumann, K. & Linden, M. (2008). *Weisheitskompetenzen und Weisheitstherapie – die Bewältigung von Lebensbelastungen und Anpassungsstörungen.* Pabst, ISBN 978-3-89967-490-3, Lengerich, Germany

Beck, A.T. (1972). *Depression.* University of Pennsylvania Press, ISBN 978-0-81227-662-7, Pennsylvania, USA

Benassi, V.A.; Sweeny, P.D. & Dufour, C.L. (1988). Is there a relation between locus of control orientation and depression? *Journal of Abnormal Psychology,* Vol. 97, No. 3, (September 1988), pp. 357-367, ISSN 0021-843X

Biebrich, R. & Kuhl, J. (2004). Handlungsfähigkeit un das Selbst. *Zeitschrift für Differentielle und Diagnostische Psychologie,* Vol. 25, No. 2, (June 2004), pp. 57-77, ISSN 0170-1789

Boltanski, L. (1976). Die soziale Verwendung des Körpers. In: *Zur Geschichte des Körpers,* D. Kamper & V. Rittner, pp. 138-183, Hanser, ISBN 978-3-44612-256-7, München, Germany

Bortz, J. & Döring, N. (2006). *Forschungsmethoden und Evaluation für Human- und Sozialwissenschaftler,* Springer, ISBN 978-3-54033-350, Berlin, Germany

Brähler, E.; Mühlan, H.; Albani, C. & Schmidt, S. (2007). Teststatistische Prüfung und Normierung der deutschen Version des EUROHIS-QOL Lebensqualität-Index und des WHO-5 Wohlbefindens-Index. *Diagnostica,* Vol. 53, No. 2, (March 2007), pp. 83-96, ISSN 0012-1924

Bullinger, M. & Pöppel, E. (1988). Lebensqualität in der Medizin: Schlagwort oder Forschungsansatz? *Deutsches Ärzteblatt,* Vol. 85, No. 32, pp. 679-680, ISSN 0012-1207

Bullinger, M.; Ravens-Sieberer, U. & Siegrist, J. (2000). Gesundheitsbezogene Lebensqualität in der Medizin - eine Einführung. In: *Lebensqualitätsforschung aus medizinpsychologischer und –soziologischer Perspektive,* M. Bullinger; J. Siegrist & U. Ravens-Sieberer, pp. 11-21, Hogrefe, ISBN 978-8-01711-726, Göttingen, Germany

Burger, J.M. (1984). Desire for control, locus of control, and proneness to depression. *Journal of Personality,* Vol. 52, No. 1, (March 1984), pp. 71-89, ISSN 1467-6494

Caraway, K.; Tucker, C.M.; Reincke, W.M. & Hall, C. (2003). Self-efficacy, goal orientation, and fear of failure as predictors of school engagement in high school students. *Psychology in Schools,* Vol. 40, No. 4, (July 2003), pp. 417-427, ISSN 1520-6807

Daig, I. & Lehmann, A. (2007). Verfahren zur Messung der Lebensqualität. *Zeitschrift für Medizinische Psychologie,* Vol. 16, No. 1-2, (April 2007), pp. 5-23, ISSN 0940-5569

Diehl, J.M. & Kohr, H.U. (1989). *Deskriptive Statistik.* Klotz, ISBN 978-3-88074-110-2, Eschborn, Germany

Diehl, V.; von Kalle, A.K.; Kruse, T. & Sommer, H. (1990). "Lebensqualität" als Bewertungskriterium in der Onkologie. In: *"Lebensqualität" als Bewertungskriterium in der Medizin.*, P. Schölmerich & G. Thews, pp. 149-167, Elsevier, ISBN 978-3-43711-360-4, München, Germany

Erikson, E.H. (1976). *Identität und Lebenszyklus.* Suhrkamp, ISBN 978-3-51827-616-7, Frankfurt a. M., Germany

Ferring, D. & Filipp, S.H. (1989). Der Fragebogen zur Erfassung gesundheitsbezogener Kontrollüberzeugungen (FEGK). Kurzbericht. *Zeitschrift für Klinische Psychologie,* Vol. 18, No. 3, pp. 285-289, ISSN 1616-3443

Filipp, S.H. & Mayer, A.K. (2005). Selbstkonzept-Entwicklung. In: *Soziale, emotionale und Persönlichkeitsentwicklung. Enzyklopädie der Psychologie, Themenbereich C: Theorie und Forschung, Serie V: Entwicklungspsychologie, Band 3,* J.B. Arsendorpf, pp. 259-334, Hogrefe, ISBN 978-3-80170-588-6, Göttingen, Germany

Flammer, A. (1990). *Erfahrung der eigenen Wirksamkeit. Einführung in die Psychologie der Kontrollmeinung,* Huber, ISBN 978-3-45681-942-6, Bern, Switzerland

Fröhlich, C.; Pinquart, M.; Silbereisen, R.K. & Wedding, U. (2007). Zusammenhänge von gesundheitsbezogenen Kontrollüberzeugungen, Alltagskompetenz und Therapieziel mit dem emotionalen Befinden bei neu diagnostizierten Krebspatienten. *Zeitschrift für Medizinische Psychologie,* Vol. 16, No. 3, (October 2007) pp. 99-104, ISSN 0940-5569

Fröhlich, M. & Pieter, A. (2009). Cohen's Effektstärke als Mass der Bewertung von praktischer Relevanz - Implikationen für die Praxis. *Schweizerische Zeitschrift für Sportmedizin und Sporttraumatologie,* Vol. 57, No. 4, (December 2009), pp. 140-143, ISSN 1422-0644

Fröhlich, M.; Pieter, A.; Emrich E. & Stark, R. (2009). Lebensqualität bei chronisch progredienten Erkrankungen. In: *Menschen in Bewegung – Sportpsychologie zwischen Tradition und Zukunft,* I. Pfeffer & D. Alfermann, pp. 57, Czwalina, ISBN 978-3-88020-529-1, Ahrensburg, Germany

Fröhlich, M.; Pieter, A.; Klein, M. & Emrich, E. (2010). Gesundheitsbezogene Lebensqualität in Abhängigkeit von sozialen Faktoren bei Personen mit neuromuskulären Erkrankungen. *Sport- und Präventivmedizin,* Vol. 40, No. 3, (October 2010), pp. 35-40, ISSN 1867-1977

Goschke, T. (2004). Vom freien Willen zur Selbstdetermination. Kognitive und volitionale Mechanismen der intentionalen Handlungssteuerung. *Psychologische Rundschau,* Vol. 55, No. 4, (December 2004), ISSN 0033-3042

Gunzelmann, T.; Albani, C.; Beutel, M. & Brähler, E. (2006). Die subjektive Gesundheit älterer Menschen im Spiegel des SF-36. Normwerte aus einer bevölkerungsrepräsentativen Erhebung. *Zeitschrift für Gerontologie,* Vol. 39, No. 2 (June 2006), pp. 109-119, ISSN 0948-6704

Hannover, B. & Kühnen, U. (2002). Der Einfluss independenter Selbstkonstruktion auf die Informationsverarbeitung im sozialen Kontext. *Psychologische Rundschau,* Vol. 53, No. 2, (June 2002), pp. 61-79, ISSN 0033-3042

Hartig, J. (2009). Kompetenzen als Ergebnisse von Bildungsprozessen. In: *Kompetenzerfassung in pädagogischen Handlungsfeldern. Theorien, Konzepte und Methoden,* N. Jude; J. Hartig & E. Klieme, pp. 13-24, Bundesministerium für Bildung und Forschung, Berlin, Germany

Helmchen, H. (1990). "Lebensqualität" als Bewertungskriterium in der Psychiatrie. In: *"Lebensqualität als Bewertungskriterium in der Medizin,* P. Schölmerich & G. Thews, pp. 93-115, Elsevier, ISBN 978-3-43711-360-4, München, Germany

Hintze, J.M. & Shapiro, E.S. (1999). School. In: *Developmental issues in the clinical treatment of children,* W.K. Silverman & T.H. Ollendick, pp. 156-170, Allyn and Bacon, ISBN 978-0-20517-001-2, Needham Heights, USA

Jerusalem, M. & Mittag, W. (1999). Selbstwirksamkeit, Bezugsnormen, Leistung und Wohlbefinden in der Schule. In: *Emotion, Motivation und Leistung,* M. Jerusalem & R. Pekrun, pp. 223-245, Hogrefe, ISBN 978-3-80170-929-7, Göttingen, Germany

Jungbauer-Gans, M. & Kriwy, P. (2003). *Soziale Benachteiligung und Gesundheit bei Kindern und Jugendlichen.* VS Verlag für Sozialwissenschaften, ISBN 978-3-53114-261-6, Wiesbaden, Germany

Kleftaras, G. (1997). Control-related beliefs and depressive symptomatology in a semi-institutionalized population of french elderly persons. *Revue Européene de Psychologie Appliquée,* Vol. 47, pp. 225-229, ISSN 1162-9088

Koch, J.W. & Burgunder, J.M. (2002). Rehabilitation bei neuromuskulären Erkrankungen: Stellenwert der medizinischen Trainingstherapie. *Schweizer Archiv für Neurologie und Psychiatrie,* Vol. 153, No. 2, (June 2002), pp. 69-81, ISSN 0036-7273

Krampen, G. (1988). *Diagnostik von Attributionen und Kontrollüberzeugungen* (FKK). Hogrefe, Test-No. 01 093 01, Göttingen, Germany

Kuhl, J. (2001). *Motivation und Persönlichkeit. Interaktion psychischer Systeme.* Hogrefe, ISBN 978-3-49917-395-0, Göttingen, Germany

Lambert, T. & Ziese, T. (2005). *Armut, soziale Ungleichheit und Gesundheit. Expertise des Robert-Koch-Instituts zum 2. Armuts- und Reichtumsbericht der Bundesregierung in Berlin.* Bundesministerium für Gesundheit, Berlin, Germany

Levenson, H. (1972). Distinction within the concept of internal-external control: Development of a new scale. *Proceedings of the 80th Annual Convention of the American Psychological Asscociation,* pp. 261-262.

Levenson, H. (1974). Activism and powerful others: Distinction within the concepts of internal-external control. *Journal of Personality Assessment,* Vol. 38, pp. 377-383, ISSN 0022-3891

Lohaus, A. & Schmitt, G.M. (1989). *Fragebogen zur Erhebung von Kontrollüberzeugungen zu Krankheit und Gesundheit (KKG).* Hogrefe, Test-No. 01 060 01, Göttingen, Germany

Lohaus, A. (1992). Kontrollüberzeugungen zu Gesundheit und Krankheit. *Zeitschrift für Klinische Psychologie und Psychotherapie,* Vol. 21, No.1, (March 1992), pp. 76-87, ISSN 1616-3443

Lulé, D.; Häcker, S.; Ludolph, A.; Birbaumer, N. & Kübler, A. (2008). Depression und Lebensqualität bei Patienten mit amyothropher Lateralsklerose. *Deutsches Ärzteblatt,* Vol. 105, No. 23, pp. 397-403, ISSN 0012-1207

Määta, S.; Häkan, S. & Nurmi, J.E. (2002). Achievement strategies at school: types and correlates. *Journal of Adolescence,* Vol. 25, No. 1, (February 2002), pp. 31-46, ISSN 0140-1971

Mielck, A. & Helmert, U. (2006). Soziale Ungleichheit und Gesundheit. In: *Handbuch Gesundheitswissenschaften.* K. Hurrelmann, U. Laaser & O. Razum, pp. 603-623, Juventa, ISBN 978-3-77990-790-9, Weinheim, Germany

Mielck, A. (2000). *Soziale Ungleichheit und Gesundheit. Empirische Ergebnisse, Erklärungsansätze, Interventionsmöglichkeiten.* Huber, ISBN 345-6-84235-X, Bern, Switzerland

Petermann, H. & Roth, M. (2006). Produktiver Umgang mit den Aufgaben einer Lebensphase. In: *Gesundheitspsychologie,* B. Renneberg & P. Hammelstein, pp. 245-263, Springer, ISBN 978-3-54025-462-1

Pieter, A.; Fröhlich, M.; Klein, M. & Emrich, E. (submitted). Bildung als Korrelat gesundheitsbezogener Kontrollüberzeugungen. Eingereicht bei *Physioscience.*

Pieter, A.; Fröhlich, M. & Klein, M. (2011). Kohärenzgefühl bei Personen mit neuromuskulären Erkrankungen. *Bewegungstherapie und Gesundheitssport,* Vol. 27, No.1, (Januar 2011), pp 22-26, ISSN 0930-1348.

Pieter, A.; Fröhlich, M.; Emrich, E. & Papathanassiou, V. (2010). Rationale Verhaltensalternativen und selbstbestimmtes Handeln als Komponenten des Gesundheitsverhaltens. *Prävention und Gesundheitsförderung,* Vol. 5, No. 4, (November 2010), pp. 300-306, ISSN 1861-6755

Radoschewski, M. (2000). Gesundheitsbezogene Lebensqualität – Konzepte und Maße. Entwicklungen und Stand im Überblick. *Bundesgesundheitsblatt –*

Gesundheitsforschung - Gesundheitsschutz, Vol. 43, No. 3 (March 2000), pp. 165-189, ISSN 14376-9990.

Raspe, H.H. (1990). Zur Theorie und Messung der "Lebensqualität" in der Medizin. In: *"Lebensqualität als Bewertungskriterium in der Medizin.*, P. Schölmerich & G. Thews, pp. 23-40 , Elsevier, ISBN 978-3-43711-360-4, München, Germany

Ravens-Sieberer, U.; Görtler, E. & Bullinger, M. (2000). Subjektive Gesundheit und Gesundheitsverhalten von Kindern und Jugendlichen - Eine Befragung Hamburger Schüler im Rahmen der schulärztlichen Untersuchung. *Gesundheitswesen,* Vol. 62, No. 3, (October 2000), pp. 148-155, ISSN 0941-3790

Reinmann, G. (2010). Mögliche Wege der Erkenntnis in den Bildungswissenschaften. In: *Konkrete Psychologie - die Gestaltungsanalyse der Handlungswelt,* G. Jüttemann & W. Mack, pp. 237-252, Pabst, ISBN 978-3-89967-492-7, Lengerich, Germany

Resetka, H.J.; Liepmann, D. & Frank, G. (1996). Qualifizierungsmaßnahmen und psychosoziale Befindlichkeiten bei Arbeitslosen. Peter Lang, ISBN 978-3-63149-223-9, Frankfurt a. M., Germany

Richter, M. (2005). *Gesundheit und Gesundheitsverhalten im Jugendalter - Der Einfluss sozialer Ungleichheit.* VS Verlag für Sozialwissenschaften, ISBN 353-1-14528-2, Wiesbaden, Germany

Robbins, B.A.; Simmons, Z.; Bremer, B.A.; Walsh, S.M. & Fischer, S. (2001). Quality of life in ALS is maintained as physical function declines. *Neurology,* Vol. 56, No. 3, (August 2000), pp. 388-392, ISSN 0028-3878

Robert Koch-Institut (2006). *Bundesweiter Telefongesundheitssurvey (4. Welle - GSTel 06).* Robert Koch-Institut, Retrieved from http://www.rki.de/cln_169/nn_201172/DE/Content/GBE/Erhebungen/Gesundheitssurveys/Geda/Cati06_inhalt.html

Robert Koch-Institut und Bundeszentrale für gesundheitliche Aufklärung (2008). *Erkennen - Bewerten - Handeln: Zur Gesundheit von Kindern und Jugendlichen in Deutschland.* Robert Koch-Institut, Berlin, Germany

Ross, C.E. & Sastry, J. (1999). The sense of personal control. Social-structural causes and emotional consequences. In: *Handbook of the sociology of mental health,* C.S. Aneshensel & J.C. Phelan, pp. 369-394, Kluwer Academic/Plenum Publishers, ISBN 978-0-30646-069-6, New York, USA

Rotter, J.B. (1966). Generalized expectancies for internal vs external control of reinforcement. *Psychological Monographs,* Vol. 80, No. 1 , (March 1966), pp. 1-28, ISSN 0096-9753

Schumacher, J.; Klaiberg, A. & Brähler, E. (2003). *Diagnostische Verfahren zu Lebensqualität und Wohlbefinden.* Hogrefe, ISBN 978-3-80171-696-7, Göttingen, Germany.

Schwarzer, R. & Fuchs, R. (1996). Self-efficacy and health behaviors. In: *Predicting health behavior: Research and practice with social cognition models,* M. Conner & P. Normann, pp. 163-196, Open University Press, ISBN 978-0-33521-176-0, Buckingham, England

Seligman, M.E.P. (1975). *Helplessness.* Freeman, ISBN 067-1-01911-2, San Francisco, USA

Seligman, M.E.P. (2010). *Der Glücks-Faktor. Warum Optimisten länger leben.* Ehrenwirth, ISBN 978-3-40360-548-5, München, Germany

Siegrist, J. (1990). Grundannahmen und gegenwärtige Entwicklungsperspektiven einer gesundheitsbezogenen Lebensqualitätsforschung. In: *"Lebensqualität" als Bewertungskriterium in der Medizin.*, P. Schölmerich & G. Thews, pp. 59-66, Elsevier, ISBN 978-3-43711-360-4, München, Germany

Staudinger, U.M. & Baltes, P.B. (1996). Interactive minds: A faciliative setting for wisdom-related performance? *Journal of Personality and Social Psychology*, Vol. 71, No. 4 (December 1999), pp. 746-762, ISSN 0022-3514

Tausch, R. (2008). *Hilfen bei Stress und Belastungen.* Rowohlt, ISBN 978-3-49960-124-8, Hamburg, Germany

Taylor, S.E. (1999). *Health psychology.* McGraw Hill, ISBN 98-0-07292-746-7, New York, USA

Weinert, F.E. (1999). Konzepte der Kompetenz. OECD, Paris, France

Weinmann, M.; Bader, J.P.; Endrass, J. & Hell, D. (2001). Sind Kompetenz- und Kontrollüberzeugungen depressionsabhängig? – Eine Verlaufsuntersuchung. *Zeitschrift für Klinische Psychologie und Psychotherapie,* Vol. 30, No.3, (October 2001), pp. 153-158, ISSN 1616-3443

WHOQOL-Group (1994).The development of the World-Health Organization quality of life assessment instrument: The WHOQOL. In: *Quality of life assessment: international perspectives.,* Orley, J. & Kuyken, W. (Eds.), pp. 41-57, Springer, ISBN 978-3-54058-205-2, Heidelberg, Germany